D1766941

Breast Pathology

Sami Shousha

Editor

Breast Pathology

Problematic Issues

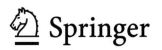

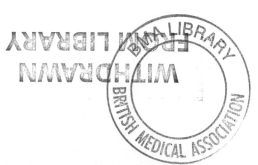

Editor
Sami Shousha
Charing Cross Hospital
Imperial College Healthcare NHS Trust & Imperial College
London
United Kingdom

ISBN 978-3-319-28653-2   ISBN 978-3-319-28655-6   (eBook)
DOI 10.1007/978-3-319-28655-6

Library of Congress Control Number: 2016959451

Printed on acid-free paper

This Springer imprint is published by Springer Nature
The registered company is Springer International Publishing AG Switzerland

To Seham, Sarah, and Susan

Introduction

This is not a textbook of breast pathology. It is rather a modern version of the late John Azzopardi's classic book, *Problems in Breast Pathology*, which was published in 1979. In fact, this book is mainly based on the annual "Hammersmith Diagnostic Histopathology of Breast Disease Course" of which Azzopardi was the main instigator and lecturer for a very long time during the 1980s. Although the course has grown enormously since, Azzopardi's spirit is still there guiding us to concentrate on tackling the problems that face us in our daily working life as diagnostic breast pathologists.

Some of the problems that faced Azzopardi's generation of pathologists are still there, and his classic book still provides needed help, but time has passed and new developments and attitudes in the diagnosis and treatment of breast diseases have arisen calling for a book that deals with added new problems. That is the aim of this book, and I hope that aim is fulfilled. All the book's authors teach in the Hammersmith course, and all are eminent practicing breast pathologists with a wide experience in that field. But as with any multiauthor book, each author has his own way of writing and of expressing his approach in solving problems. This also sometimes creates a degree of repetition, but this may be useful in confirming ideas that all agree on or providing different approaches to solving specific problems.

I hope you will find the book useful and enjoyable at the same time.

Sami Shousha
London, May 2016

Contents

1   **Dealing with the Gross Specimen** 1
Sami Shousha

2   **Handling Neoadjuvant Therapy Specimens** 11
Elena Provenzano

3   **Proliferative Breast Lesions** 33
Sarah E. Pinder

4   **Problematic Core Biopsies** 43
Sarah E. Pinder

5   **Ductal Carcinoma In Situ** 61
Jeremy Thomas

6   **Lobular Neoplasia** 77
Abeer Shaaban

7   **Grading of Invasive Carcinoma** 87
Emad A. Rakha and Ian O. Ellis

8   **Fibroepithelial Lesions** 97
Andrew H. S. Lee

9   **Mucinous Lesions of the Breast and Expression
of WT1** 109
Sami Shousha

10   **Spindle Cell Lesions** 123
Sami Shousha

11   **Papillary Carcinomas** 137
Emad Rakha

12   **Metaplastic Breast Carcinomas** 153
Emad Rakha

13   **Metastatic Lesions in the Breast** 167
Sami Shousha

14   **Axillary Lymph Node Biopsies** 175
Sami Shousha

**15 A Practical Approach to the Use of Immunohistochemistry
     in the Diagnosis and Management of Breast Disease** 189
     Colin A. Purdie

**16 Molecular Classification and Testing of Breast
     Carcinoma** 215
     Elena Provenzano and Suet-Feung Chin

17 Uncommon Benign Breast Lesions 233
     Sami Shousha

18 Uncommon Malignant Lesions 247
     Sami Shousha

19 Male Breast Lesions 265
     Abeer Shaaban

Index 275

Contributors

Suet-Feung Chin Department of Histopathology, Addenbrookes Hospital and CRUK Cambridge Research Institute, Cambridge, UK

Ian O. Ellis Department of Cellular Pathology, University of Nottingham and Nottingham University Hospitals NHS Trust, City Hospital Campus, Nottingham, UK

Andrew H.S. Lee Nottingham University Hospitals, Nottingham, UK

Sarah E. Pinder Department of Pathology, Guy's Hospital, King's College London, London, UK

Elena Provenzano Department of Histopathology, Addenbrookes Hospital and CRUK Cambridge Research Institute, Cambridge, UK

Colin A. Purdie Department of Pathology, Ninewells Hospital & Medical School, University of Dundee, Dundee, UK

Emad Rakha Department of Histopathology, Nottingham University Hospitals NHS Trust; University of Nottingham, Nottingham City Hospital, Nottingham, UK

Abeer Shaaban Department of Histopathology, Queen Elizabeth Hospital Birmingham; University of Birmingham, West Midlands, UK

Sami Shousha Department of Histopathology, Charing Cross Hospital, Imperial College Healthcare NHS Trust & Imperial college, London, UK

Jeremy Thomas Western General Hospital, Edinburgh, UK

Dealing with the Gross Specimen

1

Sami Shousha

Abstract

The main thrust of this chapter concerns dealing with the tissue removed from patients with breast carcinoma treated with conservative surgery. Dealing with other specimens is also briefly discussed as dealing with core biopsies, specimens from patients with DCIS, specimens from patients who had neoadjuvant chemotherapy, and axillary lymph node specimens are dealt with in other Chaps. (4, 5, 2, and 14, respectively). The accounts in this chapter are mainly based on the practice at Charing Cross Hospital, London.

Keywords

Core biopsies • Excision biopsies • Microcalcification • Lumpectomy • Mastectomy • Excision margins

Introduction

Good fixation is essential for proper diagnosis. In our department we prefer to receive all breast specimens, except core biopsies, fresh in a plastic bag, immediately after surgical excision whenever this is feasible and in the absence of any suspected infections. The specimen is registered, given a laboratory number, and the pathologist in charge is called to deal with it. For biopsies coming from other hospitals, we ask the surgeons to immerse it in an adequate amount of formalin and send it to us as soon as possible where it is dealt with immediately. If there is going to be a delay, we advise slicing mastectomy specimens before immersing it in formalin. Core biopsies are put in formalin straight after being removed from the patient or, in case of stereotactic biopsies, after x-raying the specimen by the radiologist to ensure the presence of calcification in the cores. The specimen container must be clearly labeled with the patient identity and side and type of specimen. It should be accompanied by a request form detailing the patient's name, date of birth, hospital number, the responsible clinician, location, date of request, and relevant clinical history. The information written on the specimen container is checked with that on the request

S. Shousha
Department of Histopathology, Charing Cross
Hospital, Fulham Palace Road, London W6 8RF, UK
e-mail: s.shousha@imperial.ac.uk

form, particularly as regards the patient's name and type and side of the biopsy. Any tissue left after sampling a specimen is retained for 4–5 weeks after authorization of the report.

Core Biopsies

These are thoroughly dealt with in Chap. 4 but will mention here a few points which we apply in our institution. In our hospital, hard copies of the x-rays of stereotactic core biopsies are not available anymore. Instead, the x-rays are sent to us as e-mail messages from the Radiology Department. They are also available via the hospital net, but we find receiving them as e-mails to be more convenient and easier to access, although the quality of the pictures can be sometimes not as good. Viewing the x-rays when reporting these core biopsies is essential to ensure the presence of the biopsied calcification in the stained sections. If no microcalcification is seen in the three stained sections, or if only fine microcalcification is present in spite of the presence of coarser calcification in the submitted x-ray, further sections have to be cut and examined.

If more than one case is received at the same time, they are not accessioned into the laboratory consecutively but separated by another type of specimen to avoid possible mix-up. The number of cores received from each case is recorded, together with their length and color. In addition to the case number, we usually write the patient's name by pencil on the side of the cassette. The specimen is entirely submitted for histological examination, preferably not more than four cores in each cassette. Three shallow levels are cut and stained with hematoxylin and eosin (H&E). Three intervening sections are kept unstained in case they are needed later for the immunohistochemical assessment of hormone receptors and HER2 status if the case proved to be an invasive carcinoma. Additional sections can be requested if more immunohistochemical or special stains are needed. For vacuum biopsies, six levels are cut and stained with H&E if the procedure was carried out for microcalcification. Otherwise, only three levels are cut with intervening spares on coated slides for immunohistochemistry if required.

Dealing with Specimens from Conservative Surgery

Many cases of breast carcinoma, invasive and in situ, are now treated by limited (conservative) surgery rather than mastectomy. These are usually relatively small mono-focal tumors that are detected by palpation or by screening mammography. If the tumor is palpable, it can be removed by a wide local excision or a quadrantectomy depending on the size of the tumor and the size of the breast. If the lesion is impalpable, it is removed by a wire-guided wide local excision. The lesion is localized by inserting a wire radiologically, either by stereotactic or ultrasound technique. The wire guides the surgeon to the site of the tumor, and the area around the tip of the wire is removed.

The size of the excised biopsy depends on the size of the tumor as determined radiologically. The surgeon orientates the specimen by attaching sutures of different lengths to the margins of the specimen. At least two margins have to be marked, and these are usually the lateral, indicated by a long suture, and the superior indicated by a short suture (Fig. 1.1). An additional looped suture maybe attached to the anterior surface for confirming the orientation. Metal clips are usually attached to the sutures to help identifying the margins when the specimen is x-rayed (see below).

If the lesion was originally detected because of the presence of microcalcification, the excised specimen is usually x-rayed by the surgeon in the operating theater, using a Faxitron, to ensure the removal of all microcalcifications, with a

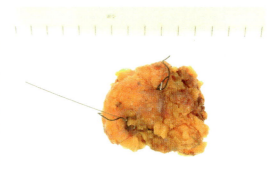

Fig. 1.1 Specimen with marking sutures

reasonable distance (around 10 mm) between the microcalcification and the margins of the specimen [1]. If this is not the case, the surgeon may have to remove more breast tissue from the biopsy cavity. A copy of the specimen x-ray is sent with the specimen or is made available for the pathologist to examine via the hospital computer system (Fig. 1.2). To be on the safe side, some surgeons take additional "bed biopsies" from different parts of the post-biopsy cavity, particularly that part of the cavity where the tumor was felt to be nearest [2]. These bed biopsies are sent to the pathologist in separate containers labeled with the side from which the biopsy was taken, lateral, medial, etc. and with a stitch attached to one, usually the outer, surface.

The role of the pathologist in these cases is not only to make a diagnosis but also to decide whether or not the lesion has been completely excised. If it has not, a re-excision biopsy, or biopsies, will be needed, to ensure the complete removal of the lesion and to minimize the possibility of recurrence.

The specimens received are described, weighed, and measured. To assess completeness of excision, ink has to be applied to the margins of the specimens. For the main specimen, different colored inks are applied to different margins. There are different ways of slicing specimens, and coloring will depend on how the specimen is going to be sliced. As we usually "bread slice" our specimens, we use four colors, for example,

black anterior, blue posterior, red superior, and yellow inferior (Fig. 1.3). A few drops of 1 % acetic acid and absolute alcohol are added to the inked areas to help the adherence of the ink to the specimen surface. A couple of minutes are allowed for the ink to dry, and excess ink is removed by blotting paper. The specimen is then sliced from one margin to the other, say from medial to lateral, into 3–4 mm thick slices. In this case, the first slice will indicate the medial margin and the last slice the lateral margin; hence there is no need to ink the medial and lateral margins with different colors. This sequence of coloring may vary according to the shape of the specimen. In the above example, if the tumor is felt to be close to the medial or lateral margin, that margin is cut into cruciate sections in order to be able to assess accurately the distance between tumor and margin.

Once the specimen is sliced, the slices are sampled and processed for microscopic examination. Fat is not trimmed off the slices, as ink usually seeps through the fat down to the surface of the more firm tissue underneath, which would give a false impression of the actual surgical resection margin if the fat is removed. The slices are laid flat on the dissecting board and inspected (Fig. 1.4). Most invasive tumors can be easily visualized by inspecting and palpating the slices, because of their grayish color and harder consistency. DCIS is more difficult to visualize but may appear as granular area(s). The gross appearance of any abnormality is described. If the specimen is small, weighing around 25 g or less, all slices are processed. For larger specimens, all slices with obvious tumor or abnormal appearance, including the site of any previous recent needle

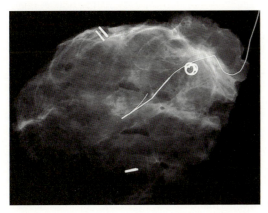

Fig. 1.2 Specimen x-ray with attached wire and orientating clips

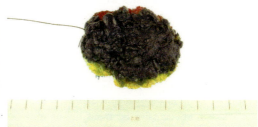

Fig. 1.3 Painted specimen

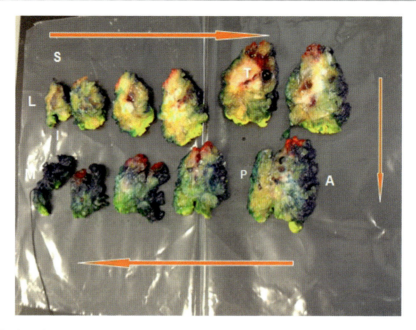

Fig. 1.4 Sliced specimen

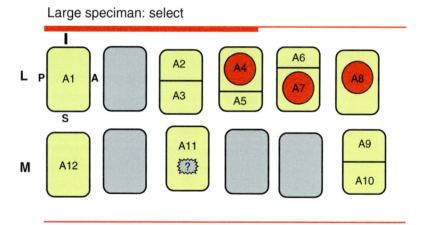

Fig. 1.5 A diagram showing slice selection for processing. The tumor is in *red*. *Yellow*-colored slices are processed. Slice 11 has an additional abnormal-looking area. *A1-A12* refer to cassette numbers. *L: lateral, M: medial, I: inferior, S: superior, A: anterior, P: posterior*

aspiration or core biopsies which is usually indicated by an area of hemorrhage or discoloration, have to be processed together with the preceding and following slices, as well as the first and last slice (Fig. 1.5). Many cases of invasive lobular carcinoma present in the form of a diffuse thickening, rather than a well-defined mass, and satellite lesions adjacent to the main tumor may be present, some being impalpable. Thorough sampling is especially required in these cases, particularly from the excision margins, to assess complete removal.

If a slice is too big to fit in a small cassette, it is divided into two or more pieces. We usually process the slice containing the main part of the tumor, with four margins, in one cassette, which in many cases is a mega-cassette (double the size of a normal cassette, Fig. 1.6). The cassettes are given consecutive numbers. A map is kept to identify where each section has come from. For

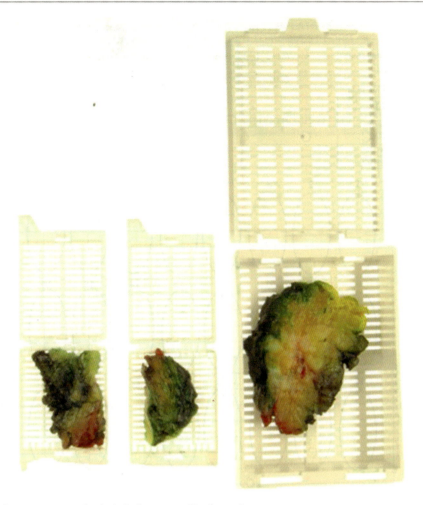

Fig. 1.6 A large cassette used to include the tumor with all margins

this purpose we use a pro forma diagram (Fig. 1.7). Alternatively, the slices can be x-rayed in a departmental Faxitron [3] or in the Radiology Department, and the x-ray image is used to identify where the sections were taken from (Fig. 1.8). We also have an additional form to list all the cassettes used with their given number, the number of samples in each and where the tissue in each has come from (Fig. 1.9).

For re-excision and bed biopsies, only one color is applied to the outer surface of the specimen and then cut into vertical slices with each slice having an outer inked surface and inner uninked surface.

In some centers, frozen sections of the biopsy margins or cytology imprints of its surface are carried out to ensure completeness of excision. This is not the practice in our hospital as we believe that these time-consuming intraoperative procedures use less than optimal microscopic methods for diagnosis and are done under pressure while the patient is still anesthetized and the surgeon waiting for the result to proceed with the operation.

Reporting Excision Margin Status

It is recommended that the histopathology report should state the distances between the tumor and all margins: medial, lateral, anterior, posterior, superior, and inferior. The actual distance in

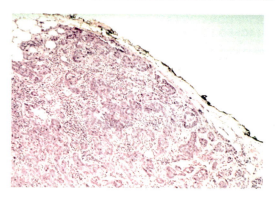

Fig. 1.11 Invasive carcinoma 0.2 mm from the inked excision margin

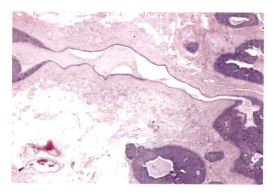

Fig. 1.12 DCIS involving parts of duct with intervening noninvolved area

tumor" is an adequate surgical margin for breast-conserving surgery in patients with invasive breast cancers [6]. This is based on the assumption that postoperative adjuvant therapy can take care of any few tumor cells that might have been left behind [4]. The situation is different for DCIS, as involved ducts can have an irregular course and involvement by DCIS can be discontinuous (Fig. 1.12). In many institutions, including ours, a re-excision is carried out if DCIS is present less than 2 mm from the margin except for the anterior and posterior margins if the excision was carried out from the skin to fascia.

Lumpectomy Specimens

These are usually done for benign lesions, e.g., fibroadenomas, which are removed with variable amount of "normal" breast tissue around them.

The biopsy is weighed, measured, and described and its surface inked, as sometimes the lesion might turn out to be malignant on microscopic examination. If orientation sutures are present, different color inks are used as explained above. According to its size, the specimen is either processed in its entirety, after being bisected, e.g., small fibroadenomas, or selectively sampled after being sliced. Sampling must be directed mainly at the nonfatty areas of the biopsy, as the likelihood of finding any epithelial lesions within pure adipose tissue is extremely low [7].

Mastectomy Specimens

The specimen is weighed, measured, and described macroscopically as a right/left breast with/without an axillary tail, and note whether any attached chest wall tissue is present. The covering skin is measured and examined for signs of previous operations or any other abnormality. If a prior biopsy site is present, the scar is described (recent, healed) and its quadrant location in the breast is noted. The quadrants are recognized by imaginary vertical and horizontal axes through the nipple or its indicated site. If present the nipple is described particularly as regards the presence or absence of retraction or evidence of inflammation or ulceration.

The posterior and anterior surfaces of the breast are painted with two different colors of ink. The specimen is then sliced. There are different ways of slicing. We slice perpendicular to the skin, with each slice being approximately 1 cm thick. The lesions are identified and described especially as regards their size, location, and distance from the nearest margin.

Tumors or the walls of previously excised biopsies are processed in their entirety if this is feasible. Sections are also taken from any other abnormal areas as well as a vertical section of the nipple. If lymph nodes are included in the specimen, these are dissected and all embedded.

Mastectomies are sometimes carried out for small impalpable tumors, because of various clinical reasons. It is essential to know the site of the lesion beforehand. This is usually indicated

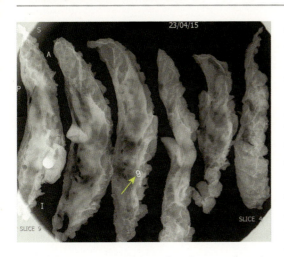

Fig. 1.13 X-ray of mastectomy slices from a patient who had preoperative neoadjuvant chemotherapy. The *arrow* points to the marker inserted by the radiologist during the chemotherapy course

calcification are processed. For neoadjuvant cases, the area around the marker is thoroughly sampled. The subject is dealt with in more details in Chap. 2.

"Prophylactic (risk-reducing) mastectomies" are dealt with in the same way, with samples taken from any suspicious areas, or in the absence of such areas, from various parts of the breast containing fibrous tissue.

Axillary Lymph Node Specimens and Specimens Received After Neoadjuvant Therapy

These are dealt with in Chaps. 14 and 2, respectively.

on the request form as two figures, for example, "5,2" which indicates that the tumor is at 5 o'clock and is 2 cm from the nipple. If such information is not provided, the surgical team should be contacted to get this information. A preoperative mammogram can also help in identifying the possible site of the lesion. The suspected slice can then be x-rayed to confirm the presence of the mammographic abnormality.

We usually x-ray the slices of mastectomies carried out for DCIS or for cases treated preoperatively by neoadjuvant therapy, particularly when there is no palpable tumor. If the approximate position of the lesion is known, we only x-ray five or six slices from the area where the lesion is expected to be. The x-ray would show any areas of calcification or, in case of neoadjuvant therapy, the marker inserted by the radiologist that indicates the tumor site (Fig. 1.13). Our radiologist would insert a marker, during the course of chemotherapy, if he/she notices that the tumor is showing a good response regardless of whether the patient is going to be treated by conservative surgery or mastectomy. We use the x-ray to indicate the sites from which samples are taken for processing. For DCIS, all areas of

References

1. Bathla L, Harris A, Davey M, Sharma P, Silva E. High resolution intra-operative two-dimensional specimen mammography and its impact on second operation for re-excision of positive margins at final pathology after breast conservation surgery. Am J Surg. 2011;202:387–94.
2. Zavagno G, Dona M, Orvieto E, Mocellin S, Pasquali S, Goldin E, Mele ML, Belardinelli V, Nitti D. Separate cavity margins excision as a complement to conservative breast cancer surgery. Eur J Surg Oncol. 2010;36:632–8.
3. Oakley KL, Going JJ. Specimen slice radiography of cancer in breast conserving excisions. J Clin Pathol. 1995;48:1028–30.
4. Morrow M, Harris JR, Schnitt SJ. Surgical margins in lumpectomy for breast cancer- bigger is not better. N Engl J Med. 2012;367:79–82.
5. Moran MS, Schnitt SJ, Giuliano AE, Harris JR, Khan SA, Horton J, et al. Society of Surgical Oncology-American Society for Radiation Oncology consensus guideline on margins for breast-conserving surgery with whole-breast irradiation in stages I and II invasive breast cancer. Ann Surg Oncol. 2014;21:704–16.
6. Harnes JK, Giuliano AE, Pockaj BA, Downs-kelly E. Margins: a status report from the annual meeting of the American Society of Breast Surgeons. Ann Surg Oncol. 2014;21:3192–7.
7. Schnitt SJ, Wang HH. Histologic sampling of grossly benign breast biopsies. How much is enough. Am J Surg Pathol. 1989;13:505–12.

Elena Provenzano

Abstract

Neoadjuvant therapy, including chemotherapy, endocrine therapy, and/or radiotherapy, has gained acceptance in the routine management of women with early breast cancer with aggressive biological and clinical features and may result in tumor downsizing allowing breast conservation in patients who would otherwise require mastectomy. Tumor response to neoadjuvant therapy is an important prognostic factor and is increasingly being used to guide clinical decisions regarding further adjuvant therapy. Specimen handling post-neoadjuvant therapy can be challenging, especially if there has been an excellent response with no residual macroscopic lesion; good multidisciplinary team communication is essential. Histological reporting includes detection and quantification of residual disease and grading of response, as well as more traditional features such as tumor grade, histological type, and the presence of in situ disease and lymphovascular invasion. This chapter discusses the issues involved in the macroscopic and microscopic assessment of breast cancer specimens following neoadjuvant therapy, including specimen handling, grading of response in the breast and axilla, receptor testing, and the role and limitations of neoadjuvant clinical trials.

Keywords

Breast cancer • Neoadjuvant chemotherapy • Histopathology • Macroscopic handling

Introduction

Neoadjuvant therapy, including chemotherapy, endocrine therapy, and/or radiotherapy, is a primary treatment given before the first curative surgical intervention. Traditionally, neoadjuvant therapy was used for large, locally advanced tumors including inflammatory cancers to convert inoperable to operable disease. More

E. Provenzano
Department of Histopathology (Box 235),
Addenbrookes Hospital, Hills Rd,
Cambridge CB2 0QQ, UK
e-mail: elena.provenzano@addenbrookes.nhs.uk

recently, neoadjuvant chemotherapy has gained acceptance in the routine management of women with early breast cancer with aggressive biological and clinical features whom would otherwise require adjuvant chemotherapy. In this context, neoadjuvant treatment can produce tumor downsizing allowing breast conservation in patients who would otherwise require mastectomy [1, 2].

Tumor response to neoadjuvant therapy is an important prognostic factor [3], and there is emerging evidence that the degree of response can be used to guide further adjuvant treatment [4]. Patients with complete regression of their tumor (pathological complete response [pCR]) may not benefit from radiotherapy, and conversely women whose tumors show a poor response may be candidates for trials of novel targeted agents. The US Food and Drug Administration has recently recognized neoadjuvant clinical trials as a means of expediting approval of novel agents for use in high-risk breast cancer, with pCR acting as a surrogate endpoint for survival [5]. For these reasons, accurate quantification of residual disease post-neoadjuvant therapy is essential [6]. Breast surgical specimens post-neoadjuvant therapy are often complicated, and intelligent specimen handling with good clinical pathological correlation to precisely localize the tumor bed is vital to histopathological assessment of these cases.

Pretreatment Diagnosis

In patients who receive neoadjuvant chemotherapy, the diagnostic core biopsy is very important, as in the event of a pCR it may represent the only tumor tissue sample available. Percutaneous image-guided core needle biopsy is the recommended modality [7]. The biopsy must contain sufficient tumor for definitive diagnosis of invasive carcinoma, as well as for the assessment of key prognostic and predictive factors including tumor grade, histological type, ER and HER2 status, as well as any additional tests used in patient selection for neoadjuvant therapy, e.g., Ki67 or multigene assays [6, 8]. Caution should

be taken if there is only limited invasive carcinoma present or if the core biopsy and/or imaging findings suggest a significant component of in situ disease.

Many neoadjuvant clinical trial protocols include designated baseline core biopsies for research, either at the time of diagnostic biopsy or as a subsequent procedure. The cores can be in addition to those required for diagnosis, or on occasion formalin-fixed cores can be re-embedded as a research block after reporting. Detailed recommendations for tissue sample collection for translational research in neoadjuvant trials have been provided elsewhere [9, 10]. Some trials also require additional on-treatment core biopsies at subsequent time points, for monitoring response and/or examining the biological changes in the tumor with treatment.

Routine axillary ultrasound should be performed, with histological assessment of morphologically abnormal nodes, either by FNA or core needle biopsy. Confirmation of axillary nodal involvement assists nodal evaluation post-treatment and may influence the type of axillary surgery. Pretreatment sentinel lymph node (SLN) biopsy precludes assessment of nodal response to neoadjuvant therapy, which is an important independent prognostic factor, and invalidates calculation of the residual cancer burden (RCB – discussed below) and ypTNM staging if node positive; it should be reserved for cases in which pretreatment lymph node status will influence systemic and/or local treatment decision-making [11].

Specimen Handling

Evaluation of surgical specimens post-neoadjuvant therapy for breast cancer can be challenging. In the event of an excellent response to therapy, there may be no visible macroscopic lesion or only a vague area of fibrosis detectable on palpation. Good multidisciplinary team communication is essential in this setting. Accurate localization and informed sampling of the tumor bed are more efficient and cost-effective than exhaustive block taking and will enable more reliable histological assessment of response.

As a minimum requirement, the request form must clearly state that neoadjuvant therapy has been given, along with location of the tumor/s and the pretreatment size [7]. A sample request form for use in a neoadjuvant clinical trial is given in Fig. 2.1. A diagram can be very useful or alternatively the clock face system with distance from the nipple. Placement of a radiopaque clip within the tumor bed at the time of diagnosis, even in patients undergoing mastectomy, is invaluable as the clip may be found macroscopically or on X-ray if the tumor bed is difficult to identify (Fig. 2.2) [12]. Ideally, the pathologist undertaking specimen dissection will have access to the previous imaging such as MRI scans to facilitate radiological-pathological correlation.

Specimens are better received fresh, if feasible, and sliced prior to fixation as per local specimen handling protocols. Good fixation with preservation of morphology is particularly important for subsequent histological assessment. Slicing the fresh specimen also enables tissue samples to be taken for translational research, either as part of a trial protocol or for institutional tissue banks.

Wide Local Excision Specimens

Wide local excision (WLE) specimens should be orientated, inked, and sliced at intervals as per local protocols. The various options for slicing are the same as in the adjuvant setting and depend upon pathologist preference. In our institution, we serially slice WLE specimens in the coronal plane at 1 cm intervals from anterior to deep (Fig. 2.3a). Coupled with the use of large tissue cassettes, this allows visualization of the entire lesion with all radial margins, often in one or two sections (Fig. 2.3b). Alternatively, the specimen may be sliced from medial to lateral in the sagittal plane.

For small specimens (less than 5 cm maximum dimension or 30 g in size), submitting the entire specimen for histological evaluation may be prudent, especially if there is no grossly visible lesion. Samples may still be taken for research, either using a punch needle biopsy (Fig. 2.3a) or by submitting trim from blocks if available.

For larger WLE specimens, more selective sampling is indicated. When there is an obvious macroscopic tumor, then blocking the lesion can proceed as per the adjuvant setting, with sampling of the tumor and all resection margins. Correlation with imaging is important, and the area sampled should include not only grossly visible residual disease but surrounding tissue to encompass the size of the involved area on pretreatment imaging [6]. Where the tumor bed cannot be identified macroscopically, more extensive sampling is required. If a clip was inserted at the time of diagnosis, then the clip site should be identified and sampling concentrated on the surrounding area.

Precise block description to enable reconstruction of the specimen on the histological

PATIENT LABEL

NAME:

DOB:

HOSPITAL NUMBER:

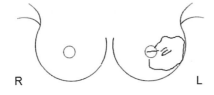

R   L

DATE OF SURGERY:

BREAST - TYPE OF OPERATION: Mastectomy / WLE

PRE TREATMENT TUMOUR DETAILS:

HISTOLOGICAL TYPE / GRADE:

ER STATUS: HER2 STATUS:

UNIFOCAL / MULTIFOCAL

TUMOUR SIZE:

CLIP PLACED: Yes / No

POST TREATMENT TUMOUR DETAILS :

UNIFOCAL / MULTIFOCAL

TUMOUR SIZE:

AXILLA - TYPE OF OPERATION: SLNB / Axillary Clearance

PRE TREATMENT LYMPH NODE STATUS: Positive / Negative / Unknown

Fig. 2.1 Sample surgical request form for use in a neoadjuvant clinical trial

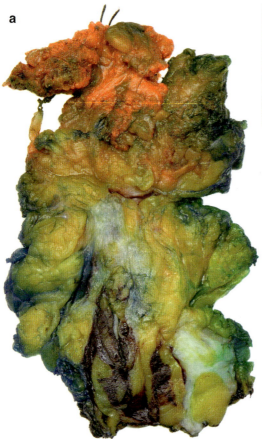

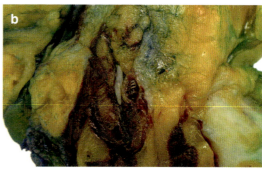

Fig. 2.2 Clip placement pre-neoadjuvant chemotherapy. (**a**) Slice from a wide local excision specimen showing an ill-defined central area of fibrosis. (**b**) A marker coil was placed pretreatment which can be identified macroscopically to localize the site of the tumor bed

sections is vital for accurate lesion measurement and to assess post-treatment tumor cellularity [6]. Diagrams with the specimen slices and location of the blocks can be very helpful for both large WLE and mastectomy specimens (see below).

Mastectomies

Mastectomy specimens in particular should be sliced when fresh at 1–2 cm intervals to ensure adequate fixation (Fig. 2.4a). The specimen should be orientated as per local protocol to enable correlation with imaging; sutures at the superior and lateral positions are preferable to a single suture in the axillary tail, as they allow more accurate orientation and localization of the tumor bed.

As with WLE specimens, if there is gross residual tumor, then sampling can proceed as per the adjuvant setting with generous blocking of the tumor and surrounding tissue to encompass the area of the tumor bed on pretreatment imaging. For example, if the residual gross lesion is 2 cm but the tumor was 5 cm on pretreatment MRI, then the sections should incorporate surrounding tissue to a dimension of 5 cm to ensure the entire tumor bed has been sampled. Routine blocks from the quadrants and nipple can also be taken as per local protocols.

If the tumor bed cannot be identified macroscopically, then close clinical and radiological correlation is essential to optimize tissue sampling. More extensive sampling is often required, although this is difficult to define from the

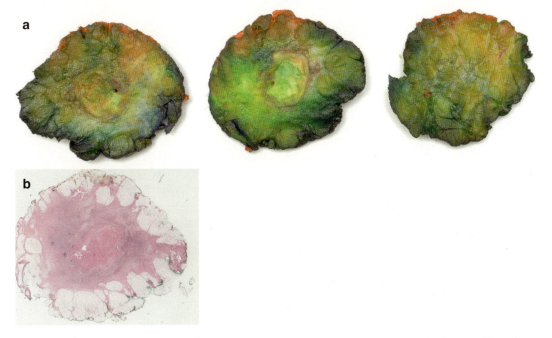

Fig. 2.3 (**a**) Wide local excision specimen sliced from anterior to deep in the coronal plane. (**b**) The use of large tissue cassettes enables representation of the entire tumor and radial margins on a single slide

literature. The US FDA guidance recommends taking ten blocks or one block for each centimeter of pretreatment tumor size, whichever is greater [5]. The BIG-NABCG Residual Disease Working Group advocates taking full-face sections from each 1 cm slice of the pretreatment tumor bed to a maximum of 25 blocks [6]. The MD Anderson group recommends 10–15 blocks in cases where there is no palpable tumor [13], and 5 blocks representing the maximum cross section of the tumor bed are required for the assessment of residual tumor cellularity [14]. If tumor bed is not identified on the first pass, returning to the specimen with submission of further tissue is advised. The pathologist should assess each case on its own merits, and common sense with intelligent sampling following clinically guided localization of the tumor bed is more cost- and time efficient than random taking of large numbers of blocks.

If a clip has been inserted, then this should be identified macroscopically, or the specimen sent for X-ray (Fig. 2.4b, c). Specimen X-ray can also be helpful if there was associated microcalcification, although this may increase, decrease, or stay stable following treatment [15–17].

When multiple lesions were present on pretreatment imaging, then each lesion should be sampled as described above, with additional blocks taken from intervening tissue to ensure they are truly separate foci.

Residual disease following neoadjuvant therapy may have a patchy distribution, and interpretation of histology slides, particularly with regard to lesion measurement, can be difficult. Detailed and accurate block description is vital to be able to reconstruct the tumor bed on subsequent H&E-stained sections. Diagrams or photographs with the relative location of the blocks can be invaluable when reviewing the slides.

Axillary Lymph Nodes

The approach to sampling axillary lymph nodes is the same as in the adjuvant setting, although lymph nodes may be more difficult to identify with lower yields following neoadjuvant chemotherapy [18, 19].

Sentinel lymph nodes should be sliced at 2–3 mm intervals perpendicular to the long axis

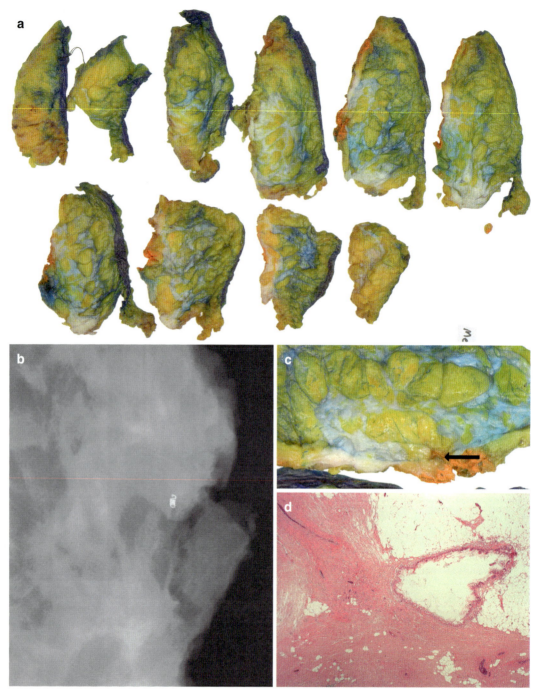

Fig. 2.4 Handling of a mastectomy specimen following neoadjuvant chemotherapy. (**a**) Serial slices of a mastectomy specimen. There was no obvious tumor mass, although an area of firmness could be palpated anteriorly (*orange ink*) in slices 4, 5, and 6. (**b**) Specimen X-ray shows marker clip toward anterior aspect of slice 6 adjacent to the area of firmness. (**c**) Corresponding close-up of slice 6 revealing the tumor clip (*arrow*). The tumor measured 5 cm in dimension on the pretreatment MRI, so blocks were taken from slices 3–8 to encompass this area. (**d**) H&E section from slice 6 showing the clip site. No residual invasive carcinoma was identified despite wide sampling indicating pCR to neoadjuvant chemotherapy

and all submitted. Routine levels and/or immuno-histochemistry are not indicated, but may be performed as per institutional protocols.

Axillary clearances should be carefully examined, and all suspected nodes submitted in their entirety. The axillary tail of mastectomy specimens should also be inspected for the presence of low axillary lymph nodes.

Histological Reporting

For reporting cancer specimens in the neoadjuvant setting, the emphasis is on identifying residual disease and quantifying response. Traditional histological variables such as tumor grade, lesion size, and the presence of lymphovascular invasion retain prognostic significance following neoadjuvant therapy; however, neoadjuvant therapy can alter tumor histology, making assessment more difficult.

Breast

Tumors of typical ductal/NST morphology pretreatment can take on a lobular appearance post-chemotherapy [20], growing as scattered single cells, cords, and small nests. In this situation, tumor typing on the pretreatment core biopsy is more accurate. Tumor grade can also change,

with increased nuclear pleomorphism or more commonly due to a reduction in mitotic count. Histological grade pre- and post-treatment both show an association with outcome, and a reduction in proliferation as reflected in a drop in mitotic index has been associated with improved survival post-neoadjuvant chemotherapy [21, 22].

In tumors that have responded to chemotherapy, the tumor cells often lie within a characteristic loose, edematous background stroma (Fig. 2.5a). There may be an associated lymphoplasmacytic inflammatory cell infiltrate and/or collections of foamy or pigmented macrophages (Fig. 2.5b). If sheets of macrophages are present, caution should be taken, as post-treatment tumor cells may have abundant vacuolated cytoplasm that histologically mimics macrophages; if in doubt immunohistochemistry for cytokeratin and CD68 can be useful to determine cell lineage. In the event of pCR, these stromal changes may be all that remains of the tumor bed. Gel foam marker clips lead to the formation of a cyst lined by histiocytes that is also a useful indicator that the tumor bed has been sampled (Fig. 2.4d).

In patients who receive neoadjuvant endocrine therapy, the pattern of response is different, with central scarring and fibrosis and preservation of tumor cells at the periphery [23].

Changes may also be seen in the background breast tissue, with atrophy and hyalinization of benign lobules with or without a perilobular

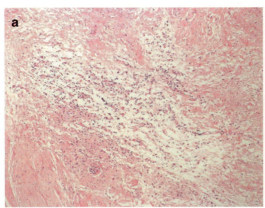
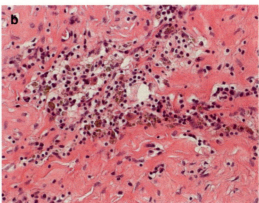

Fig. 2.5 Changes in the tumor bed post-neoadjuvant chemotherapy. (**a**) Characteristic loose myxoid stroma with patchy lymphocytic inflammatory infiltrate. (**b**) Collections of pigmented macrophages with associated chronic inflammatory cells

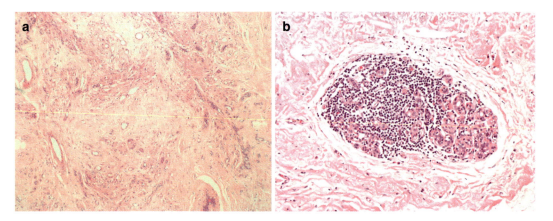

Fig. 2.6 (**a**) Background benign breast tissue showing marked atrophy with sclerosis and hyalinization of lobules. (**b**) Benign breast lobule with a prominent lymphocytic infiltrate

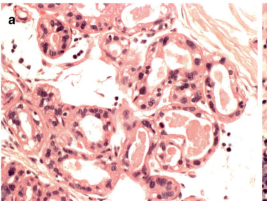 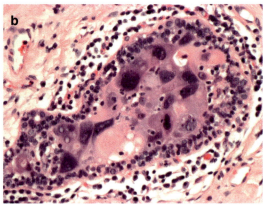

Fig. 2.7 (**a**) Benign lobule with reactive nuclear changes. There is a spectrum of change with occasional enlarged bizarre-looking nuclei among smaller more regular nuclei. These changes may be seen some distance from the tumor bed. (**b**) High-grade DCIS where all the nuclei are markedly pleomorphic

lymphocytic infiltrate (Fig. 2.6) [24, 25]. There may be reactive cytological atypia within benign lobules that may be mistaken for DCIS; this often occurs as scattered bizarre cells or as a spectrum of atypia within an otherwise benign lobule, in contrast to DCIS where all the cells appear "uniformly" atypical (Fig. 2.7) [8].

Two main patterns of response to chemotherapy have been described radiologically, and this is often mirrored by the histological findings (Fig. 2.8). The first is "concentric shrinking," where the tumor remains as a solitary mass lesion but shrinks in size. The second pattern is termed the "scatter pattern," where the tumor melts away in a nonuniform way, leaving scattered deposits

of tumor across the tumor bed. The latter pattern is associated with an increased risk of local recurrence following breast-conserving surgery [26, 27]. The scatter pattern can be particularly difficult to assess histologically, as there may be widely separated residual islands of tumor cells making accurate measurement impossible. If there was a single lesion on pretreatment imaging and the residual nests of tumor cells all lie within a reactive stromal background, then it is best to regard this as a single lesion and give a descriptive report providing the maximum dimension of the individual residual tumor foci as well as the maximum dimension of the entire tumor bed [6]. To calculate the residual cancer burden (RCB),

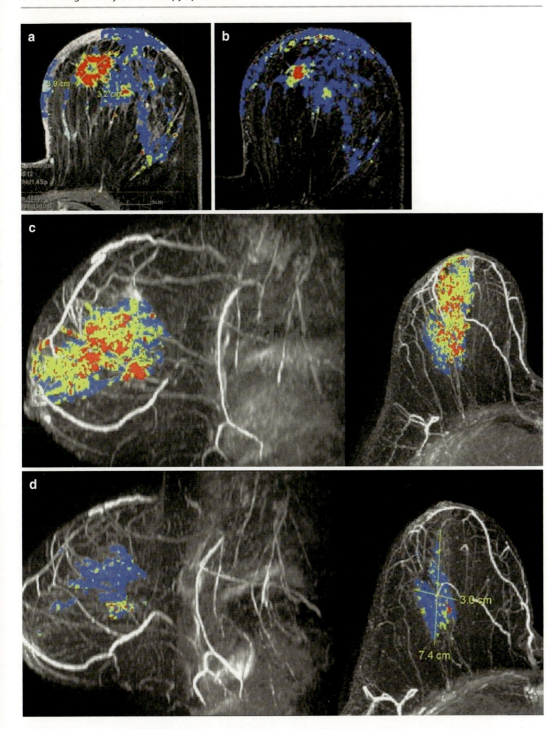

Fig. 2.8 Two main MRI response patterns following neoadjuvant chemotherapy. (**a, b**) Concentric shrinking pattern. The pretreatment MRI shows two adjacent tumor foci (**a**). Follow-up MRI after the fourth cycle of chemotherapy shows the presence of two discrete foci with a reduction in size of both (**b**). (**c, d**) Scatter pattern. The pretreatment MRI shows a large area of enhancement (**c**). The post-treatment MRI shows tumor extending over the same area, with patchy residual foci of enhancement (MRI images courtesy of Dr F Kilburn-Toppin)

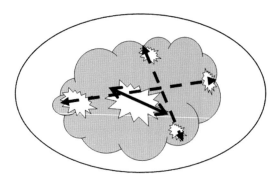

Fig. 2.9 Schematic of size measurement when there are multiple residual deposits spread over the tumor bed (*gray*). To calculate the RCB, the size of the entire lesion with intervening fibrosis should be measured in two dimensions (*black dotted line*). In contrast, the seventh edition of the TNM staging system uses the size of the largest single contiguous deposit (*black solid line*)

the size of the entire tumor bed with residual cancer including non-contiguous foci is measured in two dimensions (Fig. 2.9). This approach correlates well with radiological findings, and several studies have shown a relationship between residual tumor size and cellularity measured in this way and outcome post-neoadjuvant chemotherapy [28–30]. It should be noted that the seventh edition of the TNM defines tumor size as the dimension of the largest contiguous group of tumor cells (Fig. 2.9), with addition of the (m) classifier to indicate multiple foci [31]. There are no studies as yet that show a relationship between sizes measured in this way with outcome.

If there were multiple lesions on initial imaging, with normal breast or adipose tissue between residual tumor foci, then this is best regarded as true multifocal disease.

Neoadjuvant therapy often has a marked effect on tumor cellularity. Tumor size may not decrease; however, there may be a significant reduction in overall cellularity, making residual cellularity an important indicator of response [32]. The RCB website includes an online cellularity standard [14], and the images accompanying the description of the Miller-Payne score also provide a useful guide for estimating cellularity [33]. Changes in tumor cellularity resulting from neoadjuvant therapy can be heterogeneous; hence adequate sampling is important for accurate

assessment of overall response (Fig. 2.10). Variation in response may reflect clonal heterogeneity, and if areas of differing morphology and grade are present, this should be commented on; retesting of receptor status should be considered in this setting (see below).

Assessment of residual cellularity forms the basis of several grading systems described below, either in terms of absolute residual cellularity expressed as a percentage of the tumor bed (RCB) [30] or the degree of change in cellularity pre- and posttreatment (e.g., Pinder, Miller-Payne, Sataloff, and Chevallier systems) [25, 33–35]. The descriptions of the latter scoring systems do not explicitly state how to deal with heterogeneity, and there may be a tendency to only assess the most cellular areas of the tumor. The RCB system does not look at pretreatment cellularity but proposes standardized sampling with assessment of average cellularity across five slides representing the largest two-dimensional area of residual tumor bed.

A rare pattern of residual disease has been described where foci of lymphovascular invasion are identified in the absence of an invasive tumor focus. In this situation, the tumor bed must be well sampled to ensure that the invasive tumor has not been missed. As in the adjuvant setting, the presence of lymphovascular invasion post-neoadjuvant therapy is a marker of poor prognosis. One series suggested that patients with extensive residual lymphovascular invasion in the absence of invasive disease have a particularly poor outcome; however numbers were small and many patients had nodal involvement confounding the results [36]. Given this association with worse outcome, recent guidelines published by an international working group recommend that patients with residual lymphovascular invasion alone be regarded as not having had a pCR [6].

Axillary Lymph Nodes

Post-treatment axillary lymph node status is an important determinant of disease-free and overall survival post-neoadjuvant therapy, independent of response within the breast [3]. In two studies,

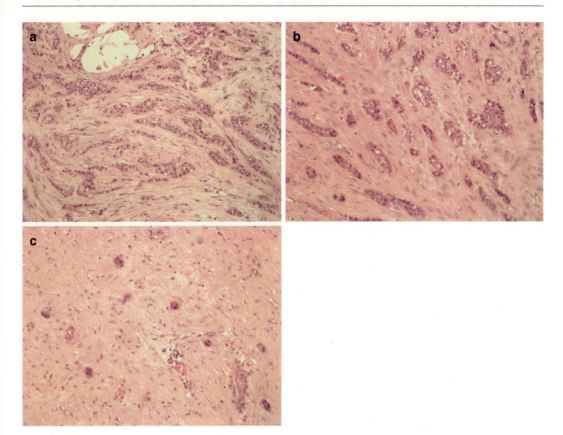

Fig. 2.10 Change in cellularity following neoadjuvant chemotherapy. (**a**) Pretreatment core biopsy showing approximately 60 % tumor cellularity. (**b**) Post-treatment resection specimen showing a mild reduction in tumor cellularity to approximately 40 % in one area. (**c**) Another area from the post-treatment resection specimen showing more marked response with less than 10 % residual cellularity. The residual cancer burden system deals with heterogeneity in response by taking the average cellularity from five slides representing the maximum tumor cross section

around 5 % of patients had residual nodal disease despite a pCR in the breast [37, 38]. This may represent a more chemoresistant subclone within the metastatic disease, but may also reflect an element of sampling error as the tumor bed in the breast is much more extensive than the nodes (Fig. 2.11). The number of involved nodes, the size of the largest metastasis, and the presence of treatment effect all show an association with survival outcomes [37, 39]. If positive nodes are removed at pretreatment SLN, this valuable information is lost.

As in the adjuvant setting, lymph node staging is either performed by SLN biopsy or axillary dissection. The accuracy of SLN in the neoadjuvant setting is the focus of ongoing investigation.

Several large series have shown that in patients with clinically negative axillary lymph nodes pretreatment, the detection rate and sensitivity of SLN are comparable to that in the adjuvant setting [40–42]. However, in patients with proven nodal disease pretreatment, the results are more variable, with an unacceptably high false-negative rate up to 40 % in some series [42, 43]. There is some evidence to suggest that the false-negative rate is lower in patients who show a clinical response in the axilla post-treatment [44]. The ACOSOG Z1071 trial examined the accuracy of post-treatment SLNB in patients with proven axillary metastases pretreatment [45]. The patients underwent pre- and post-treatment axillary ultrasound, and the biopsied node was

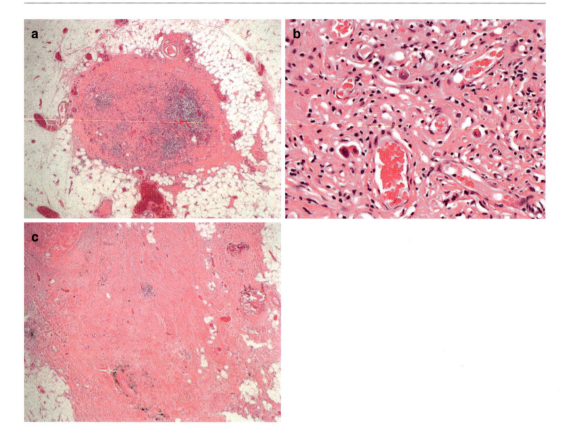

Fig. 2.11 (**a**) Lymph node showing extensive fibrosis following neoadjuvant chemotherapy. (**b**) High-power examination shows the presence of residual tumor cells. (**c**) Examination of the breast in this case showed pCR with no residual invasive tumor identified

clipped. Overall, 41 % of patients had a nodal pCR. The false-negative rate was 12.6 %; however this was 9 % for patients who had three or more nodes examined compared with 21 % in patients who had two nodes examined. The study concluded that changes in patient selection that result in greater sensitivity are necessary to support the use of SLN in this patient population, and SLN should be avoided in patients who have clinically evident residual nodal disease and/or a poor response to therapy.

Reporting of lymph nodes is similar to the adjuvant setting, and the number of positive nodes and the size of the largest metastasis should be documented. In addition, the presence of treatment effect in the lymph nodes should be recorded. If metastases are present, there should be a comment as to whether they show any evidence of treatment effect such as fibrosis; this may be heterogeneous between different nodal metastases

(Fig. 2.12). In cases where there has been a nodal pCR, there may be wedge-shaped areas of fibrosis, aggregates of foamy macrophages, or mucin pools. In the presence of these changes, the node should be closely examined for residual tumor cells; routine immunohistochemistry is not indicated but may be useful if suspicious cells are identified [46]. Small fibrous scars may be seen in the absence of neoadjuvant therapy, and it may be impossible to distinguish biopsy site changes from treatment effect. Patients with axillary downstaging have a prognosis intermediate between patients that are truly node negative and those with residual metastatic disease [47]. An estimate of the pretreatment nodal burden, as indicated by the number of nodes showing fibrosis, may be used in adjuvant decision-making such as the need for supraclavicular radiotherapy.

A particular area of controversy is the interpretation of isolated tumor cells (ITCs) in the

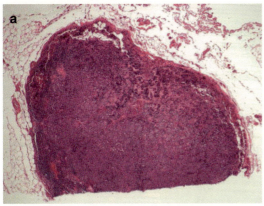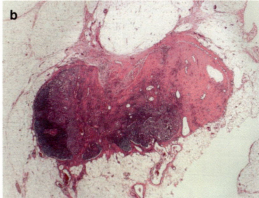

Fig. 2.12 Two lymph nodes from the same patient following neoadjuvant chemotherapy. (**a**) Lymph node with macrometastasis showing no evidence of chemotherapy response. (**b**) Another lymph node with metastatic tumor associated with marked fibrosis consistent with partial response to therapy

neoadjuvant setting [2]. These often occur as single cells scattered throughout an area of reactive stromal changes and most likely represent previous macrometastatic disease that has regressed with chemotherapy, the nodal equivalent of minimal residual disease. In this circumstance the size of the entire deposit including intervening fibrosis should be measured, not just the size of the largest cell cluster [6]. ITCs identified post-neoadjuvant therapy have been associated with a worse prognosis and if present should not be designated as pCR [37]. The TNM staging system regards ITCs as node negative post-neoadjuvant therapy (ypN0(i)) but states that they should not be called pCR [31]. In contrast, the WHO advises that they should be regarded as node positive [48].

Some centers use molecular assays such as OSNA to assess SLN without any morphological examination. There is some evidence to suggest that this technique can be applied in the neoadjuvant setting [49]; however sensitivity may be reduced [50], and it is not recommended as it precludes assessment of nodal response and is not calibrated to detect ITCs [6, 51].

of axillary lymph node status (ypT0ypNx). Current definitions, endorsed by the FDA for use in neoadjuvant clinical trials, require the absence of invasive disease in the breast and axillary lymph nodes, with or without the presence of DCIS (ypT0/isypN0 or ypT0ypN0). Whether the presence of residual DCIS should preclude pCR is a matter of controversy. The meta-analysis of 12 large neoadjuvant clinical trials undertaken by the CTNeoBC found similar event-free and overall survival in patients without residual invasive disease in the breast, regardless of the presence or absence of DCIS [3]. The rate of pCR according to the three definitions was 22% for ypT0/is, 18% for ypT0/isypN0, and 13% for ypT0ypN0. In contrast, a pooled analysis of seven neoadjuvant trials by the German and Austrian Breast Group found that patients with residual DCIS had a significantly worse event-free survival, with no significant difference in overall survival [52]. The definition of pCR used should be clearly stated in the report, and the presence of residual DCIS should be recorded and measured.

Definition of pCR

Several definitions of pCR have been used in the literature making comparisons of clinical trial results difficult. Many early studies regarded response in the breast only, without consideration

Grading of Response

There have been numerous systems developed for grading of response following neoadjuvant chemotherapy. Some of the more commonly used systems are summarized in Table 2.1. Early

Table 2.1 Summary of key grading systems of response following neoadjuvant chemotherapy for breast cancer

Grading system	Breast	Lymph nodes	Comment
AJCC ypTNM [31]	Size categories as per TNM	Nodal stages as per TNM. ITCs called node negative [pN0(i+)], but not regarded as pCR	pCR no invasive disease, CIS allowed
	Tis carcinoma in situ. T1 ≤20 mm, T2 20–50 mm, T3 >50 mm, T4 extension to the skin or chest wall		No evaluation of response
			Seventh edition size = largest contiguous focus of tumor cells with (m) if multiple foci across tumor bed
Modified NPI [53]	Size of invasive cancer and post-therapy tumor grade	Number of involved nodes	pCR no invasive disease, CIS allowed
	$0.2 \times$ size + grade + LN stage		No evaluation of response
			Association with outcome on univariate analysis [54]
Chevallier [34]	1. Disappearance of tumor on either macroscopic or microscopic assessment	Classes 1 and 2 include no metastatic tumor in the nodes	Classes 1 and 2 regarded as pCR (i.e., CIS allowed)
	2. CIS present, no residual invasive tumor		
	3. Invasive carcinoma present with stromal changes		Association with DFS and OS [55, 56]
	4. Few modifications in the appearance of the tumor		
Sataloff [35]	T-A. Total or near total therapeutic effect (scattered cells <5% of tumor surface)	N-A. Therapeutic effect, no metastatic disease	T-A includes pCR and minimal residual disease
	T-B. >50% therapeutic effect but less than T-A	N-B. No nodal metastasis or therapeutic effect	Association with DFS and OS [56]
	T-C. <50% therapeutic effect	N-C. Therapeutic effect, metastasis present	
	T-D. No therapeutic effect evident	N-D. Metastatic disease, no therapeutic effect	
Miller-Payne [33]	1. No change or some alteration in tumor cells but no reduction in overall cellularity	Not graded	pCR no invasive disease, CIS allowed
	2. Minor loss of tumor cells (up to 30%)		Comparison of pre- and posttreatment cellularity
	3. 30–90% reduction in cellularity		Significant association with DFS and OS
	4. >90% loss of tumor cells		
	5. No malignant cells identifiable. DCIS allowed		
RCB [30]	Size of tumor in two dimensions, percentage cellularity of residual tumor and percentage that is DCIS	Number of involved nodes and size of the largest metastasis	pCR no invasive disease, CIS allowed
	Results entered into an online algorithm giving a continuous numerical index divided into four grades (0–3)	Cannot be applied if there is a positive pretreatment SLN	Cellularity posttreatment – no comparison with pretreatment biopsy
			Validated in several series
			Good reproducibility

RPCB [57]	Combination of RCB with posttreatment Ki67 index	As above	The addition of Ki67 improved prognostic power of RCB Further model including grade and ER status provided further prognostic information Requires external validation
Pinder [25]	1. pCR. (i) No residual carcinoma, (ii) residual invasive tumor but DCIS present	1. No metastasis, no evidence of response	pCR no invasive disease, CIS allowed
	2. Partial response. (i) MRD, <10% tumor remaining, (ii) 10–50% tumor remaining, (iii) >50% tumor remaining	2. No metastasis, evidence of response	Comparison of pre- and posttreatment cellularity
	3. No evidence of response	3. Metastasis with response	No data regarding association with survival
		4. Metastasis, no response	
NRI [58]	Initial clinical stage based on pretreatment MRI minus the posttreatment ypT stage based on pathological tumor measurement. An additional one point is given for near pCR and two points for pCR	Axillary staging by US and FNA or pretreatment SLN	Comparison of pretreatment clinical and radiological measurements and posttreatment pathological measurements
	Breast response score plus axillary response score/by maximum score if pCR is achieved. 0=no response to 1=pCR	Pre-Rx clinical axillary node stage minus posttreatment pathology stage – pA3, ≥1 palpable node positive; pA2, ≥1 non-palpable node positive for macrometastasis; pA1, ≥1 non-palpable node positive for micrometastasis; pA0, no metastasis	Based on residual invasive disease only, CIS permitted Association with survival in triple-negative breast cancer [59]
CPS-EG [60]	Combination of presenting clinical stage (score 0–2), posttreatment pathological stage (score 0–2), ER negativity (score 1) and nuclear grade 3 (score 1)		Association with DFS Internal and external validation [61]
NPRI [62]	Formula includes the presence of fibrosis (0,1), presence of LVI (0/1), number of positive lymph nodes and planned hormonal therapy NPRI-PG1 – no trace of residual disease	Calculation includes number of positive lymph nodes and the presence of fibrosis in nodes	pCR defined as the absence of invasive disease, CIS permitted
	NPRI-PG2 – good		
	NPRI-PG3 – moderate		Association with DFS and BCSS
	NPRI-PG4 – poor prognosis		Requires external validation

systems, such as the Sataloff, Chevallier, and Miller-Payne systems, rely on a comparison between tumor cellularity in the pretreatment core biopsy and post-treatment resection specimen. The grade of response is a reflection of the relative decrease in cellularity induced by chemotherapy. These systems have been validated in clinical trials and shown to correlate with patient outcome.

An alternative method, the RCB, has been proposed by the team at the MD Anderson Cancer Center [30]. The RCB is a measure of the volume of residual disease in the breast and axillary lymph nodes, without reference to pretreatment tumor cellularity. The RCB score is determined based on maximum size of the tumor bed measured in two dimensions, average residual invasive tumor cellularity, the number of positive lymph nodes, and the size of the largest lymph node metastasis. These values can be entered into an online calculator [14] which determines the RCB score as a continuous variable and the RCB class with 0 being pCR, (1) representing minimal residual disease, (2) representing an intermediate residual disease volume, and (3) representing extensive residual tumor with poor outcome. Patients showing excellent response with minimal residual disease (RCB class 1) have an equivalent outcome to patients with pCR. The RCB has been validated in several studies and was shown to be reproducible with good correlation with long-term outcome [29, 63, 64]. It has been advocated as the preferred method for use in clinical trials as it quantifies partial response; however it can be quite labor intensive until one becomes familiar with its use.

Traditional staging systems, such as the Nottingham Prognostic Index (NPI) and TNM stage, also correlate with outcome post-neoadjuvant therapy [54, 65]. There are more complex systems that include a combination of pretreatment clinical stage and post-treatment pathological findings, such as the NRI and CPS + EG score [58, 60, 61]. The latter combines pretreatment clinical stage, ER status, and histological grade with post-treatment pathological stage. The Nottingham group has proposed the Nottingham Clinico-Pathological Response Index (NPRI), which includes the presence of fibrosis, LVI status, and administration of post-treatment hormonal therapy [62].

The likelihood of pCR, and the strength of correlation between chemotherapy response and outcome, is closely associated with tumor biology. Novel classification systems are being developed that include a combination of pathological response and biological tumor markers. One example is the residual proliferative cancer burden, which combines the RCB with post-treatment Ki67 index [57].

The above scoring systems are purely used in patients who receive neoadjuvant chemotherapy. The Preoperative Endocrine Prognostic Index (PEPI) has been developed for patients who receive neoadjuvant endocrine therapy [66]. The PEPI score is calculated using pathological tumor stage, nodal status, and post-treatment ER status and Ki67 index. Each of these variables is given a score of 0–3, with a total score of four or more associated with an increased risk of relapse. Patients in the low-risk group (score 0) have a very low risk of relapse so they do not require any adjuvant therapy other than hormonal agents, whereas the high-risk group may benefit from additional therapy such as chemotherapy.

Retesting of Tumor Markers Post-neoadjuvant Therapy

Reassessment of hormone receptors and HER2 status post-neoadjuvant therapy is currently not routine in many centers [6]. Several studies have compared ER, PR, and HER2 status pre- and post-neoadjuvant chemotherapy, and two meta-analyses of published series have reported discordance for ER in 13 and 18 %, PR in 32 and 26 %, and HER2 in 9 and 6 % of cases [67, 68]. Sources of discordance may include technical artifacts such as fixation, intratumoral heterogeneity, and changes in expression induced by treatment.

Results of repeat receptor testing are of biological interest in the clinical trial setting. In the majority of patients, receptor status does not change; however conversion to a positive result would indicate eligibility for targeted therapy. In routine practice, the decision to retest markers may be influenced by pretreatment receptor status and histological findings in the post-treatment resection specimen [6]. There is current uncertainty as to whether change in receptor status should influence the choice of future adjuvant therapies [69–71]. Loss of HER2 amplification was identified in 32 % of tumors in one series following neoadjuvant therapy that included trastuzumab, and patients with tumors that retained HER2 amplification had a better recurrence-free survival [72]. Several studies have looked at changes in hormone receptor (HR) status with conflicting results. Chen et al. found conversion from HR-positive to HR-negative status in 15 % of patients, and this was associated with worse overall and disease-free survival [69]. Tacca et al. found a change in HR status in 23 % of patients; patients whose tumors changed from ER-negative to ER-positive had a better overall survival than patients who remained ER-negative, whereas patients who switched from ER-positive to ER-negative disease showed no survival difference from patients with stable ER-positive disease but better survival than patients with stable ER-negative disease [71]. In contrast, Jin et al. found a change in HR status in 18 % of patients, with stable HR-positive patients having the best overall survival and patients whose tumors switched from HR-spositive to HR-negative the worst [73]. In a more recent series, Lim et al. found that stable HR-positive patients had the best prognosis, followed by HR-negative patients who convert to HR-positive, with patients who were HR-negative post-chemotherapy having the worst outcomes regardless of pretreatment HR status [74]. Reassessment should be considered if receptor results are unknown, if results on the pretreatment core biopsy were equivocal or there was insufficient invasive tumor represented and tumoral heterogeneity with morphologically distinct areas present in the excision specimen, or if there has been poor/no response to therapy [6].

Neoadjuvant Therapy and Clinical Trials

Adjuvant clinical trials giving long-term survival outcomes remain the gold standard in determining the efficacy of new therapeutic agents; however they require large numbers of patients and are expensive to run, and the outcome data takes years to mature. Using this traditional approach, there is a very long delay between the discovery of new agents and their introduction into routine clinical practice. An example is trastuzumab, which has revolutionized the management of HER2-positive breast cancer. The HER2 protein was first discovered in 1984 [75], and the first animal studies of trastuzumab took place in 1990 with phase II clinical trials following in 1996 [76, 77]. Trastuzumab was approved for use in metastatic breast cancer in 1998; however the first randomized adjuvant trial in early breast cancer did not occur until 2000, and it was not until 2006 that trastuzumab received FDA approval for use in the adjuvant setting and was accepted as standard of care [78, 79]. This is a delay of 10 years from phase II trials to adjuvant use.

Neoadjuvant clinical trials, using pCR as a surrogate for survival outcome, have the advantage of being smaller and cheaper and provide faster results. The neoadjuvant approach has recently been approved by the FDA to support accelerated approval of novel agents in patients with high-risk subtypes of breast cancer, i.e., high-grade hormone receptor-negative and/or HER2-positive breast cancer [5]. The early NOAH trial looking at neoadjuvant trastuzumab in HER2-positive breast cancer found double the pCR rate in patients given chemotherapy plus trastuzumab compared with chemotherapy alone (38 % versus 19 %, respectively); this translated into an overall survival benefit of similar magnitude in the subsequent adjuvant trials [80–82]. However, more recent adjuvant trials have failed to show an overall survival benefit despite significant differences in pCR rate in the matching neoadjuvant trials. For example, the NeoALTTO trial, comparing lapatinib versus trastuzumab versus combined therapy in HER2-positive patients, found a significant difference in pCR rate between the combination arm and both of the single-agent arms (47 % combined, 20 % lapatinib alone, 28 % trastuzumab alone) [83]. However the ALTTO trial, a randomized phase III study addressing the same question, found a longer disease-free survival in the combination therapy arm, but this was not statistically significant [84]. This leads to questions regarding the validity of neoadjuvant trials and the use of pCR as a marker of outcome; however caveats apply when comparing outcome results from neoadjuvant and adjuvant trials [85].

The first explanation for differences between pCR rates and survival outcomes is based on tumor biology. Different tumor subtypes have different pCR rates, with high pCR rates in triple-negative (27–36%) and HER2-positive/HR-negative (26–55%) disease, compared with low rates in HR-positive/HER2-negative (<10%) disease [3, 52, 86]. However, despite the low pCR rate, women with HR-positive/HER2-negative disease still have good survival outcomes. The association between pCR and survival is not significant in women with low-grade ER-positive/HER2-negative breast cancer, compared with grade 3 ER-positive/HER2-negative, HER2-positive, or triple-negative disease where there is a much stronger association [3]. Even among HER2-positive patients, ER-negative patients have higher pCR rates (39% and 19%, respectively) [86] and a stronger association between pCR and survival than ER-positive patients [3]. This means that the correlation between pCR rates in neoadjuvant trials and survival outcomes in the adjuvant setting will be influenced by the trial eligibility criteria and the biological characteristics of the breast cancers included in the trial. The neoadjuvant model using pCR as an endpoint is most relevant for high-risk triple-negative or HER2-positive disease and may be best suited to trials of novel agents in specified molecular subpopulations. This does not mean neoadjuvant trials cannot be applied to other breast cancer subtypes, but alternative measures of response may need to be used.

In a similar vein, the outcome in neoadjuvant trials is sharply divided between pCR and non-pCR. The non-pCR subgroup includes a continuum of response from patients who have an excellent response with only a few residual tumor cells to patients who have no response or indeed progress on therapy. Long-term survival analyses using the RCB system show that patients with RCB class 1 (minimal residual disease) have similar survival outcomes to patients who have pCR [30]. Hence the survival benefit of a drug may be underestimated by including patients who have an excellent response in the nonresponder (non-pCR) group.

The design of neoadjuvant and adjuvant clinical trials themselves may also confound the association between pCR and survival outcomes. In many neoadjuvant trials, patients also receive additional adjuvant therapy, such as radiotherapy following breast conservation, hormone therapy for ER-positive patients, and continuation of trastuzumab or other anti-HER2 agents in HER2-positive patients. This adjuvant therapy presumably has an additional survival benefit and could reduce the size of the effect of pCR on survival outcome.

In summary, neoadjuvant clinical trials play an important role in facilitating the approval of new drugs and targeted agents and expediting their introduction into routine clinical use. The opportunity to observe tumor response, and take tumor samples before, during, and after treatment, also provides a unique and valuable means of improving our understanding of the biology of breast cancer and interrogating the molecular mechanisms underlying sensitivity and resistance to treatment. However, neoadjuvant trials must be carefully designed with attention to precisely defined patient populations, rigorous pathology protocols, and consideration of the impact of additional adjuvant therapy on survival outcomes.

References

1. Buchholz TA, Mittendorf EA, Hunt KK. Surgical considerations after neoadjuvant chemotherapy: breast conservation therapy. J Natl Cancer Inst Monogr. 2015;51:11–4.
2. King TA, Morrow M. Surgical issues in patients with breast cancer receiving neoadjuvant chemotherapy. Nat Rev Clin Oncol. 2015;12:335–43.
3. Cortazar P, Zhang L, Untch M, Mehta K, Costantino JP, Wolmark N, et al. Pathological complete response and long-term clinical benefit in breast cancer: the CTNeoBC pooled analysis. Lancet. 2014;384: 164–72.
4. Mamounas EP, Anderson SJ, Dignam JJ, Bear HD, Julian TB, Geyer Jr CE, et al. Predictors of locoregional recurrence after neoadjuvant chemotherapy: results from combined analysis of national surgical adjuvant breast and bowel project B-18 and B-27. J Clin Oncol. 2012;30:3960–6.

5. Guidance for industry pathological complete response in neoadjuvant treatment of high-risk early-stage breast cancer: use as an endpoint to support accelerated approval. Administration USDoFaD, editor. 2014. http://www.fda.gov/downloads/Drugs/Guidance ComplianceRegulatoryInformation/Guidances/ UCM305501.pdf

6. Provenzano E, Bossuyt V, Viale G, Cameron D, Badve S, Denkert C, et al. Standardization of pathologic evaluation and reporting of postneoadjuvant specimens in clinical trials of breast cancer: recommendations from an international working group. Mod Pathol. 2015;28:1185–201.

7. Bossuyt V, Provenzano E, Symmans WF, Boughey JC, Coles C, Curigliano G, et al. Recommendations for standardized pathological characterization of residual disease for neoadjuvant clinical trials of breast cancer by the BIG-NABCG collaboration. Ann Oncol. 2015;26:1280–91.

8. Pinder SE, Rakha EA, Purdie CA, Bartlett JM, Francis A, Stein RC, et al. Macroscopic handling and reporting of breast cancer specimens pre- and post-neoadjuvant chemotherapy treatment: review of pathological issues and suggested approaches. Histopathology. 2015;67:279–93.

9. Leyland-Jones BR, Ambrosone CB, Bartlett J, Ellis MJ, Enos RA, Raji A, et al. Recommendations for collection and handling of specimens from group breast cancer clinical trials. J Clin Oncol. 2008;26: 5638–44.

10. Loi S, Symmans WF, Bartlett JM, Fumagalli D, Van't Veer L, Forbes JF, et al. Proposals for uniform collection of biospecimens from neoadjuvant breast cancer clinical trials: timing and specimen types. Lancet Oncol. 2011;12:1162–8.

11. Kuehn T, Bauerfeind I, Fehm T, Fleige B, Hausschild M, Helms G, et al. Sentinel-lymph-node biopsy in patients with breast cancer before and after neoadjuvant chemotherapy (SENTINA): a prospective, multicentre cohort study. Lancet Oncol. 2013;14: 609–18.

12. Oh JL, Nguyen G, Whitman GJ, Hunt KK, Yu TK, Woodward WA, et al. Placement of radiopaque clips for tumor localization in patients undergoing neoadjuvant chemotherapy and breast conservation therapy. Cancer. 2007;110:2420–7.

13. Buzdar AU. Preoperative chemotherapy treatment of breast cancer – a review. Cancer. 2007;110: 2394–407.

14. Residual cancer burden calculator and associated documents (guide for measuring cancer cellularity, examples of gross and microscopic evaluation, pathology protocol for macroscopic and microscopic assessment of RCB). http://ww3.mdanderson.org/app/medcalc/ index.cfm?pagename=jsconvert3. Cited 11 Sep 2015.

15. Adrada BE, Huo L, Lane DL, Arribas EM, Resetkova E, Yang W. Histopathologic correlation of residual mammographic microcalcifications after neoadjuvant chemotherapy for locally advanced breast cancer. Ann Surg Oncol. 2015;22(4):1111–7.

16. Li JJ, Chen C, Gu Y, Di G, Wu J, Liu G, et al. The role of mammographic calcification in the neoadjuvant therapy of breast cancer imaging evaluation. PLoS One. 2014;9(2):e88853. Clinical Trial, Phase II.

17. Weiss A, Lee KC, Romero Y, Ward E, Kim Y, Ojeda-Fournier H, et al. Calcifications on mammogram do not correlate with tumor size after neoadjuvant chemotherapy. Ann Surg Oncol. 2014;21:3310–6.

18. Belanger J, Soucy G, Sideris L, Leblanc G, Drolet P, Mitchell A, et al. Neoadjuvant chemotherapy in invasive breast cancer results in a lower axillary lymph node count. J Am Coll Surg. 2008;206:704–8.

19. Neuman H, Carey LA, Ollila DW, Livasy C, Calvo BF, Meyer AA, et al. Axillary lymph node count is lower after neoadjuvant chemotherapy. Am J Surg. 2006;191(6):827–9.

20. Carder P. Typing breast cancer following primary chemotherapy. Histopathology. 1999;35:584–5.

21. Diaz J, Stead L, Shapiro N, Newell R, Loudig O, Lo Y, et al. Mitotic counts in breast cancer after neoadjuvant systemic chemotherapy and development of metastatic disease. Breast Cancer Res Treat. 2013;138:91–7.

22. Penault-Llorca F, Abrial C, Raoelfils I, Chollet P, Cayre A, Mouret-Reynier MA, et al. Changes and predictive and prognostic value of the mitotic index, Ki-67, cyclin D1, and cyclo-oxygenase-2 in 710 operable breast cancer patients treated with neoadjuvant chemotherapy. Oncologist. 2008;13:1235–45.

23. Thomas JS, Julian HS, Green RV, Cameron DA, Dixon MJ. Histopathology of breast carcinoma following neoadjuvant systemic therapy: a common association between letrozole therapy and central scarring. Histopathology. 2007;51(2):219–26.

24. Aktepe F, Kapucuoglu N, Pak I. The effects of chemotherapy on breast cancer tissue in locally advanced breast cancer. Histopathology. 1996;29:63–7.

25. Pinder SE, Provenzano E, Earl H, Ellis IO. Laboratory handling and histology reporting of breast specimens from patients who have received neoadjuvant chemotherapy. Histopathology. 2007;50:409–17.

26. Akay CL, Meric-Bernstam F, Hunt KK, Grubbs EG, Bedrosian I, Tucker SL, et al. Evaluation of the MD Anderson prognostic index for local-regional recurrence after breast conserving therapy in patients receiving neoadjuvant chemotherapy. Ann Surg Oncol. 2012;19:901–7.

27. Chen AM, Meric-Bernstam F, Hunt KK, Thames HD, Outlaw ED, Strom EA, et al. Breast conservation after neoadjuvant chemotherapy. Cancer. 2005;103: 689–95.

28. Peintinger F, Kuerer HM, McGuire SE, Bassett R, Pusztai L, Symmans WF. Residual specimen cellularity after neoadjuvant chemotherapy for breast cancer. Br J Surg. 2008;95:433–7.

29. Peintinger F, Sinn B, Hatzis C, Albarracin C, Downs-Kelly E, Morkowski J, et al. Reproducibility of residual cancer burden for prognostic assessment of breast cancer after neoadjuvant chemotherapy. Mod Pathol. 2015;28:913–20.

30. Symmans WF, Peintinger F, Hatzis C, Rajan R, Kuerer H, Valero V, et al. Measurement of residual breast cancer burden to predict survival after neoadjuvant chemotherapy. J Clin Oncol. 2007;25: 4414–22.

31. Edge SB, Byrd DR, Compton CC, Fritz AG, Greene FL, Trotti A, editors. AJCC cancer staging handbook. 7th ed. New York: Springer; 2010.

32. Rajan R, Poniecka A, Smith TL, Yang Y, Frye D, Pusztai L, et al. Change in tumor cellularity of breast carcinoma after neoadjuvant chemotherapy as a variable in the pathologic assessment of response. Cancer. 2004;100:1365–73.

33. Ogston KN, Miller ID, Payne S, Hutcheon AW, Sarkar TK, Smith I, et al. A new histological grading system to assess response of breast cancers to primary chemotherapy: prognostic significance and survival. Breast. 2003;12:320–7.

34. Chevallier B, Roche H, Olivier JP, Chollet P, Hurteloup P. Inflammatory breast cancer. Pilot study of intensive induction chemotherapy (FEC-HD) results in a high histologic response rate. Am J Clin Oncol. 1993;16:223–8.

35. Sataloff DM, Mason BA, Prestipino AJ, Seinige UL, Lieber CP, Baloch Z. Pathologic response to induction chemotherapy in locally advanced carcinoma of the breast: a determinant of outcome. J Am Coll Surg. 1995;180:297–306.

36. Rabban JT, Glidden D, Kwan ML, Chen YY. Pure and predominantly pure intralymphatic breast carcinoma after neoadjuvant chemotherapy: an unusual and adverse pattern of residual disease. Am J Surg Pathol. 2009;33:256–63.

37. Hennessy BT, Hortobagyi GN, Rouzier R, Kuerer H, Sneige N, Buzdar AU, et al. Outcome after pathologic complete eradication of cytologically proven breast cancer axillary node metastases following primary chemotherapy. J Clin Oncol. 2005;23: 9304–11.

38. Provenzano E, Vallier AL, Champ R, Walland K, Bowden S, Grier A, et al. A central review of histopathology reports after breast cancer neoadjuvant chemotherapy in the neo-tango trial. Br J Cancer. 2013;108:866–72.

39. Klauber-DeMore N, Ollila DW, Moore DT, Livasy C, Calvo BF, Kim HJ, et al. Size of residual lymph node metastasis after neoadjuvant chemotherapy in locally advanced breast cancer patients is prognostic. Ann Surg Oncol. 2006;13:685–91.

40. Classe JM, Bordes V, Campion L, Mignotte H, Dravet F, Leveque J, et al. Sentinel lymph node biopsy after neoadjuvant chemotherapy for advanced breast cancer: results of Ganglion Sentinelle et Chimiotherapie Neoadjuvante, a French prospective multicentric study. J Clin Oncol. 2009;27:726–32.

41. Hunt KK, Yi M, Mittendorf EA, Guerrero C, Babiera GV, Bedrosian I, et al. Sentinel lymph node surgery after neoadjuvant chemotherapy is accurate and reduces the need for axillary dissection in breast cancer patients. Ann Surg. 2009;250:558–66.

42. van Deurzen CH, Vriens BE, Tjan-Heijnen VC, van der Wall E, Albregts M, van Hilligersberg R, et al. Accuracy of sentinel node biopsy after neoadjuvant chemotherapy in breast cancer patients: a systematic review. Eur J Cancer. 2009;45:3124–30.

43. Straver ME, Rutgers EJ, Russell NS, Oldenburg HS, Rodenhuis S, Wesseling J, et al. Towards rational axillary treatment in relation to neoadjuvant therapy in breast cancer. Eur J Cancer. 2009;45:2284–92.

44. Alvarado R, Yi M, Le-Petross H, Gilcrease M, Mittendorf EA, Bedrosian I, et al. The role for sentinel lymph node dissection after neoadjuvant chemotherapy in patients who present with node-positive breast cancer. Ann Surg Oncol. 2012;19:3177–84.

45. Boughey JC, Suman VJ, Mittendorf EA, Ahrendt GM, Wilke LG, Taback B, et al. Sentinel lymph node surgery after neoadjuvant chemotherapy in patients with node-positive breast cancer: the ACOSOG Z1071 (alliance) clinical trial. JAMA. 2013;310:1455–61.

46. Loya A, Guray M, Hennessy BT, Middleton LP, Buchholz TA, Valero V, et al. Prognostic significance of occult axillary lymph node metastases after chemotherapy-induced pathologic complete response of cytologically proven axillary lymph node metastases from breast cancer. Cancer. 2009;115:1605–12.

47. Newman LA, Pernick NL, Adsay V, Carolin KA, Philip PA, Sipierski S, et al. Histopathologic evidence of tumor regression in the axillary lymph nodes of patients treated with preoperative chemotherapy correlates with breast cancer outcome. Ann Surg Oncol. 2003;10:734–9.

48. Lakhani SR, Ellis IO, Schnitt SJ, Tan PH, Van de Vijver MJ, editors. WHO classification of tumours of the breast. 4th ed. Lyon: IARC; 2012.

49. Navarro-Cecilia J, Duenas-Rodriguez B, Luque-Lopez C, Ramirez-Exposito MJ, Martinez-Ferrol J, Ruiz-Mateas A, et al. Intraoperative sentinel node biopsy by one-step nucleic acid amplification (OSNA) avoids axillary lymphadenectomy in women with breast cancer treated with neoadjuvant chemotherapy. Eur J Surg Oncol. 2013;39:873–87.

50. Takamoto K, Shimazu K, Naoi Y, Shimomura A, Shimoda M, Kagara N, et al. One-step nucleic acid amplification assay for detection of axillary lymph node metastases in breast cancer patients treated with neoadjuvant chemotherapy. Ann Surg Oncol. 2015. doi:10.1245/s10434-015-4693-y9.

51. Feldman S, Krishnamurthy S, Gillanders W, Gittleman M, Beitsch PD, Young PR, et al. A novel automated assay for the rapid identification of metastatic breast carcinoma in sentinel lymph nodes. Cancer. 2011;117:2599–607.

52. von Minckwitz G, Untch M, Blohmer JU, Costa SD, Eidtmann H, Fasching PA, et al. Definition and impact of pathologic complete response on prognosis after neoadjuvant chemotherapy in various intrinsic breast cancer subtypes. J Clin Oncol. 2012;30:1796–804.

53. Abrial C, Thivat E, Tacca O, Durando X, Mouret-Reynier MA, Gimbergues P, et al. Measurement of

residual disease after neoadjuvant chemotherapy. J Clin Oncol (Comment Lett). 2008;26:3094; author reply 3095.

54. Chollet P, Amat S, Belembaogo E, Cure H, de Latour M, Dauplat J, et al. Is Nottingham prognostic index useful after induction chemotherapy in operable breast cancer? Br J Cancer. 2003;89:1185–91.

55. Chollet P, Amat S, Cure H, de Latour M, Le Bouedec G, Mouret-Reynier MA, et al. Prognostic significance of a complete pathological response after induction chemotherapy in operable breast cancer. Br J Cancer. 2002;86:1041–6.

56. Penault-Llorca F, Abrial C, Raoelfils I, Cayre A, Mouret-Reynier MA, Leheurteur M, et al. Comparison of the prognostic significance of Chevallier and Sataloff's pathologic classifications after neoadjuvant chemotherapy of operable breast cancer. Hum Pathol. 2008;39:1221–8.

57. Sheri A, Smith IE, Johnston SR, A'Hern R, Nerurkar A, Jones RL, et al. Residual proliferative cancer burden to predict long-term outcome following neoadjuvant chemotherapy. Ann Oncol. 2015;26:75–80.

58. Rodenhuis S, Mandjes IA, Wesseling J, van de Vijver MJ, Peeters MJ, Sonke GS, et al. A simple system for grading the response of breast cancer to neoadjuvant chemotherapy. Ann Oncol. 2010;21:481–7.

59. Jebbink M, van Werkhoven E, Mandjes IA, Wesseling J, Lips EH, Vrancken Peeters MJ, et al. The prognostic value of the neoadjuvant response index in triple-negative breast cancer: validation and comparison with pathological complete response as outcome measure. Breast Cancer Res Treat. 2015;153:145–52.

60. Jeruss JS, Mittendorf EA, Tucker SL, Gonzalez-Angulo AM, Buchholz TA, Sahin AA, et al. Combined use of clinical and pathologic staging variables to define outcomes for breast cancer patients treated with neoadjuvant therapy. J Clin Oncol. 2008;26:246–52.

61. Mittendorf EA, Jeruss JS, Tucker SL, Kolli A, Newman LA, Gonzalez-Angulo AM, et al. Validation of a novel staging system for disease-specific survival in patients with breast cancer treated with neoadjuvant chemotherapy. J Clin Oncol. 2011;291956–1962.

62. Abdel-Fatah TM, Ball G, Lee AH, Pinder S, MacMilan RD, Cornford E, et al. Nottingham Clinico-Pathological Response Index (NPRI) after neoadjuvant chemotherapy (Neo-ACT) accurately predicts clinical outcome in locally advanced breast cancer. Clin Cancer Res. 2015;21:1052–62.

63. Nahleh Z, Sivasubramaniam D, Dhaliwal S, Sundarajan V, Komrokji R. Residual cancer burden in locally advanced breast cancer: a superior tool. Curr Oncol. 2008;15:271–8.

64. Romero A, Garcia-Saenz JA, Fuentes-Ferrer M, Lopez Garcia-Asenjo JA, Furio V, Roman JM, et al. Correlation between response to neoadjuvant chemotherapy and survival in locally advanced breast cancer patients. Ann Oncol. 2013;24:655–61.

65. Carey LA, Metzger R, Dees EC, Collichio F, Sartor CI, Ollila DW, et al. American Joint Committee on cancer tumor-node-metastasis stage after neoadjuvant chemotherapy and breast cancer outcome. J Natl Cancer Inst. 2005;97:1137–42.

66. Ellis MJ, Tao Y, Luo J, A'Hern R, Evans DB, Bhatnagar AS, et al. Outcome prediction for estrogen receptor-positive breast cancer based on postneoadjuvant endocrine therapy tumor characteristics. J Natl Cancer Inst. 2008;100:1380–8.

67. Jabbour MN, Massad CY, Boulos FI. Variability in hormone and growth factor receptor expression in primary versus recurrent, metastatic, and post-neoadjuvant breast carcinoma. Breast Cancer Res Treat. 2012;135:29–37.

68. Zhang N, Moran MS, Huo Q, Haffty BG, Yang Q. The hormonal receptor status in breast cancer can be altered by neoadjuvant chemotherapy: a meta-analysis. Cancer Invest. 2011;29:594–8.

69. Chen S, Chen CM, Yu KD, Zhou RJ, Shao ZM. Prognostic value of a positive-to-negative change in hormone receptor status after neoadjuvant chemotherapy in patients with hormone receptor-positive breast cancer. Ann Surg Oncol. 2012;19:3002–11.

70. Hirata T, Shimizu C, Yonemori K, Hirakawa A, Kouno T, Tamura K, et al. Change in the hormone receptor status following administration of neoadjuvant chemotherapy and its impact on the long-term outcome in patients with primary breast cancer. Br J Cancer. 2009;101:1529–36.

71. Tacca O, Penault-Llorca F, Abrial C, Mouret-Reynier MA, Raoelfils I, Durando X, et al. Changes in and prognostic value of hormone receptor status in a series of operable breast cancer patients treated with neoadjuvant chemotherapy. Oncologist. 2007;12:636–43.

72. Mittendorf EA, Wu Y, Scaltriti M, Meric-Bernstam F, Hunt KK, Dawood S, et al. Loss of HER2 amplification following trastuzumab-based neoadjuvant systemic therapy and survival outcomes. Clin Cancer Res. 2009;15:7381–8.

73. Jin X, Jiang YZ, Chen S, Yu KD, Shao ZM, Di GH. Prognostic value of receptor conversion after neoadjuvant chemotherapy in breast cancer patients: a prospective observational study. Oncotarget. 2015;6:9600–11.

74. Lim SK, Lee MH, Park IH, You JY, Nam BH, Kim BN, et al. Impact of molecular subtype conversion of breast cancers after neoadjuvant chemotherapy on clinical outcome. Cancer Res Treat. 2016;48(1):133–41.

75. Schechter AL, Stern DF, Vaidyanathan L, Decker SJ, Drebin JA, Greene MI, et al. The neu oncogene: an erb-B-related gene encoding a 185,000-Mr tumour antigen. Nature. 1984;312:513–6.

76. Baselga J, Tripathy D, Mendelsohn J, Baughman S, Benz CC, Dantis L, et al. Phase II study of weekly intravenous recombinant humanized anti-p185 HER2 monoclonal antibody in patients with HER2/neu-overexpressing metastatic breast cancer. J Clin Oncol. 1996;14:737–44.

77. Shepard HM, Lewis GD, Sarup JC, Fendly BM, Maneval D, Mordenti J, et al. Monoclonal antibody therapy of human cancer: taking the HER2 protooncogene to the clinic. J Clin Immuno. 1991;11:117–1127.

78. Baselga J, Perez EA, Pienkowski T, Bell R. Adjuvant trastuzumab: a milestone in the treatment of HER-2-positive early breast cancer. Oncologist. 2006;11 Suppl 1:4–12.

79. Braga S, dal Lago L, Bernard C, Cardoso F, Piccart M. Use of trastuzumab for the treatment of early stage breast cancer. Expert Rev Anticancer There. 2006; 6:1153–64.

80. Gianni L, Eiermann W, Semiglazov V, Manikhas A, Lluch A, Tjulandin S, et al. Neoadjuvant chemotherapy with trastuzumab followed by adjuvant trastuzumab versus neoadjuvant chemotherapy alone, in patients with HER2-positive locally advanced breast cancer (the NOAH trial): a randomised controlled superiority trial with a parallel HER2-negative cohort. Lancet. 2010;375:377–84.

81. Perez EA, Romond EH, Suman VJ, Jeong JH, Sledge G, Geyer Jr CE, et al. Trastuzumab plus adjuvant chemotherapy for human epidermal growth factor receptor 2-positive breast cancer: planned joint analysis of overall survival from NSABP B-31 and NCCTG N9831. J Clin Oncol. 2014;32:3744–52.

82. Smith I, Procter M, Gelber RD, Guillaume S, Feyereislova A, Dowsett M, et al. 2-year follow-up of trastuzumab after adjuvant chemotherapy in HER2-positive breast cancer: a randomised controlled trial. Lancet. 2007;369:29–36.

83. Baselga J, Bradbury I, Eidtmann H, Di Cosimo S, de Azambuja E, Aura C, et al. Lapatinib with trastuzumab for HER2-positive early breast cancer (NeoALTTO): a randomised, open-label, multicentre, phase 3 trial. Lancet. 2012;379:633–40.

84. Piccart-Gebhart M, Holmes AP, Baselga J, Azambuja ED, Dueck AC, Viale G. First results from the phase III ALTTO trial (BIG 2–06; NCCTG [Alliance] N063D) comparing one year of anti-HER2 therapy with lapatinib alone (L), trastuzumab alone (T), their sequence (T!L), or their combination (TþL) in the adjuvant treatment of HER2-positive early breast cancer (EBC) [abstract]. J Clin Oncol. 2014;32:LBA4.

85. DeMichele A, Yee D, Berry DA, Albain KS, Benz CC, Boughey J, et al. The neoadjuvant model is still the future for drug development in breast cancer. Clin Cancer Res. 2015;21:2911–5.

86. Houssami N, Macaskill P, von Minckwitz G, Marinovich ML, Mamounas E. Meta-analysis of the association of breast cancer subtype and pathologic complete response to neoadjuvant chemotherapy. Eur J Cancer. 2012;48:3342–54.

Proliferative Breast Lesions

Sarah E. Pinder

Abstract

This chapter deals with ductal and lobular proliferative lesions with an emphasis on the benign and atypical ones including in particular usual and atypical ductal hyperplasia, columnar cell lesions, and flat epithelial atypia. In situ malignant lesions are mentioned briefly, and criteria for distinguishing them from benign and atypical proliferative lesions are discussed.

Keywords

Usual epithelial hyperplasia • Columnar cell lesions • Flat epithelial atypia • Atypical lobular hyperplasia • Lobular carcinoma in situ • Ductal carcinoma in situ

Introduction

Proliferation lesions in the breast are classically subdivided into intraductal and intralobular epithelial proliferations. Although this is somewhat arbitrary, and it is known that there are molecular and genetic similarities between some of the ductal and the lobular lesions, this classification is based on typical topographical patterns and will be maintained in this chapter.

The intraductal epithelial proliferations include usual epithelial hyperplasia (also called usual ductal hyperplasia or hyperplasia of usual type), atypical ductal hyperplasia (ADH), and ductal carcinoma in situ (DCIS). The intralobular lesions include atypical lobular hyperplasia (ALH) and lobular carcinoma in situ (LCIS), together categorized as lobular neoplasia, and also the columnar cell lesions. The latter range from columnar cell change and columnar cell hyperplasia to flat epithelial atypia (FEA) and to flat high-grade DCIS.

In broad terms the clinical significance of intraductal and intralobular epithelial proliferations lies with the increased risk of some of these lesions for subsequent development of carcinoma, either ipsilaterally (i.e., true precursors) and/or contralaterally (i.e., risk lesions). There is

S.E. Pinder
Division of Cancer Studies, Guy's Hospital,
King's College London,
3rd Floor, Bermondsey Wing, Great Maze Pond,
London SE1 9RT, UK
e-mail: sarah.pinder@kcl.ac.uk

© Springer International Publishing Switzerland 2017
S. Shousha (ed.), *Breast Pathology*, DOI 10.1007/978-3-319-28655-6_3

now a greater understanding of the genetic changes in the various epithelial proliferations [1], and the various different pathways of progression to subtypes of invasive breast carcinoma are being explored [2].

Ductal Lesions

Usual Epithelial Hyperplasia

Usual epithelial hyperplasia is regarded as one component of fibrocystic change, along with fibrosis, cysts, and apocrine change, and can be subcategorized as mild, moderate, or marked (florid) depending on the degree within the duct space. Moderate and florid usual epithelial hyperplasia confers a 1.5–2 times increased risk of developing carcinoma in either breast [3]. As this level of risk is minimal and is not regarded as requiring increased radiological surveillance or follow-up, this subclassification is of limited value clinically.

Usual epithelial hyperplasia is a nonneoplastic and non-clonal proliferation within the breast ducts. This can generally be identified as a cytologically mixed process with nuclei of varying size and, in particular, shape. Very often elongated nuclei are admixed with rounder forms and the nuclei may overlap. The cells may be arranged in a streaming pattern. Architecturally, while occasionally florid forms may present with a solid proliferation pattern, typically there are rather ill-formed, irregular, slit-like peripheral spaces (Fig. 3.1).

Rarely there may be necrosis within the ducts bearing usual epithelial hyperplasia (Figs. 3.1 and 3.2), although this is most commonly seen when the hyperplasia is present within a coexisting lesion, such as a complex sclerosing lesion, papilloma, or fibroadenoma, and particularly if there has been a prior needling procedure, such as fine-needle aspiration cytology (FNAC) or needle core biopsy. Clearly, the presence of a prominent epithelial proliferation with central necrosis will raise concerns about the differential diagnosis of DCIS. The appearances of usual epithelial hyperplasia do not generally mimic

low-grade DCIS, where there are regular, small, evenly spaced nuclei, but intermediate-grade DCIS may be mistaken for usual epithelial hyperplasia, particularly DCIS of neuroendocrine type, where a streaming pattern is common [4].

A form of hyperplasia resembling that seen in the male breast in gynecomastia may be seen [5, 6]. This may have rudimentary micropapillary architecture within lobules and terminal ducts but is formed from cells without the monotony of low-grade DCIS. Additional features that may be helpful in the identification of gynecomastoid-type

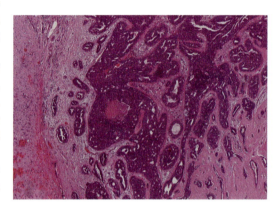

Fig. 3.1 Usual epithelial hyperplasia within a complex sclerosing papillary lesion. Branching spaces are filled with an epithelial proliferation within a mass lesion. Even at this magnification, the irregular shape of peripheral fenestrations can be seen

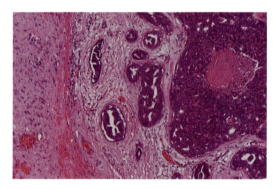

Fig. 3.2 Usual epithelial hyperplasia within a complex sclerosing papillary lesion (higher magnification of lesion in Fig. 3.1). Although there is one space with central necrosis, the overall architecture of this intraductal epithelial proliferation demonstrates the slit-like spaces and impression of streaming typical of florid usual epithelial hyperplasia

usual epithelial hyperplasia are that the nuclei are often arranged around the periphery of the micropapillary structures and the central core may thus appear somewhat empty. Also, the nuclei are typically somewhat hyperchromatic, and the abnormal cells do not involve the entire space but are admixed with normal cuboidal/columnar cells [6].

Where usual epithelial hyperplasia shows worrisome features, immunohistochemistry can be helpful. This non-clonal process shows a mosaic, heterogeneous pattern in the epithelial proliferation with the basal cytokeratin markers, cytokeratin 5 (Ck5 or Ck5/6) and cytokeratin 14 (Ck14) [7] (Fig. 3.3). However, other markers, such as estrogen receptor (ER), may also be valuable; ER similarly may show a heterogeneous pattern with nuclei in usual epithelial hyperplasia ranging from negative through mild and moderate to strong positivity (Fig. 3.4). It should be noted, however, that the proportion of ER-positive cells increases with age and also that occasionally contiguous positive cells are seen in some cases [8]. Conversely non-high-grade DCIS is almost invariably Ck5 and Ck14 negative and uniformly ER strongly positive. The algorithm does not usefully apply to high-grade DCIS, as basal-like DCIS may not infrequently show heterogeneous reactivity with basal cytokeratin markers.

Atypical Ductal Hyperplasia

The term atypical ductal hyperplasia (ADH) should not be used to describe cases of usual epithelial hyperplasia where the pathologist is concerned about the presence of a few superimposed cells with intermediate- or high-grade atypia. ADH is a specific and rare entity, and to maintain any clinical significance, the diagnosis should be applied only to microfocal cases of a low-grade proliferation resembling low-grade DCIS. Indeed this similarity to low-grade DCIS forms the basis of the diagnostic criteria both qualitatively and quantitatively [9]. The *qualitative* assessment is based on cytological features as well as architectural pattern (Figs. 3.5, 3.6, and 3.7). These include:

- A uniform, regular, small cell, luminal epithelial cell population (Ck5, Ck14 homogeneously negative)
- Even spacing of the nuclei
- Secondary luminal spaces, some of which are rigid, whereas others are tapering
- Hyperchromatic, typically small, round, uniform nuclei with sparse mitoses
- Cribriform, micropapillary, or, less commonly, solid growth pattern

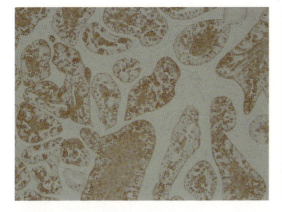

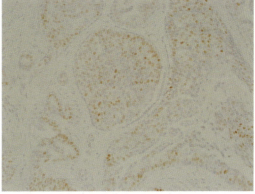

Fig. 3.3 Usual epithelial hyperplasia within a complex sclerosing papillary lesion (same lesion as Figs. 3.1 and 3.2), cytokeratin 14. The heterogeneous pattern of immunoreactivity with cytokeratin 14 indicates the non-clonality of this epithelial proliferation

Fig. 3.4 Usual epithelial hyperplasia within a complex sclerosing papillary lesion (same lesion as Figs. 3.1, 3.2, and 3.3), estrogen receptor. A heterogeneous pattern of staining and range of intensity from negative to moderate in this case is helpful as reassurance of non-clonality

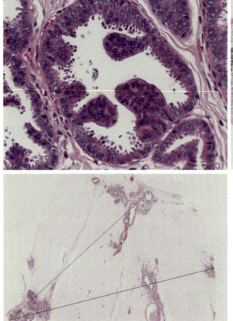

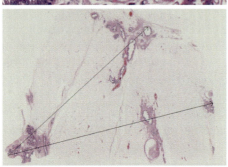

Figs. 3.5, 3.6, and 3.7 Differential diagnosis of atypical ductal hyperplasia (ADH) and low-grade ductal carcinoma in situ (DCIS). Figure 3.5 shows architectural atypia, in the form of well-formed micropapillae (with narrow stalks and wider tips) in an acinar space with prominent apical snouts in the adjacent lining epithelium. Distinguishing ADH from low-grade DCIS on this image (of a single space) is not possible, as extent cannot be determined. In Figs. 3.6 and 3.7, the extent of the micropapillary architectural atypia is more apparent at lower magnification. This cytologically low-grade and architecturally atypical epithelial proliferation is extensive and is therefore be categorized as low-grade DCIS

The *quantitative* assessment is *based on assessment of lesion* size:

- Areas of ADH are usually small, involving less than two complete membrane-bound spaces.

As the diagnosis of ADH lays with the recognition of some of the features of low-grade DCIS and is regarded by some as an early form of this process, one could question the value of the diagnosis. It has been retained in the lexicon of breast diagnostic entities because of the data from studies indicating that this lesion confers a subsequent increased risk of the development of invasive breast cancer but that this risk applies to both breasts and is not purely ipsilateral and at the same site [10]. In other words, ADH does not behave as a classical precursor of invasive disease.

Differential diagnosis of ADH includes low-grade DCIS and also flat epithelial atypia (FEA). Indeed, FEA and ADH may coexist (Fig. 3.8) and cause particular problems in diagnosis as there may be incomplete architectural atypia within membrane-bound spaces, for example, in the form of micropapillae or bridges. These can potentially extend over several millimeter, and consideration then has to be given to a diagnosis of low-grade DCIS. Such cases have to be assessed on a case-by-case basis according to the degree and extent of the architectural atypia, and if such a lesion extends widely, the diagnosis of ADH should be questioned (Fig. 3.7).

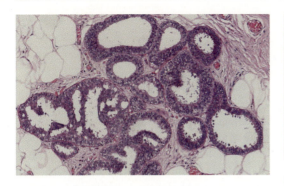

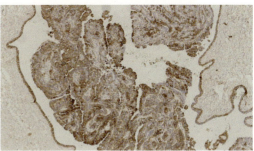

Fig. 3.8 Flat epithelial atypia with superimposed architectural atypia. This terminal duct lobular unit is composed of mildly dilated acini, lined by a flat epithelium with prominent apical snouts. The nuclei are uniform and round, rather than columnar in shape. In addition to this flat epithelial atypia, however, there are ill-formed bridges and rudimentary micropapillae indicating that atypical ductal hyperplasia/low-grade ductal carcinoma in situ should be considered in the diagnosis and levels/further sections examined

Fig. 3.9 Usual epithelial hyperplasia in an intraductal papilloma, cytokeratin 5. Cytokeratin 5 reactivity, with a mosaic, heterogeneous pattern, confirms the non-clonal nature of this epithelial proliferation within a benign papillary lesion

Ductal Carcinoma In Situ

DCIS is considered to be a precursor of invasive breast carcinoma. There is, however, very limited data on the frequency of progression and the time taken to presentation as invasive disease. Historical series of "comedo" carcinoma include cases of mixed DCIS and invasive carcinoma, and older nomenclature makes evaluation of such descriptions problematic [11]. DCIS was first recognized in 1893 (reviewed in [12]). Despite the name, most DCIS is generally considered to arise from the junction of the terminal duct and the lobular units. Typically, however, it then extends within the duct system. Interestingly, unlike some other precursor lesions at other sites, DCIS is, in the vast majority of cases, a unicentric proliferation of epithelial cells within a single duct system [13, 14]. DICS should not be misinterpreted as multifocal because it is not seen contiguously in two-dimensional histological sections and it is important that pathologists understand the breast duct distribution and anatomy [15].

It is now clear that, just like invasive breast cancer, DCIS is not a single entity but can be categorized as a range of subtypes, based on a range of features. The subject is dealt with in more details in Chap. 5.

Epithelial Proliferation (Hyperplasia, Atypia, and DCIS) Within Papillary Lesions

Comment should be made here on the problematic, but not uncommon, area of epithelial proliferation within a papillary lesion (see also Chap. 11). When the coexisting papillary lesion is benign (i.e., an intraductal papilloma), the underlying architecture and immunohistochemical pattern confirms that the fibrovascular fronds are typically wide with a myoepithelial layer between the epithelium and the stroma, unlike papillary carcinoma in situ [16]. Assessment of the epithelial proliferation should be undertaken as for any other intraductal epithelial proliferation, including the cytology and architecture. Usual epithelial hyperplasia, often with benign apocrine change, is common in papillomas. As elsewhere, the hyperplasia will show variation in nuclear size and shape but without overtly malignant features, for example, mitoses or marked pleomorphism. Immunohistochemistry can be used to confirm the mosaic pattern of expression with Ck5, Ck14, and ER, as above (Fig. 3.9). If the epithelial proliferation in a papillary lesion is of low-grade, monotonous, and clonal appearance, the extent of the atypical epithelial proliferation should be determined and the lesion categorized as atypia within a papilloma if less than 3 mm or as low-grade DCIS within a papilloma if more than 3 mm in extent [17] (Fig. 3.10).

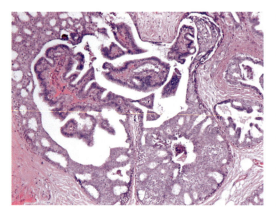

Fig. 3.10 Low-grade ductal carcinoma within a papilloma. An architecturally atypical (largely cribriform) low-grade epithelial proliferation is seen contained within this expanded space. Centrally, wide fibrovascular cores with overlying columnar-shaped epithelium are seen as part of the preexisting papilloma. The extent of the atypical proliferation was more than 3 mm, and this was therefore regarded as low-grade DCIS in a papilloma

This author regards papillomas bearing DCIS as distinct from papillary carcinoma in situ, which are lesions with thin fibrovascular fronds and overlying perpendicularly arranged columnar-shaped neoplastic epithelial cells but without an interspersed myoepithelial layer. The term atypical papilloma is not recommended in either situation, as this is clinically unhelpful.

Paget's Disease of the Nipple

Paget's disease of the nipple is diagnosed when malignant cells, usually of high cytonuclear grade, infiltrate along the basement membrane of the underlying ducts to the skin surface and are seen within the epidermis of the nipple [18]. These cells are typically Cam5.2 and HER2 (3+ and/or amplified) positive. With careful and thorough examination, underlying high-grade DCIS is almost always identified, although this may be small and present only in superficial duct spaces and may not be detected radiologically or clinically. There may be associated invasive disease, but this is less frequent than in older series in the literature.

Lobular Lesions

Atypical Lobular Hyperplasia and Classical Lobular Carcinoma In Situ (In Situ Lobular Neoplasia)

Distinguishing ALH from LCIS relies on assessment of the amount of expansion of the acini in the lobular unit, both in terms of the proportion of acini involved and the extent of expansion of each space. In ALH there is minimal extension of less than half of the acini, while in LCIS more than half of the acini within the TDLU are distended by an expansion of the typical cells (eight or more cells across each acinus). The subject is dealt with in detail in Chap. 6.

Columnar Cell Lesions

Columnar cell lesions [19] have had a range of names in the literature, including non-exhaustively, blunt duct adenosis, columnar cell change, columnar cell hyperplasia, unfolded lobules, and columnar alteration with prominent snouts and secretions (CAPSSs). This includes a spectrum of lesions ranging from columnar cell change through columnar cell hyperplasia to flat epithelial atypia [20, 21]. These lesions of the terminal duct lobular unit have become increasingly identified as a consequence of rigorous investigation of low suspicion radiological calcification identified through digital screening mammography and include:

- Columnar cell change
- Columnar cell hyperplasia
- Flat epithelial atypia

Columnar Cell Change and Columnar Cell Hyperplasia

Columnar cell change is diagnosed when the acini are lined by tall columnar-shaped epithelial cells, typically with apical snouts (Figs. 3.11 and 3.12). There may be mild dilatation of the acini, which often contain luminal secretions that may

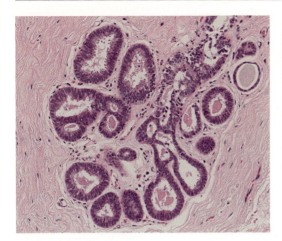

Fig. 3.11 Columnar cell change. A terminal duct lobular unit is formed from mildly dilated acini, lined by cells with columnar-shaped nuclei. Apical snouts are seen. There is no cytological atypia and this represents columnar cell change

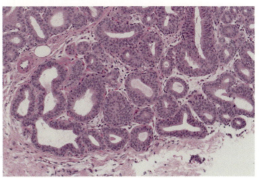

Fig. 3.13 Flat epithelial atypia (FEA). A terminal duct lobular unit formed from mildly dilated acini, lined by cells with round, bland, and uniform nuclei. Although this case does not show the typical rounded and smooth internal luminal aspect, the cytological features indicate that this should be regarded as FEA

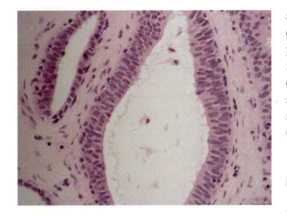

Fig. 3.12 Columnar cell change. High-power magnification shows the bland cytological features and the elongated columnar-shaped nuclei in columnar cell change

bear microcalcification. There is variation in the "tallness" of the cells between cases, and some lesions may be more cuboidal than columnar. Columnar cell change is diagnosed if there is a single layer of cells lining the acini, while columnar cell hyperplasia is identified if there is multilayering around the space with humps and tufts (broader at the base and not micropapillary in pattern). Care should be taken that this is not artifactual due to crosscutting of the acinar space, for example, if this is seen along only one edge of lobule.

True micropapillae and rigid epithelial bridges are not seen in columnar cell change or columnar cell hyperplasia. If architectural atypia, for example, in the form of micropapillary structures, is identified, the process should be assessed for extent and degree within the membrane-bound spaces and classified as atypical ductal hyperplasia or low-grade DCIS, accordingly (see above) (Fig. 3.8).

Flat Epithelial Atypia

If low-grade cytological atypia is seen lining the terminal duct lobular unit, the lesion is classified as flat epithelial atypia (FEA). On low power the terminal duct lobular unit may appear darker than other adjacent units, and there is sometimes an associated mild to moderate lymphoid cell population in the stroma. The cells in this process are cytologically akin to those of low-grade DCIS but are present in a flat layer (one or more) lining mildly dilated acini (Fig. 3.13). These acini typically have a smooth internal luminal aspect and bear secretions, with or without microcalcification. The nuclei are round, monotonous, and evenly spaced (Fig. 3.14). The cells may have clumped chromatin or vesicular nuclei or prominent multiple nucleoli, but mitoses are infrequent. There is an increased nuclear-cytoplasmic ratio.

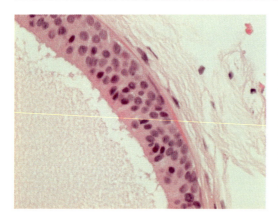

Fig. 3.14 Flat epithelial atypia (FEA). High-power magnification of an expanded acinar space lined by multilayered (but flat and non-architecturally atypical) epithelium formed from uniform cells with round, monotonous nuclei

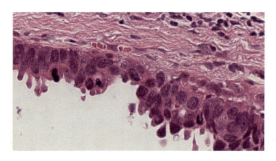

Fig. 3.15 Flat high-grade ductal carcinoma in situ. The epithelial cells lining this space are large and atypical, with nuclei more than 3× the diameter of the adjacent erythrocytes. Apical snouts remain prominent

However, if there is marked cytological atypia, the diagnosis of flat high-grade DCIS should be considered (Fig. 3.15). Historically this latter entity was described as one form of "clinging carcinoma" (reviewed in [22]). It typically involves both lobules and ducts and is formed from one or more flat layers of malignant cells with pleomorphic, large, and atypical nuclei (grade 3 nuclei).

Immunohistochemistry is of relatively little assistance in diagnosis; the columnar cell lesions are typically homogeneously estrogen receptor positivity and uniformly basal cytokeratin negative. This latter finding may be helpful in distinguishing cases of columnar cell change from microcysts with a flattened apocrine epithelial lining; the latter is typically uniformly ER negative.

Columnar cell change and columnar cell hyperplasia are regarded as benign and require no further investigation when identified in a core biopsy (see Chap. 4). Flat epithelial atypia is often seen in association with other lesions of the low-grade neoplasia family, including lobular neoplasia and ADH/low-grade DCIS [23], and these should be carefully sought if FEA is seen in any specimen. The columnar cell lesions overall confer a minimal increased risk of development of invasive carcinoma, but this is not independent of associated epithelial proliferation in some series [23]. However, even when identified as the sole lesion in a core biopsy specimen, FEA appears to confer an, albeit small, risk of upgrade, and adjacent DCIS or invasive carcinoma is reported in 9 % of cases (confidence intervals 5–14 %) in one systematic review [24].

Conclusion

Although the epithelial proliferations can usefully be regarded as intraductal or intralobular, they may coexist, and the recognition of anyone in any tissue sample should prompt the careful examination for other forms. Although the genetic features of the various epithelial proliferations are not described in detail here, it is clear that there are biological, molecular, and genetic similarities between, for example, FEA, ADH/low-grade DCIS, and LCIS and that these frequently show loss of 16q, while this is uncommon in high-grade processes [25, 26]. It is now widely believed that those low-grade and high-grade epithelial proliferations with a precursor risk follow different pathways to progression to invasive carcinoma and that the carcinomas that arise have differing histological features, biology, and prognosis.

References

1. Bombonati A, Sgroi DC. The molecular pathology of breast cancer progression. J Pathol. 2011;223(2):307–17.
2. Simpson PT, Reis-Filho JS, Gale T, Lakhani SR. Molecular evolution of breast cancer. J Pathol. 2005;205(2):248–54.

3. Cui Y, Page DL, Lane DS, Rohan TE. Menstrual and reproductive history, postmenopausal hormone use, and risk of benign proliferative epithelial disorders of the breast: a cohort study. Breast Cancer Res Treat. 2009;114(1):113–20.

4. Tan PH, Lui GG, Chiang G, Yap WM, Poh WT, Bay BH. Ductal carcinoma in situ with spindle cells: a potential diagnostic pitfall in the evaluation of breast lesions. Histopathology. 2004;45:343–51.

5. Rosai J. Ackerman's surgical pathology. 8th ed. St Louis: Mosby; 1996. p. 1583–7.

6. Tham K, Dupont WD, Page DL, Gary GF, Rogers LW. Micro-papillary hyperplasia with atypical features in female breast, resembling gynecomastia. Prog Surg Pathol. 1989;10:101–10.

7. Bánkfalvi A, Ludwig A, De-Hesselle B, Buerger H, Buchwalow IB, Boecker W. Different proliferative activity of the glandular and myoepithelial lineages in benign proliferative and early malignant breast diseases. Mod Pathol. 2004;17(9):1051–61.

8. Shoker BS, Jarvis C, Sibson DR, Walker C, Sloane JP. Oestrogen receptor expression in the normal and pre-cancerous breast. J Pathol. 1999;188(3):237–44.

9. Page DL. Atypical hyperplasia, narrowly and broadly defined. Hum Pathol. 1991;22:631–2.

10. Fitzgibbons PL, Henson DE, Hutter RV. Benign breast changes and the risk for subsequent breast cancer: an update of the 1985 consensus statement. Cancer Committee of the College of American Pathologists. Arch Pathol Lab Med. 1998;122(12):1053–5.

11. Bloodgood JC. Comedo carcinoma (or comedo-adenoma) of the female breast. Am J Cancer. 1934;22:842–53.

12. Bijker N, Donker M, Wesseling J, den Heeten GJ, Rutgers EJ. Is DCIS breast cancer, and how do I treat it? Curr Treat Opt Oncol. 2013;14(1):75–87.

13. Holland R, Hendriks JH. Microcalcifications associated with ductal carcinoma in situ: mammographic-pathologic correlation. Semin Diagn Pathol. 1994;11:181–92.

14. Holland R, Hendriks JH, Vebeek AL, Mravunac M, Schuurmans Stekhoven JH. Extent, distribution, and mammographic/histological correlations of breast ductal carcinoma in situ. Lancet. 1990;335:519–22.

15. Going JJ, Moffat DF. Escaping from Flatland: clinical and biological aspects of human mammary duct anatomy in three dimensions. J Pathol. 2004;203(1):538–44.

16. Tse GM, Tan PH, Moriya T. The role of immunohistochemistry in the differential diagnosis of papillary lesions of the breast. J Clin Pathol. 2009;62(5):407–13.

17. Page DL, Salhany KE, Jensen RA, Dupont WD. Subsequent breast carcinoma risk after biopsy with atypia in a breast papilloma. Cancer. 1996;78(2):258–66.

18. Sandoval-Leon AC, Drews-Elger K, Gomez-Fernandez CR, Yepes MM, Lippman ME. Paget's disease of the nipple. Breast Cancer Res Treat. 2013;141(1):1–12.

19. Schnitt SJ, Vincent-Salomon A. Columnar cell lesions of the breast. Adv Anat Pathol. 2003;10(3):113–24.

20. Pinder SE, Reis-Filho JS. Non-operative breast pathology: columnar cell lesions. J Clin Pathol. 2007;60(12):1307–12.

21. Jara-Lazaro AR, Tse GM, Tan PH. Columnar cell lesions of the breast: an update and significance on core biopsy. Pathology. 2009;41(1):18–27.

22. Schnitt SJ. Clinging carcinoma: an American perspective. Semin Diagn Pathol. 2010;27(1):31–6.

23. Abdel-Fatah TM, Powe DG, Hodi Z, Lee AH, Reis-Filho JS, Ellis IO. High frequency of coexistence of columnar cell lesions, lobular neoplasia, and low grade ductal carcinoma in situ with invasive tubular carcinoma and invasive lobular carcinoma. Am J Surg Pathol. 2007;31(3):417–26.

24. Verschuur-Maes AH, van Deurzen CH, Monninkhof EM, van Diest PJ. Columnar cell lesions on breast needle biopsies: is surgical excision necessary? A systematic review. Ann Surg. 2012;255(2):259–65.

25. Bürger H, de Boer M, van Diest PJ, Korsching E. Chromosome 16q loss – a genetic key to the understanding of breast carcinogenesis. Histol Histopathol. 2013;28(3):311–20.

26. Go EM, Tsang JY, Ni YB, Yu AM, Mendoza P, Chan SK, Lam CC, Lui PC, Tan PH, Tse GM. Relationship between columnar cell changes and low-grade carcinoma in situ of the breast – a cytogenetic study. Hum Pathol. 2012;43(11):1924–31.

Problematic Core Biopsies

4

Sarah E. Pinder

Abstract

This chapter deals with practical problems in the handling and reporting of breast core biopsy specimens, including approaches for identification of histological microcalcifications. The use of reporting categories ("B" codes) is recommended, and the chapter largely concentrates on those entities causing diagnostic difficulties, such as the B3 lesions, of uncertain malignant potential, as well as potentially problematic malignant lesions, albeit these make up a minority of a pathologist's routine practice.

Keywords

Core biopsy • B3, lesion of uncertain malignant potential • Atypical intraductal epithelial proliferation • Flat epithelial atypia • Radial scar • Papillary lesions • Spindle cell lesions

Introduction

The increased use of the needle core biopsy technique for sampling lesions in the breast since the development of core biopsy "guns" in the 1990s has resulted in an improved non-operative diagnosis of lesions over and above that achieved with fine needle aspiration cytology (FNAC). It is now, therefore, recommended that needle core

biopsy, or vacuum-assisted biopsy, is used for assessment of mammographic screen-detected abnormalities. Evidence suggests that core biopsy has greater sensitivity and specificity in evaluating microcalcification, asymmetry, and architectural distortion than does FNAC. In addition, for certain types of mammographic abnormality, particularly low to moderate suspicious microcalcification, a larger volume of tissue improves accuracy of diagnosis [1].

The definitive diagnosis of malignancy allows a planned *therapeutic* surgical procedure (with or without axillary surgery, as appropriate), as opposed to a *diagnostic* excision, with patient involvement in the decision-making process. Conversely, lesions that are definitively diagnosed as a specific benign lesion can be left in

S.E. Pinder
Division of Cancer Studies,
Guy's Hospital, King's College London,
3rd Floor, Bermondsey Wing, Great Maze Pond,
London SE1 9RT, UK
e-mail: sarah.pinder@kcl.ac.uk

© Springer International Publishing Switzerland 2017
S. Shousha (ed.), *Breast Pathology*, DOI 10.1007/978-3-319-28655-6_4

situ according to patient choice. There remain, however, a small proportion of diseases that are problematic to diagnose on core biopsy. These are often the same as those that cause diagnostic difficulties in definitive surgical excision specimens, but there are additional considerations and challenges because of the inherent nature of the core biopsy sampling technique such that only a small portion of the lesion is received for assessment.

The proportion of cases classified as "borderline" is fewer than assigned as such with FNAC, but these cause particular difficulties in subsequent clinical management. Recent guidelines for handling these lesions (categorized as B3, of uncertain malignant potential) have also been developed, and these, along with the diagnosis of these indeterminate lesions, are one of the most difficult issues for the breast pathologist and the multidisciplinary team.

Macroscopic Specimen Handling

The number of cores received for histological diagnosis will vary depending on the nature of the lesion, the method for targeting (free-hand, ultrasound, or stereotactic), and the gauge of the needle used. However, the same approach for reporting should be applied whether the specimen is an 18-, 16-, or 14-gauge or wider-bore sample (as may be obtained with a vacuum-assisted technique) such as an 11-, 8-, or 7-gauge needle.

The tissue, as soon as sampled, should be immediately fixed in an adequate amount of formalin. There is established data that a delay to fixation impairs assessment of hormone receptors and HER2 in breast cancer [2, 3]; however, there is relatively little robust data on the optimum length of fixation. In general it is widely recommended that core biopsy specimens are fixed for at least 6 h prior to processing, albeit some groups have reported excellent concordance between core biopsy samples for specimens fixed for approximately 45 min with the subsequent excised tumor [4]. Given the drive for same-day diagnostics, this has implications for the labora-

tory scheduling of processing of core biopsy samples, and more research regarding fixation is required [5]. In particular, laboratories must therefore optimize and validate their immunohistochemical results on breast core biopsy specimens that have been fixed for only short periods of time. Conversely, there may be potential issues for specimen fixed for longer periods of time, both with regard to biomarker assessment and to the evaluation of microcalcifications. It has been reported that microcalcifications disappear radiologically within 3 days in core biopsy specimens fixed in solutions with high water content [6], although this is not generally an issue in routine practice.

Full microscopic interpretation of core biopsies requires accurate and complete details of the clinical history and the radiological findings; this must be provided on the histology request form. Information including patient demographics, the side and site of the biopsy, and the radiological details such as the nature of the lesion(s), such as well-defined, or spiculate, mass, asymmetric deformity, calcification, etc. should be provided, ideally as well as the radiologist's impression/suspicion of the lesion (e.g., U4, M5, to indicate a lesion suspicious on ultrasound and malignant on mammogram).

There is no uniformity regarding the approach to the macroscopic description of core biopsies and vacuum-assisted biopsies on receipt in the laboratory. Some record the number of cores and their length, so that the details recorded in the clinic can be confirmed and also checked on the histological slide. There is increasingly a move to weigh vacuum-assisted biopsies to evaluate the amount of tissue obtained, akin to surgical specimens. Other radiology departments place the cores into capsules/containers in the clinic and then put these into the formalin pot, so that these can be directly transferred to cassettes in the laboratory, without further handling. This reduces the risk of loss of small biopsy specimens, but macroscopic description is not available for comparison or assessment.

As for all histopathology samples, it is important to ensure that the biopsy is properly embedded flat after processing and that the block is trimmed adequately (but not excessively) when the sections are taken. In general, while one hematoxylin and eosin (H&E)-stained section (i.e., one level) is usually sufficient for breast cores from mass lesions, many laboratories cut three levels for all breast cores. Cores from radiological calcifications should routinely have a minimum of three levels examined. However, it is worthwhile reserving some of the levels in between the three H&E sections for immunohistochemistry, if subsequently required, so that the block is not exhausted and the area of concern potentially discarded.

A radiograph of the core biopsies will be taken from cases of microcalcification so that the radiologist can determine if they have adequately sampled the lesion of concern. It is essential that they provide a comment regarding the presence of representative microcalcification to the pathologist, along with access to the images, either as hard copy or digitally. This will enable the pathologist to assess the amount and site of microcalcification for which they are searching, for example, if this lies in one, or several, of the cores sampled. Further H&E levels can be examined if the calcification is not adequately represented (either in terms of amount or distribution) in the initial levels. It is not infrequent that additional levels are required for identification, particularly from wider-bore needle cores, and, on occasions, multiple further sections are necessary, particularly from larger, vacuum-assisted, cores (e.g., 7 g). This can become somewhat of a search for a needle in a haystack, and alternative solutions, such as undertaking x-ray of the paraffin wax-embedded cassettes, can be performed; this can both confirm the presence of calcifications and indicate the portion of tissue requiring further levels. One additional approach can be for the radiologist to place the portion or core containing the calcification into either a separate formalin pot or capsule or wrapping it in filter paper, to distinguish the portion of the tissue that requires the most thorough examination from those which are free of calcification. The laboratory can thus separately block the most relevant fragment and cut deeper sections, if needed, on this portion of the sample.

Calcification Problems

On occasions, even though calcification has been seen radiologically in the specimen, this is not identified in the tissue sample; this situation was reported in 22 % of cases in one series [7]. This may be because the calcification has been "trimmed out" in initial preparation or has not been retained in the tissue during fixation and processing and section cutting. Conversely, even if the cores have been sampled for radiological calcification, and none is seen on x-ray of the tissue, the specimen should be processed and examined, and a specific diagnosis will be made in 38 % of cases [7]. On the other hand, in 13 % of cases in this series by Lieberman et al. when calcifications were not present on specimen radiographs, they were identified histologically; particular care must be taken in this situation so that false reassurance of small benign microcalcifications, for example, in atrophic lobules, is not taken to explain radiologically suspicious microcalcifications that have not been adequately sampled.

Lesions commonly associated with microcalcification include not only ductal carcinoma in situ (DCIS) but a variety of benign processes, such as fibrocystic and columnar cell changes, sclerosing adenosis, fibroadenomas and fibroadenomatoid hyperplasia, and stromal changes, such as fat necrosis (Fig. 4.1). Weddellite (calcium oxalate) may be difficult to see on routine examination of H&E sections, but can be

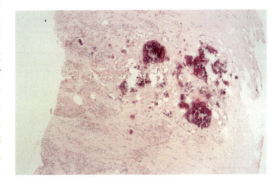

Fig. 4.1 Vacuum-assisted core biopsy with microcalcification within fat necrosis and scarring (hematoxylin and eosin)

identified with polarized light, and specimens should be examined with particular concentration on microcysts and apocrine change where this form of microcalcification is most common.

Reporting Categories

Diagnostic core biopsy samples (of any gauge) should be reported not only with a text description of the histological features of the specimen but also a reporting category. This approach allows the independent opinion from each specialist member of the multidisciplinary team to provide input into the "triple assessment," comprising imaging (e.g., mammography and ultrasound), clinical examination, and needle biopsy with histological examination. It is essential that core biopsy results are not interpreted in isolation. Multidisciplinary discussion is required to determine whether the biopsy findings are concordant with the radiological and clinical findings and whether the biopsy is representative of the lesion. If there is discordance, then further management must be discussed; providing a category (B1–B5) facilitates this process [8].

B1, Normal Tissue

This category should be used when the histological features are of normal tissue, whether or not breast parenchymal structures are present. Thus a B1 classification is appropriate for a core including normal breast ducts and lobules or one composed of mature adipose tissue only. The report should include description of the components present. While a normal histology may indicate that the lesion has not been sampled, other benign lesions such as hamartomas and lipomas can provide normal microscopic features.

The pathologist should assign the reporting (B1 to B5) category they provide based on the histological features they see, not on the radiological or clinical characteristics [8]. Specifically the histological category should not be amended after multidisciplinary discussion, even if the collaborative results are then interpreted as

consistent. This appears somewhat contentious, with some pathologists being requested to alter the "B" category of a lesion after discussion if the radiological and pathology findings are in concordance (e.g., change a B1 to a B2 if all the findings are in keeping with a hamartoma). It is this author's opinion that this is a question of communication and education and that it is acceptable for not all categories to "match" exactly, but to record the overall view of the multidisciplinary outcome.

Clearly, the multidisciplinary discussion will influence whether the pathologist elects to undertake examination of additional levels or immunohistochemistry (e.g., if minimal changes only are seen from a lesion interpreted radiologically as suspicious). However, features such as minor degrees of fibrocystic change are usually best categorized as B1, and it is again the remit of the multidisciplinary team meeting to determine if the lesion of interest has been sampled, if the core biopsy is representative, and if the B1 result explains the clinical and radiological findings.

One other area of possible disagreement is whether cores with microcalcification, particularly if of sufficient size to be radiologically visible, for example, within intralobular secretions and involutional lobules or in the stroma, should be regarded as B1 or B2 (Fig. 4.2). It is important

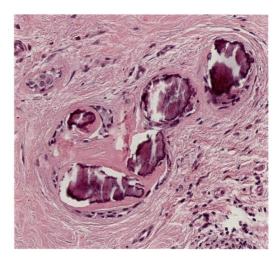

Fig. 4.2 Island of microcalcification, in a sub-epithelial position within dense fibrous stroma (hematoxylin and eosin)

to assess the size of such microcalcification seen histologically; mammograms do not demonstrate microcalcification, either singly or in clusters, less than 100 μm in diameter [9], and tiny islands of microcalcification within involutional lobules that are relatively common cannot be seen mammographically and should not lead to misleading or false reassurance of benignity. As with all non-operative core biopsy specimens, discussion between pathology and radiology colleagues must be undertaken to confirm whether the microcalcification in the histological specimen is representative of that seen on the mammogram.

It is also the case that the pathologist should not categorize a biopsy as B1 simply because it may not reflect the clinical or radiological abnormality. The pathologist should describe the histological features they see and base the B category on this. While judicious use of the B1 category for minimal changes avoids false reassurance that the lesion has been sampled, for example, minor fibrocystic changes (B1) from a well-defined mass lesion, additional comment in the report that the biopsy may not be representative of the lesion can emphasize this. It remains the role of the multidisciplinary meeting to judge whether the core biopsy is "adequate."

B2, Benign

A core is classified as B2, benign, when it contains a specific benign lesion. This category therefore includes a wide variety of benign breast lesions including fibroadenomas, fibrocystic change, and sclerosing adenosis but also incorporates non-parenchymal lesions such as acute inflammation/abscesses and fat necrosis (Fig. 4.1).

B5, Malignant

The B5 category should be used for lesions of definite malignant nature and is subdivided into B5a, B5b, and B5c.

B5a, in situ carcinoma, should be reported when features of unequivocal ductal carcinoma in situ (DCIS) are seen (any grade) and for cases of pleomorphic, but not classical type, lobular carcinoma in situ (LCIS). This category is also used for fragments of unequivocally malignant in situ papillary lesions (papillary carcinoma in situ and/or encysted/encapsulated papillary carcinoma). If there is unequivocal DCIS present in the cores with features suspicious, but not diagnostic of invasion, the B5a category is the most appropriate. The B5b category should be applied to all invasive primary breast carcinomas and also to other rare primary malignancies including malignant phyllodes and lymphomas and to metastatic tumors to the breast. B5c should be used when it is not possible to say whether the carcinoma is invasive or in situ. This category is used rarely, but most often when fragments of carcinoma are seen without surrounding stroma, and it is impossible to be certain if these are derived from an invasive or an in situ lesion.

Category B5a: In Situ Carcinoma

One of the benefits of core biopsy compared to FNAC is the definitive diagnosis of a greater proportion of cases of DCIS non-operatively. Diagnostic excision biopsy for diagnosis of DCIS is now uncommon in the United Kingdom. However, inherent in the small sample one obtains with core biopsy, foci of invasive carcinoma within an area of DCIS may be missed; the rate of "upgrade" to invasive carcinoma depends at least in part on the size and number of cores sampled. Vacuum-assisted core biopsies are "upgraded" to invasive disease in approximately 10 % of cases, while this is approximately 20–30 % of patients with a smaller-gauge core biopsy sample [10].

The nuclear grade of the DCIS should be indicated on the core biopsy. There is evidence that high-grade lesions are associated with increased risk of there being a missed focus of invasive carcinoma [11]. The architectural growth pattern of the DCIS and the presence of comedo-type necrosis should also be noted. Clearly the presence or absence of associated calcifications (in secretions in the lumen or in comedo-type necrosis) should be reported for radiological correlation.

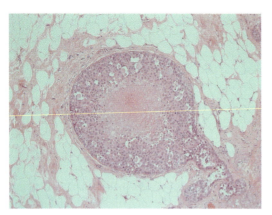

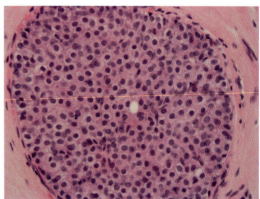

Fig. 4.3 Pleomorphic lobular carcinoma in situ with central comedo-type necrosis. Note the discohesion of the malignant cells within the membrane-bound space (hematoxylin and eosin)

Fig. 4.4 Differential diagnosis of this monotonous, small cell solid epithelial proliferation lies between low-grade ductal carcinoma in situ (*DCIS*) and lobular neoplasia (hematoxylin and eosin). The well-defined cell membranes and absence of prominent intracytoplasmic vacuoles favor DCIS, but E-cadherin immunophenotyping may prove valuable

Pleomorphic LCIS can mimic high-grade DCIS. There is frequently associated comedo-type necrosis (Fig. 4.3) with microcalcification, and the lesion may therefore present mammographically [12]. As clinical management, albeit based on scanty data, is at present largely similar to that of DCIS, these lesions should also be categorized as B5a. Similarly, while an absence, or weak expression, of E-cadherin can help differentiate between high-grade DCIS and pleomorphic LCIS, pragmatically (and reassuringly) this is of limited clinical value, if one is certain that the disease has nuclei equivalent to the pleomorphism/atypia score of 3 as applied to invasive carcinoma grading.

More problematic are the rare cases where lobular neoplasia is difficult or impossible to distinguish from low- or intermediate-grade solid architecture DCIS (Fig. 4.4). In these cases E-cadherin immunostaining can be helpful [13] (in conjunction with p120 catenin or beta-catenin, if available). Membrane expression of E-cadherin is typically absent (or weaker than adjacent normal ducts and lobules) in lobular neoplasia but is present in DCIS. If the histology and the pattern of immunohistochemistry is unclear (as is not infrequent in these "borderline" cases), and definite distinction between classical lobular neoplasia and DCIS is not possible, or the lesion has a mixed DCIS/LCIS phenotype, then a B4 categorization (see below) is prudent.

Literature has shown that encysted papillary carcinomas (encapsulated papillary carcinomas) lack a peripheral, as well as internal, myoepithelial layer and probably represent an indolent form of invasive carcinoma [14]. Regardless of whether these are truly invasive or in situ lesions, the prognosis of patients with these carcinomas is equivalent to those with DCIS alone. The current recommendation is therefore that these lesions should be categorized as B5a, rather than B5c. However, the pathology report should provide details of the histological appearance and the grade of the lesion; some units choose to recommend sentinel lymph node biopsy for large, high-grade encysted papillary carcinoma in patients undergoing breast-conserving therapy.

Category B5b: Invasive

A significant advantage of core biopsy is the ability to definitively diagnose invasive carcinoma. However, in some cases only very small foci (<1 mm) of invasion may be seen, and it is not possible to distinguish microinvasive from invasive disease. If the core biopsy shows one or more foci of invasion less than 1 mm, additional levels should be examined to see if the area is larger than 1 mm and thus meet the criteria for invasive disease. Immunohistochemistry for myoepithelial markers can be applied to confirm the extent of the invasive focus from H&E. However, rare cases can be difficult to categorize (i.e., as B5a versus B5b); clarification in the text portion of the report (e.g., that the histological features are those of DCIS with a tiny focus of invasion (B5a) compared to cases with no DCIS and only a tiny focus of invasion (where B5b may be more appropriate)) is essential to enable informed multidisciplinary discussion regarding subsequent repeat investigation or therapeutic excision with, or without, axillary surgery. The category of B5c should not be used for microinvasive carcinoma.

Assessment of Prognostic and Predictive Factors in Invasive Carcinoma in Core Biopsy

Invasive carcinoma in a core biopsy should be graded and the histological subtype provided if possible. Concordance between histological grade on core biopsy and the subsequent tumor in surgical excision is achieved in approximately 70 % of cases [15]. The provisional (core) grade more often underestimates (25 %) the final definitive grade than overestimates it (8%), predominantly because the mitotic count (because of the inherent nature of sampling) may be lower in the core biopsy. Thus, accuracy is greater with lesions defined as provisional grade 3, with 77 % of such tumors on core biopsy confirmed as high-grade invasive carcinomas on excision [15]. This may be valuable in the selection of patients for neoadjuvant chemotherapy, and conversely may be the only source of assessment in those who have had complete pathological response to such treatment.

Assessment of histological type is useful to identify patients with invasive lobular carcinomas (ILC), who may be offered MRI if they are considering breast-conserving surgery, to identify multifocal disease. Recent analysis has shown that of 1,112 lesions categorised as having an ILC component on core biopsy, 471 (93 %)

interpreted as pure ILC had an ILC component on excision. Of cores diagnosed as mixed ILC plus another type on core, complete agreement between core and excision was 46 %, with 27 % cases of pure ILC, whilst 26 % non-concordant [16].

Estrogen and progesterone receptors and HER2 assessment of invasive carcinoma in core biopsies correlate well with that in the subsequent surgical excision specimens [17], and the core biopsy is the recommended specimen for the assessment of these biomarkers.

Problematic Malignant Lesions

Some, relatively common, subtypes of invasive breast carcinoma may cause diagnostic problems in core biopsy specimens, just as in surgical excisions. Tubular carcinomas may mimic radial scars/complex sclerosing lesions (CSLs) or even sclerosing adenosis, and care should be taken to identify the stromal reaction typical in association with this form of carcinoma (Fig. 4.5) and the presence of tubular structures throughout the lesion, not only centrally (Fig. 4.6). However, immunohistochemical staining for myoepithelial markers can be useful in this situation. Invasive lobular carcinomas may be subtle and mimic chronic inflammatory changes or be missed entirely. The targetoid infiltrative pattern of invasive lobular carcinoma may be helpful, but a reactive lymphocyte process can have a similar distribution. Cytokeratin immunohistochemistry will highlight the malignant epithelial cells, but

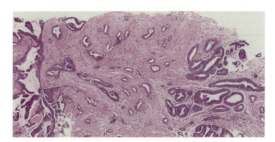

Fig. 4.5 Angulated tubules within immature-type fibrous stroma are seen in this core of invasive carcinoma. This has features of tubular carcinoma and is of provisional (core) grade 1 (hematoxylin and eosin)

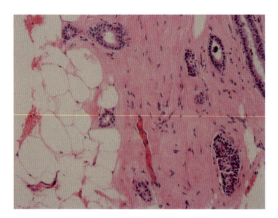

Fig. 4.6 Although the stroma in this case is relatively paucicellular, the presence of tubular structures at the junction of the fat and collagenous areas raises concern for the diagnosis of invasive carcinoma (rather than, e.g., radial scar), despite the blandness of the nuclei (hematoxylin and eosin). Immunohistochemistry for myoepithelial markers (smooth muscle myosin and p63) showed an absence of myoepithelium around the glands and confirmed the diagnosis of malignancy

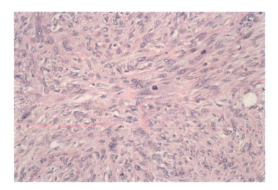

Fig. 4.7 This spindle cell lesion is formed from moderately sized spindle-shaped cell with moderate pleomorphism and conspicuous mitoses. Immunohistochemistry confirmed that this was metaplastic carcinoma

recognition of the abnormal cell proliferation requires vigilance, as the features can be subtle.

Other less common and unusual lesions may be difficult to recognize simply because of their rarity; recognition rests on the pathologist considering the diagnosis. Spindle cell and metaplastic carcinomas (Fig. 4.7) include a range of lesions from low-grade spindle cell lesions resembling fibromatosis through to forms resembling primary sarcoma. In such cases an antibody panel of a range of anti-cytokeratin antibodies (high and low molecular weight cytokeratins and broad

spectrum) will assist in diagnosis. It should also be remembered that primary breast sarcomas are rare and most commonly originate in association with a (malignant) phyllodes tumor, although the epithelial component may not be present in the core biopsy. Malignant lymphomas in the breast are rare; they are most commonly of high-grade B-cell morphology and may mimic carcinoma. The discohesion may mimic invasive lobular carcinomas, but the typical single-file growth pattern of a lobular lesion is not seen. Correct diagnosis requires a high index of suspicion and judicious use of immunohistochemistry (CD45, CD20, CD3, CD30, etc.) to differentiate the lesion from either an invasive carcinoma or other, metastatic, malignancy. Indeed, metastasis to the breast from primary malignancies elsewhere is not uncommon, although it might not be always biopsied unless it is the first presentation of the disease. A wide range of carcinomas can metastasize to the breast, including lesions from the lung, ovary (serous papillary), kidney, and prostate and malignant melanoma [18]. The diagnosis of a metastasis in the breast should be considered if the features are not typical of a specific histological subtype of invasive breast carcinoma. A prior clinical history should be sought from the referring clinical team, and if the patient has a known previous malignancy, comparison of the histological features should be undertaken. Immunohistochemistry is also often helpful, although no marker is completely sensitive or specific. Breast carcinoma usually expresses cytokeratin 7 and 18 (and not cytokeratin 20) [19], and epithelial membrane antigen. It should be remembered, however, that even "breast" biomarkers such as ER and HER2 may be misleading; ER positivity is seen in a wide range of carcinomas other than invasive breast cancers and is strongly positive in some (not just only gynecological carcinomas) and cannot be used for identification of the primary site of a malignancy.

B3, Lesion of Uncertain Malignant Potential

While most core biopsy samples can be readily categorized as normal, benign, or malignant, a small proportion (7.8 % (range 4.0–13.2 % for different units) of samples cannot and are categorized as of uncertain malignant potential (B3) or suspicious (B4) (UK NHSBSP Pathology audit 2015, unpublished data), most of these (median 6.7 % (range 3.3–12.6 %)) are categorized as B3. Series have identified a wide range (e.g., 4–22 % [20] to 2.3–7.9 % [21]) in the proportion of B3 diagnoses, with a consequent range of positive predictive values between 14.3 and 28.3 % [21], indicating some degree of diagnostic variation between pathologists/institutions.

The B3 category includes a range of lesions, classified as such either because (a) they are entities known to be heterogeneous (and the area sampled by needle core, while benign per se, may not be representative of the whole), or (b) they are lesions known to be associated with carcinoma (either in situ or invasive), or (c) both lesional heterogeneity and the association with malignancy may apply. The group of B3 lesions thus includes some lesions with epithelial atypia and some without, and this should be identified and reported separately.

The B3 lesions are known to be associated with differing risks of "upgrade" (i.e., ductal carcinoma in situ (DCIS) or invasive carcinoma at the same time and at the same site in the breast as the B3 diagnosis). This is not equivalent to "risk" in the sense of development of subsequent invasive carcinoma in any site in either breast, although some lesions that are regarded as B3, of uncertain malignant potential, such as lobular carcinoma in situ and atypical ductal hyperplasia, confer an increased risk of subsequent carcinoma, as well as having a risk of upgrade.

The lesions classified as B3 include:

- Atypical intraductal epithelial proliferation (AIDEP)
- Non-pleomorphic/classical lobular in situ neoplasia (ALH or LCIS)
- Flat epithelial atypia (FEA)
- Radial scar, with or without epithelial atypia
- Papillary lesion, with or without epithelial atypia
- Cellular fibroepithelial lesion, where phyllodes tumor cannot be excluded
- Mucocele-like lesion
- Other rare appearances, for example, some spindle cell lesions

Atypical Intraductal Epithelial Proliferations (AIDEPs)

One can see a range of severity of atypical intraductal epithelial proliferations in core biopsy that fall short of the diagnosis of ductal carcinoma in situ and which are best classified as B3. Different patterns of atypia may be seen; lesions may resemble atypical ductal hyperplasia (ADH), flat epithelial atypia, apocrine atypia, or atypia that does not conform to one of these patterns.

The term atypical intraductal epithelial proliferation (AIDEP) is preferred over atypical ductal hyperplasia (ADH) in core biopsy samples as the latter refers to a specific small lesion that is not assessable in the limited sample provided by this technique (see Chap. 3) (Fig. 4.8). ADH is a

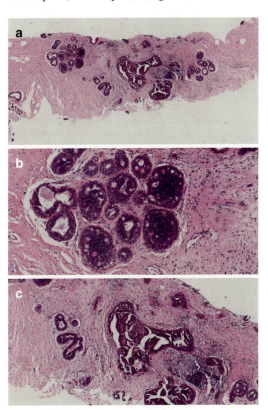

Fig. 4.8 This hematoxylin and eosin-stained vacuum-assisted core biopsy (**a**) bears a small central papilloma (**c**); as this is contained within the width of the core, this focus of the sample may be regarded as B2, benign. However, on either side of the papillary lesion, there is an epithelial proliferation with a rudimentary cribriform growth pattern (**b**); this is formed from regular, small cells and is regarded as an atypical intraductal epithelial proliferation (AIDEP). Overall, therefore, the core should be reported as B3, of uncertain malignant potential, with epithelial atypia

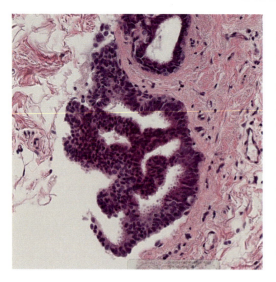

Fig. 4.9 Part of a membrane-bound space with architectural atypia in the form of wide, ill-formed bridges at one edge of a core biopsy (hematoxylin and eosin). The cells in these structures are relatively uniform, although the peripheral population is more columnar in shape with apical snouts. Additional level proved unhelpful and this was reported as B3, of uncertain malignant potential

microfocal lesion, less than 2 mm or less than two complete spaces in extent, composed of a uniform, small cell, atypical epithelial proliferation that either is present admixed with a non-uniform process such as usual epithelial hyperplasia or is too small for diagnosis of low-grade DCIS [22]. ADH therefore cannot be definitively diagnosed on the limited sampling provided by core biopsy, as the extent of the lesion cannot be determined with accuracy (Fig. 4.9).

The published literature consistently demonstrates that the upgrade rate of AIDEP to malignancy is greater with small samples compared to primary larger vacuum-assisted biopsies. The upgrade rate described for AIDEP varies from 18 to 87 % for 14g needles compared to 10–39 % with 11g or 9g samples with a pooled positive predictive value of 20.9 % from vacuum-assisted sampling [23]. In essence, unsurprisingly, if a greater amount of tissue is provided, there is a lower chance of "missing" a diagnosis of DCIS or invasive cancer. This reflects the more extensive sampling that is achieved with vacuum-assisted biopsy in this group of lesions in which there is a moderate chance of coexisting malignancy.

Lesser degrees of atypia may also necessarily be categorized as B3, but immunohistochemistry for basal cytokeratins, such as CK5 and CK14, can play a useful role in assessing epithelial proliferations, as can estrogen receptor. Low-grade DCIS, ADH, and other members of the low-grade neoplasia family are uniformly negative for basal cytokeratins and uniformly homogeneously ER positive, whereas usual-type epithelial hyperplasia shows a mosaic pattern of heterogeneous reactivity. Gynecomastoid-type usual epithelial hyperplasia, with micropapillary architecture, should not be mistaken for micropapillary ADH/DCIS, and immunohistochemistry can similarly be helpful in difficult cases (see Chap. 3).

Care should in particular be taken not to overdiagnose intraductal epithelial proliferations, for example, within fibroepithelial lesions (where they may be "telescoping" of epithelium within the duct spaces), as showing minor degrees of atypia, or to overinterpret occasional enlarged nuclei in an otherwise normal duct or lobule as atypical and record these as B3. The absence of mitoses and definite cytological atypia is helpful. Overdiagnosis of mild atypia as a B3 lesion could potentially result in patients undergoing unnecessary surgical diagnostic biopsy. New recommendations are for wider, more thorough, sampling of B3 lesions (whether diagnosed on needle core or vacuum-assisted biopsy in the first instance) with subsequent thorough vacuum-assisted sampling, akin to a diagnostic surgical excision. In such cases, the findings in subsequent specimens should be reported in conjunction with the core biopsy findings (e.g., with regard to extent of an atypical intraductal epithelial proliferation) and include a comment as to whether similar changes are present in both and whether there are signs of previous biopsy to indicate sampling of the appropriate site.

Lobular Neoplasia

As with atypical intraductal epithelial proliferations, the pathologist cannot accurately assess the extent of an atypical intralobular epithelial proliferation in core biopsy samples. For this reason the term lobular (in situ) neoplasia (LN) is preferred in core biopsy specimens rather than

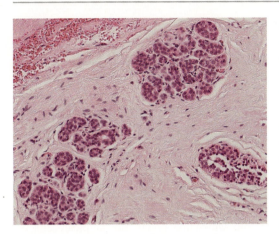

Fig. 4.10 Lobular units bearing an atypical population of moderately sized, discohesive cells which fill the acini but do not expand these spaces. In a core biopsy specimen, where the extent of the process is not assessable, this should be reported as lobular neoplasia (rather than an atypical lobular hyperplasia)

attempting to distinguish atypical lobular hyperplasia (ALH) from lobular carcinoma in situ (LCIS) [24], although these are biologically and genetically similar [25]. Classical LN is seen as a uniform, intralobular epithelial proliferation of medium-sized discohesive cells, often with prominent intracytoplasmic lumina within lobular units (Fig. 4.10). Pagetoid spread under the normal cuboidal ductal epithelium within ducts may be noted. Immunohistochemistry may be assessed on such samples with reduced or negative E-cadherin frequently (but not invariably) seen [13]. This classical form of LN should be described as B3 in core biopsy. As noted above, pleomorphic LCIS, on the other hand, is formed from cells with larger, more variable nuclei and often abundant cytoplasm but with similar discohesion and growth pattern and is recorded as B5a, in situ carcinoma (Fig. 4.3). Difficult forms of LN may rarely be seen that is not pleomorphic, but which has comedo-type necrosis or is mass forming (and which some regard as a variant of pleomorphic LCIS). These, as well as lesions which cannot be accurately classified as LCIS or DCIS, should also be categorized as B4, suspicious.

Mild atypia of epithelium within lobular units is a relatively common problem encountered in core biopsy samples. Care must be taken not to overdiagnose such minimal degrees of atypia, which may represent usual epithelial hyperplasia, apocrine change, or reactive changes (e.g., adjacent to previous sampling procedure).

Lobular neoplasia (LN) is most frequently a coincidental finding in a core biopsy, and multidisciplinary discussion is essential, as the abnormality identified clinically or radiologically may not be represented. However, there is evidence that there is an upgrade of these lesions with coexisting or adjacent DCIS and/or invasive carcinoma, whether the lesion appears coincidental or where there is, for example, microcalcification in the disease itself; there is no good evidence that lesions which are seemingly coincidentally identified histologically can be dismissed. There is significant variation in the proportion of lesions that have been surgically excised in series in the literature, and there is also variation in terminology used. However, the upgrade rate overall (with the caveats as above) is 27 % (range 0–60 %) from literature review [26]. Some groups have attempted to distinguish ALH from LCIS on core, but the range for the former remains wide (0–43 %) compared to the latter (0–60 %) and attempting to subclassify classical LN based on extent of disease in core biopsy appears fruitless [26].

Flat Epithelial Atypia

The terminology for columnar cell lesions has changed over time, causing confusion and some difficulties in review of the literature. As described in Chap. 3, columnar cell lesions arise in the terminal duct lobular unit, not the larger ducts. Originally described as columnar alteration with prominent snouts and secretions (CAPPS) [27], the benign, non-clonal forms of columnar cell lesions are now categorized as columnar cell change and columnar cell hyperplasia. Most columnar cell change, with or without hyperplasia, shows no atypia and does not cause diagnostic problems and are thus categorized as B2.

The accepted term for columnar cell lesions with cytological atypia, not of high cytonuclear grade, is flat epithelial atypia (FEA), and this

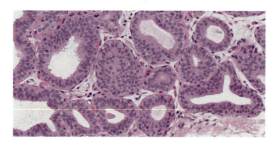

Fig. 4.11 Flat epithelial atypia (hematoxylin and eosin). Acini are lined by one or two layers of uniform cells, for the most part with round nuclei. In some areas apical snouts can be seen

should be reported as B3 (Fig. 4.11). When high cytonuclear grade is, rarely, present, the process is regarded as flat high-grade DCIS (B5a). The acini in FEA are typically moderately dilated with smooth, rounded internal luminal aspects with secretions. These secretions may bear microcalcification. In the classical form of FEA, the acini are lined by regular, uniform epithelial cells in one or more layers, without any architectural atypia, for example, as micropapillary structures or roman bridges. The nuclei are also most commonly uniform and round, sometimes with speckled chromatin and small nucleoli. Mitoses are not conspicuous.

If there is architectural atypia, for example, in the form of true micropapillary structures (with narrow stalk and wider tip) or bridges (rather than the tufts/humps which may be present in columnar cell hyperplasia), the lesion should be considered within the spectrum of AIDEP (or low-grade DCIS) in core biopsy, rather than FEA (see Chap. 3).

As with several of the entities in the B3 category, published series are biased with some, but not all, lesions being surgically excised, and others followed up mammographically. Although initial reports indicated a high upgrade for FEA, later series recorded a lower rate. In systemic review including 22 studies of patients with columnar cell atypia and subsequent surgical excision, 17 % of 389 patients developed carcinoma (37 DCIS, 10 %; 20 invasive carcinoma, 4 %) [28]. For this reason, further sampling, by vacuum-assisted biopsy is recommended.

Apocrine Lesions

Apocrine atypia, particularly in association with a sclerosing lesion such as sclerosing adenosis, may be difficult to identify in non-operative diagnostic samples as well as in surgical samples [29]. In core biopsy in particular, large nuclei, often with prominent nucleoli and a degree of pleomorphism, may be misdiagnosed as DCIS, unless the apocrine nature of the cells is correctly identified. The granular eosinophilic cytoplasm of apocrine cells should be sought as well as an accurate assessment of the nature of the spaces within which the potentially atypical cells are seen. When the apocrine proliferation is seen within ducts in a core biopsy, rather than in lobules, additional features such as more marked pleomorphism, comedo-type necrosis, and the presence of mitoses, as well as multiple duct involvement indicating a more extensive lesion, should be sought. However, moderate degrees of apocrine pleomorphism should be assessed with caution and should be regarded as atypia, B3, of uncertain malignant potential. Importantly, papillary apocrine change should not be regarded other than benign.

In a core biopsy specimen, as well as any other specific lesion, it is important that any epithelial atypia is recorded, even if there is another reason for a B3 categorization, as the risk of malignancy associated with atypical intraductal epithelial proliferations is relatively high. For this reason, for all B3 diagnoses, additional comment should be made about whether epithelial atypia is present or not.

Papillary Lesions

Intraductal papillary lesions are composed of finger-like projections of fibrovascular cores with overlying epithelium extending into a duct lumen. They are typically classified as B3 as they may show intralesional heterogeneity and the limited sampling with core biopsy may miss areas of invasive carcinoma or DCIS. Uncommonly, a very small papilloma will be entirely removed within the width of a core biopsy (particularly a wide-bore vacuum-assisted sample) and can be classified as B2, benign (Fig. 4.8c). For larger papillary lesions, which very frequently fragment

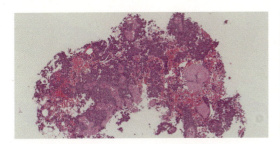

Fig. 4.12 Core of a papillary lesion showing fragmentation (hematoxylin and eosin). In this particular case, hyalinized fibrovascular cores are present with a solid overlying epithelial proliferation. Immunohistochemistry confirmed the absence of an intervening myoepithelial layer (between the fibrovascular cores and the epithelium), and this represents the solid variant of papillary carcinoma in situ (B5a)

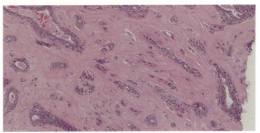

Fig. 4.13 Entrapped tubular structures in the central portion of a radial scar. Note the absence of immature-type fibroblastic reaction, lack of cytological atypia, and angulation of the epithelial elements (hematoxylin and eosin)

in core biopsy specimens (Fig. 4.12), immunohistochemistry can be helpful [14, 30]; confirmation of the absence of a myoepithelial layer between the fronds and the epithelial layer may assist in the identification of papillary carcinoma in situ, and the additional absence peripherally (if the periphery of the lesion is present in the core) in association with portions of pseudocapsule, chronic inflammation, and hemosiderin deposition may enable diagnosis of encysted papillary carcinoma. Thus, some papillary lesions may warrant categorization as B4, suspicious, or even B5a. For distinguishing usual epithelial hyperplasia from clonal proliferations within a papillary lesion, basal cytokeratins and estrogen receptors can be valuable.

The most important predictor of upgrade to malignancy in a papillary lesion on core biopsy is the presence of associated epithelial atypia, and this should be carefully sought and recorded. When a papillary lesion is seen without any epithelial atypia, the chance of malignancy in the subsequent excision specimen is relatively low (9.0 %). When atypia is also present, the upgrade rate is 36.0 % [31]. Papillary lesions are known to fragment and to show heterogeneity. While this is true of other B3 lesions, the histopathological assessment of papillary lesions with atypia requires the pathologist to assess the extent of the area of atypical epithelial proliferation present. If this is present in multiple cores, even in large samples, the area cannot be measured, and

distinguishing atypical epithelial proliferation within a papilloma (<3 mm in extent) from low-grade DCIS within a papilloma (3 mm or more) may not be possible [32]. For this reason, it is recommended that such lesions undergo diagnostic surgical excision.

Radial Scar/Complex Sclerosing Lesion (CSL)

These terms are used for lesions of essentially similar appearance but differing in size, with a radial scar being less than 10 mm and complex sclerosing lesion (CSL) larger than that. Histologically, there is central fibroelastosis containing entrapped benign compressed tubules (Fig. 4.13), typically with more dilated microcystic and fibrocystic changes seen peripherally. Very small, occult radial scars, like tiny papillomas, which are entirely excised, for example, by core biopsy or vacuum-assisted biopsy, can be classified as B2, benign, rather than as B3. However, radial scars may be associated with epithelial proliferation. This is most commonly usual epithelial hyperplasia, but atypical hyperplasia, in situ carcinoma, and invasive carcinoma are identified on diagnostic excision more often than one would anticipate by chance. It is therefore anticipated that most such lesions will be categorized as B3.

Differential diagnosis of radial scar includes tubular carcinoma; both bear entrapped tubular structures, but typically in the former, there is associated stromal reaction (Fig. 4.5). In addition, the tubular structures in radial scar are seen only within the central portion of the fibroelastosis

(Fig. 4.13), usually with peripheral microcysts and benign changes, while in tubular carcinoma, the angulated glandular structures extend into adjacent fat and fibrous tissue (Fig. 4.6). In difficult cases myoepithelial markers, for example, smooth muscle myosin heavy chain and p63, can be valuable; as the entrapped tubules in a radial scar bear surrounding myoepithelial cells. Any associated epithelial proliferation can be assessed for clonality with basal cytokeratin and estrogen receptor as for usual epithelial hyperplasia vs. neoplasia out with the setting of a sclerosing lesion.

The upgrade rate of radial scars in core biopsy is largely dependent on the presence of associated atypical epithelial proliferation; where no epithelial atypia is seen, there generally is a low rate of upgrade (<10 %) reported. For example, of 410 radial scars without atypia on core biopsy in a large UK series, 9 % had a malignant outcome (DCIS or invasive), while those with atypia had an upgrade rate of 36 % (comparable to the 39.5 % rate seen with forms of epithelial atypia in the same study) [31].

Phyllodes Tumor

The vast majority of fibroepithelial lesions on core biopsy can be definitively classified as B2, e.g., benign fibroadenoma, and do not require further management, unless the patient wishes to have the lesion excised. A small proportion has a more cellular stroma raising concern that the lesion may represent a phyllodes tumor (Fig. 4.14a). Features such as stromal overgrowth, fragmentation (defined as a stromal fragment with epithelium at one or both ends), and the presence of mitoses may be identified [33] but are not specific for the diagnosis. Marked atypia of stromal cells is uncommon in cores (Fig. 4.14b), even in lesions that have more overt features of a phyllodes tumor in the excision. Thus, histological features on which one can definitively make a diagnosis of phyllodes are uncommon, and more often differential diagnosis lies between a cellular fibroadenoma and a benign phyllodes tumor; such lesions should also be designated B3 with text comment in the histology report to indicate that "a phyllodes tumor cannot be excluded."

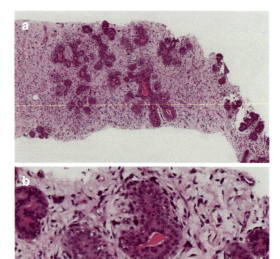

Fig. 4.14 Core biopsy from a phyllodes tumor (hematoxylin and eosin) (**a**). An increase in stromal cellularity is seen surrounding benign ductal elements. There is stromal cell atypia and pleomorphism (**b**) allowing diagnosis of this biphasic lesion as a phyllodes tumor rather than as a "cellular fibroepithelial lesion" and thus definitive surgical management (excision with a margin of surrounding normal tissue), despite the necessary categorization as B3, of uncertain malignant potential

Repeat core biopsy or vacuum-assisted biopsy of such lesions is unhelpful, and these should undergo diagnostic excision.

A lesion which is definitively diagnosed as a phyllodes tumor potentially warrants different clinical management to those where differential lies between a cellular fibroadenoma and a phyllodes tumor, although both are classified as B3 lesions. The former merits surgical excision with a margin (locally designated) of normal tissue. However, it should be noted that only a very small proportion of lesions diagnosed as cellular fibroepithelial lesion are malignant in the excision specimen. A more useful measure of the "upgrade rate" is the proportion that is a phyllodes tumor on excision; the figures in the literature show wide variation even in the larger series between 16 and 76 % [21, 34]. This implies some variation in the application of diagnostic criteria. One typical study found that 37 % of cellular fibroepithelial lesions on core were phyllodes

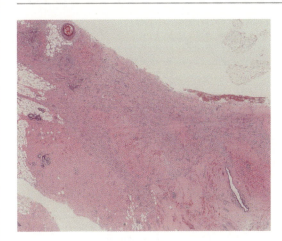

Fig. 4.15 Vacuum-assisted biopsy from an area of radiologically detected microcalcification which had previously been sampled. There is a large area of fibroblastic reaction (*central*) and a small squamous epithelial-lined inclusion (*top left*) as a result of this prior needling. Other associated changes, such as hemosiderin deposition and fat necrosis, should be sought to confirm the cause of this area of spindle cell reaction, which can then be regarded as benign, B2

tumors on excision, but it is noteworthy that only one of the 52 lesions was a malignant phyllodes tumor [31].

Spindle Cell Lesions

Spindle cell proliferations may cause difficulties in diagnosis in core biopsy samples, as in surgical specimens. The commonest lesion seen on core biopsy is scarring, sometimes as a result of prior needling procedure (e.g., FNAC or core biopsy), but usually there are associated changes such as fat necrosis or hemosiderin-laden macrophages to enable a diagnosis and categorization as B2 (Fig. 4.15). However, other spindle cell lesions are more problematic and may require categorization as B3. For example, a benign myofibroblastoma is composed of bundles of bland spindle cells with intervening eosinophilic collagen fibers mimicking those seen in keloid scars, sometimes along with adipose tissue. Immunohistochemistry typically demonstrates CD34 and desmin. Fibromatosis is a bland spindle cell proliferation that is best categorized as B3. Nuclear expression of β-catenin is frequently seen, but is not specific. Cytokeratins and CD34 are not expressed. Both these entities should be

classified as B3, but both should be distinguished from spindle cell/metaplastic carcinomas, which need to be considered in the differential diagnosis of any spindle cell lesion of the breast on core biopsy.

Spindle cell carcinomas vary from bland spindle cell forms such as fibromatosis-like metaplastic carcinoma through to high-grade malignant sarcoma-like lesions (Fig. 4.7). In these lesions, morphological evidence of epithelial differentiation must be sought as many are mixed with foci of no special type/invasive ductal carcinoma; islands may range from small scattered cohesive foci to areas of conventional carcinoma, of course these latter may not be present in the core biopsy specimen. Immunohistochemistry for a panel of cytokeratins including both luminal and basal cytokeratins should be performed. Other differential diagnoses of spindle cell lesions include a phyllodes tumor, with just the spindle cell component present. In such cases evidence for an epithelial component should be sought, for example, by performing additional levels on the core biopsy. Positive CD34 expression supports the diagnosis of phyllodes tumor. When a definitive histological diagnosis cannot be made, the abnormality should be reported as a spindle cell lesion of uncertain nature and classified as B3.

Mucocele-Like Lesions

A mucocele-like lesion is seen as mucin in the stroma and can be associated with benign cysts, ADH, DCIS, or invasive carcinoma. The risk of malignancy appears to be very low if there is no atypia on the core biopsy [35]. However, the potential pitfall in diagnosis of mucocele-like lesion is largely in distinguishing this entity from invasive mucinous carcinoma; the latter will similarly bear pools of mucin in the stroma, but these will also bear islands of neoplastic carcinoma cells, while in a mucocele-like lesion, the pools will be devoid of associated epithelial cells. Thorough examination with additional H&E levels should be performed to assess whether there is an associated atypical epithelial proliferation and whether there are epithelial cells in the mucin pools.

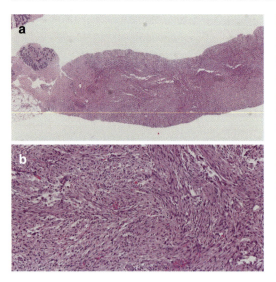

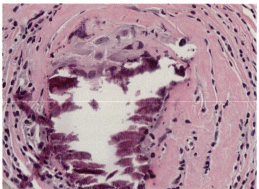

Fig. 4.17 An island of microcalcification is seen with surrounding fibrosis and chronic inflammation. A few enlarged nuclei, with single nucleoli, are seen superior to the calcification, of uncertain histogenesis, and it is not entirely clear if this represents a duct space. Additional levels and immunohistochemistry proved unhelpful, and repeat biopsy was recommended

Fig. 4.16 A spindle cell lesion is seen in these cores, adjacent to normal breast tissue (*left*) (hematoxylin and eosin). High-power magnification shows the interweaving fascicles of the lesion, with red cell extravasation. Immunohistochemistry favored a diagnosis of nodular fasciitis, and this was reported as B3, of uncertain malignant potential, and the lesion excised when the diagnosis was confirmed

Other Rare Lesions

There are a small number of other rare lesions that are usually best classified as B3 on core biopsy such as adenomyoepithelioma and microglandular adenosis, as well as spindle cell lesions either of uncertain diagnosis on core or those with definitive diagnosis, such as fibromatosis and myofibroblastoma as described above. Other very uncommon spindle cell lesions such as nerve sheath tumors, nodular fasciitis (Fig. 4.16a, b), and vascular lesions are also problematic on core and in general are classified as being of uncertain malignant potential and diagnostic excision recommended, even with thorough examination and immunohistochemical assessment.

B4, Suspicious

A B5 category should be provided for cases where there is no doubt regarding the malignant diagnosis and indicates that definitive therapeutic surgical excision, such as mastectomy, may be performed. Technical problems such as crushed core biopsies with suspicious features of DCIS or invasive carcinoma, but in which definite diagnosis cannot be made, are best classified as B4. Similarly, small groups of apparently neoplastic cells contained within blood clot or adherent to the outer aspect of the sample should be classified as suspicious. Very small foci suspicious of invasive carcinoma in which there is insufficient material to allow immunocytochemical studies, for example, to confirm the absence of a myoepithelial layer, may also be assigned to this category. A complete single duct space bearing an unequivocal high-grade atypical epithelial proliferation can be classified as B5a, DCIS. However, if one or only part of a duct space is seen containing a highly atypical epithelial process (particularly if no necrosis is present), care should be taken in providing a B5a definitive diagnosis and a B4 suspicious diagnosis considered as alternative (Fig. 4.17). Indeed "suspicious of DCIS" is the commonest cause of a B4 diagnosis in the UK [36]. On occasions, dystrophic calcification is seen histologically without unequivocal epithelial cell population but which appear to lie within a membrane-bound space. Surrounding fibrosis and chronic inflammation may be seen, and the appearances are suspicious of DCIS. In such circumstances, additional levels can be helpful but a categorization of B4 should be considered.

The management of cases classified as B4 will usually be repeat core biopsy or vacuum-assisted biopsy to obtain definitive diagnosis although in a few cases, diagnostic excision biopsy of the area may be appropriate.

References

1. Ciatto S, Houssami N, Ambrogetti D, Bianchi S, Bonardi R, Brancato B, Catarzi S, Risso GG. Accuracy and underestimation of malignancy of breast core needle biopsy: the Florence experience of over 4000 consecutive biopsies. Breast Cancer Res Treat. 2007;101:291–7.
2. Rhodes A, Jasani B, Balaton AJ, Miller KD. Immunohistochemical demonstration of oestrogen and progesterone receptors: correlation of standards achieved on in-house tumors with that achieved on external quality assessment material in over 150 laboratories from 26 countries. J Clin Pathol. 2000;53(4):292–301.
3. Lee AH, Key HP, Bell JA, Kumah P, Hodi Z, Ellis IO. The effect of delay in fixation on HER2 expression in invasive carcinoma of the breast assessed with immunohistochemistry and in situ hybridisation. J Clin Pathol. 2014;7:573–5.
4. Kalkman S, Barentsz MW, Witkamp AJ, van der Wall E, Verkooijen HM, van Diest PJ, Kalkman S, Barentsz MW, van Diest PJ. The effects of under 6 hours of formalin fixation on hormone receptor and HER2 expression in invasive breast cancer: a systematic review. Am J Clin Pathol. 2014;142(1):16–22. h.
5. Kalkman S, Barentsz MW, Witkamp AJ, van der Wall E, Verkooijen HM, van Diest PJ. Brief fixation does not affect assessment of hormone receptor expression in invasive breast carcinoma biopsies: paving the road for same-day tissue diagnostics. Am J Surg Pathol. 2014;38(8):1071–8.
6. Moritz JD, Luftner-Nagel S, Westerhof JP, Oestmann JW, Grabbe E. Microcalcifications in breast core biopsy specimens: disappearance at radiography after storage in formaldehyde. Radiology. 1996;200(2):361–3.
7. Liberman L, Evans 3rd WP, Dershaw DD, Hann LE, Deutch BM, Abramson AF, Rosen PP. Radiography of microcalcifications in stereotaxic mammary core biopsy specimens. Radiology. 1994;190(1):223–5.
8. Ellis IO, Humphreys S, Michell M, Pinder SE, Wells CA, Zakhour HD. *Best Practice No 179*. Guidelines for breast needle core biopsy handling and reporting in breast screening assessment. J Clin Pathol. 2007;60(12):1297–9.
9. Dahlstrom JE, Sutton S, Jain S. Histologic-radiologic correlation of mammographically detected microcal-cification in stereotactic core biopsies. Am J Surg Pathol. 1998;22:256–9.
10. Brennan ME, Turner RM, Ciatto S, Marinovich ML, French JR, Macaskill P, Houssami N. Ductal carcinoma in situ at core-needle biopsy: meta-analysis of underestimation and predictors of invasive breast cancer. Radiology. 2011;260:119–28.
11. Bagnall MJ, Evans AJ, Wilson AR, Pinder SE, Denley H, Geraghty JG, Ellis IO. Predicting invasion in mammographically detected microcalcification. Clin Radiol. 2001;56(10):828–32.
12. Masannat YA, Bains SK, Pinder SE, Purushotham AD. Challenges in the management of pleomorphic lobular carcinoma in situ of the breast. Breast. 2013;22(2):194–6.
13. Jacobs TW, Pliss N, Kouria G, Schnitt SJ. Carcinomas in situ of the breast with indeterminate features: role of E-cadherin staining in categorization. Am J Surg Pathol. 2001;25(2):229–36.
14. Collins LC, Carlo VP, Hwang H, Barry TS, Gown AM, Schnitt SJ. Intracystic papillary carcinomas of the breast: a reevaluation using a panel of myoepithelial cell markers. Am J Surg Pathol. 2006;30(8):1002–7.
15. Harris GC, Denley HE, Pinder SE, Lee AH, Ellis IO, Elston CW, Evans A. Correlation of histologic prognostic factors in core biopsies and therapeutic excisions of invasive breast carcinoma. Am J Surg Pathol. 2003;27(1):11–5.
16. Naidoo K, Beardsley B, Carder PJ, Deb R, Fish D, Girling A, Hales S, Howe M, Wastall LM, Lane S, Lee AHS, Philippidou M, Quinn C, Stephenson T, Pinder SE. Accuracy of classification of invasive lobular carcinoma on needle core biopsy of the breast. J Clin Pathol 2016. In press. doi:10.1136/jclinpath-2016-203886.
17. Arnedos M, Nerurkar A, Osin P, A'Hern R, Smith IE, Dowsett M. Discordance between core needle biopsy (CNB) and excisional biopsy (EB) for estrogen receptor (ER), progesterone receptor (PgR) and HER2 status in early breast cancer (EBC). Ann Oncol. 2009;20:1948–52.
18. Lee AHS. The histological diagnosis of metastases to the breast from extramammary malignancies. J Clin Pathol. 2007;60:1333–41.
19. Tot T. Cytokeratins 20 and 7 as biomarkers: usefulness in discriminating primary from metastatic adenocarcinoma. Eur J Cancer. 2002;38(6):758–63.
20. Bianchi S, Caini S, Renne G, Cassano E, Ambrogetti D, Cattani MG, Saguatti G, Chiaramondia M, Bellotti E, Bottiglieri R, Ancona A, Piubello Q, Montemezzi S, Ficarra G, Mauri C, Zito FA, Ventrella V, Baccini P, Calabrese M, Palli D, VANCB Study Group. Positive predictive value for malignancy on surgical excision of breast lesions of uncertain malignant potential (B3) diagnosed by stereotactic vacuum-assisted needle core biopsy (VANCB): a large multi-institutional study in Italy. Breast. 2011;20(3):264–70.
21. El-Sayed ME, Rakha EA, Reed J, Lee AH, Evans AJ, Ellis IO. Predictive value of needle core biopsy diag-

noses of lesions of uncertain malignant potential (B3) in abnormalities detected by mammographic screening. Histopathology. 2008;53(6):650–7.

22. Page DL, Rogers LW. Combined histologic and cytologic criteria for the diagnosis of mammary atypical ductal hyperplasia. Hum Pathol. 1992;23(10):1095–7.

23. Yu YH, Liang C, Yuan XZ. Diagnostic value of vacuum-assisted breast biopsy for breast carcinoma: a meta-analysis and systematic review. Breast Cancer Res Treat. 2010;120(2):469–79.

24. Page DL, Kidd Jr TE, Dupont WD, Simpson JF, Rogers LW. Lobular neoplasia of the breast: higher risk for subsequent invasive cancer predicted by more extensive disease. Hum Pathol. 1991;22(12):1232–9.

25. Mastracci TL, Shadeo A, Colby SM, Tuck AB, O'Malley FP, Bull SB, Lam WL, Andrulis IL. Genomic alterations in lobular neoplasia: a microarray comparative genomic hybridization signature for early neoplastic proliferation in the breast. Genes Chromosomes Cancer. 2006;45(11):1007–17.

26. Hussain M, Cunnick GH. Management of lobular carcinoma in situ and atypical lobular hyperplasia of the breast – a review. Eur J Surg Oncol. 2011;37(4):279–89.

27. Fraser JL, Raza S, Chorny K, Connolly JL, Schnitt SJ. Columnar alteration with prominent apical snouts and secretions: a spectrum of changes frequently present in breast biopsies performed for microcalcifications. Am J Surg Pathol. 1998;22(12):1521–7.

28. Verschuur-Maes AH, van Deurzen CH, Monninkhof EM, van Diest PJ. Columnar cell lesions on breast needle biopsies: is surgical excision necessary? A systematic review. Ann Surg. 2012;255(2):259–65.

29. O'Malley FP, Bane A. An update on apocrine lesions of the breast. Histopathology. 2008;52(1):3–10.

30. Tse GM, Tan PH, Moriya T. The role of immunohistochemistry in the differential diagnosis of papillary lesions of the breast. J Clin Pathol. 2009;62(5):407–13.

31. Rakha EA, Lee AH, Jenkins JA, Murphy AE, Hamilton LJ, Ellis IO. Characterization and outcome of breast needle core biopsy diagnoses of lesions of uncertain malignant potential (B3) in abnormalities detected by mammographic screening. Int J Cancer. 2011;129(6):1417–24.

32. Page DL, Salhany KE, Jensen RA, Dupont WD. Subsequent breast carcinoma risk after biopsy with atypia in a breast papilloma. Cancer. 1996;78:258–66.

33. Lee AHS, Hodi Z, Ellis IO, Elston CW. Histological features useful in the distinction of phyllodes tumor and fibroadenoma on needle core biopsy of the breast. Histopathology. 2007;51:336–44.

34. Abdulcadir D, Nori J, Meattini I, Giannotti E, Boeri C, Vanzi E, Vezzosi V, Bianchi S. Phyllodes tumors of the breast diagnosed as B3 category on image-guided 14-gauge core biopsy: analysis of 51 cases from a single institution and review of the literature. Eur J Surg Oncol. 2014;40(7):859–64.

35. Rakha EA, Shaaban AM, Haider SA, Jenkins J, Menon S, Johnson C, Yamaguchi R, Murphy A, Liston J, Cornford E, Hamilton L, James J, Ellis IO, Lee AHS. Outcome of pure mucocele-like lesions diagnosed on breast core biopsy. Histopathology. 2013;62:894–8.

36. Rakha EA, Ho BC, Naik V, Sen S, Hamilton LJ, Hodi Z, Ellis IO, Lee AH. Outcome of breast lesions diagnosed as lesion of uncertain malignant potential (B3) or suspicious of malignancy (B4) on needle core biopsy, including detailed review of epithelial atypia. Histopathology. 2011;58(4):626–32.

Ductal Carcinoma In Situ

5

Jeremy Thomas

Abstract

This chapter deals with the main issues that the pathologist faces when dealing with cases of ductal carcinoma in situ. These include methods of handling various types of specimens, problems encountered on reporting core and excision specimens of DCIS, diagnosing microinvasion, and the use of immunohistochemistry to confirm the diagnosis in certain situations. There is also a discussion of rare types of DCIS as well as DCIS arising in the context of columnar cell change and following neoadjuvant therapy.

Keywords

Ductal carcinoma in situ • Specimen handling • Grading DCIS • Special types of DCIS • Immunohistochemistry

Introduction

In the past 20 years, ductal carcinoma in situ has become a major issue in breast cancer diagnosis and management because of the worldwide introduction of breast screening programs and increasingly sensitive imaging techniques. Prior to this it was an uncommon lesion encountered in the symptomatic setting. The disease gives rise to considerable challenges for the pathologist both in terms of core biopsy diagnosis and also specimen handling. This chapter covers some of the more problematic aspects of this disease. The author has been fortunate to have access to data from the Sloane Project, a UK audit of screen-detected DCIS accruing more than 12,000 patients between 2004 and 2012. Reference to this audit is made on a number of occasions in the text.

Specimen Handling

The majority of patients with ductal carcinoma in situ (DCIS) will be diagnosed through breast screening. Whether the disease is screen detected or symptomatic, specimen handling and diagnostic approaches are identical. The majority of DCIS-containing excision specimens will follow a

J. Thomas
Western General Hospital, Edinburgh EH4 2XU, UK
e-mail: jeremy.thomas@nhslothian.scot.nhs.uk

© Springer International Publishing Switzerland 2017
S. Shousha (ed.), *Breast Pathology*, DOI 10.1007/978-3-319-28655-6_5

nonoperative diagnostic core biopsy that will have given either a firm diagnosis of DCIS or a qualified diagnosis of an atypical intraductal epithelial proliferation (AIEP). The specimen types range from small to large volume core biopsy, diagnostic and therapeutic excision biopsy, re-excisions, therapeutic mammoplasties, and mastectomy specimens which increasingly are modified due to cosmetic/reconstruction considerations.

General principles should direct the pathologist toward maximum diagnostic efficiency with the goal of sampling as much of the disease as possible so that the true extent can be measured and the possibility of missing invasive disease minimized.

Diagnostic Core Biopsies

The most recent UK guidelines were published in 2001 [1]. Although the principles of specimen handling have not changed since then, imaging techniques have and the challenge for pathologists is now very much greater. Much more subtle calcification is detected with modern equipment, and this may be associated with more diagnostically challenging proliferative lesions. Furthermore, the increasing use of magnetic resonance imaging (MRI) will detect non-calcified parenchymal distortions which may present difficulties when trying to locate the lesion in the excision specimen. The core biopsy, whether small or large volume, should be handled as follows:

1. Good fixation is essential with a minimum of 6 h in neutral buffered formalin, a requirement for satisfactory histology and optimal preservations of antigens for subsequent receptor testing or molecular studies.
2. The cores must be x-rayed at the time they are taken so that the diagnostic chain of mammographic abnormality – core biopsy – histological section is unbroken and that a confident statement can be made whether the histological section can be reasonably regarded as representative of the original mammographic abnormality.

3. When dealing with multisite diseas, x-rays must be labeled clearly so that each core biopsy can be correctly correlated with the relevant imaging abnormality.
4. The 2001 guidelines recommend hematoxylin and eosin (H&E) stained sections from three levels as a starting point for examination of a core biopsy – small or large volume. In our laboratory we start with two and then direct further examination of the tissue from there. It is important to understand how exactly the laboratory sections are blocked and how deep each level is cut. I would recommend that the block is sectioned cautiously because the lesion in question may be quite transient appearing in level 8 and disappearing again in level 12, for example.
5. After the initial levels, the pathologist may be in a position to know what sort of lesion he/she is dealing with, whether immunohistochemistry will be helpful to tease out the details of an epithelial proliferation, whether invasive disease is looking likely, and whether receptor testing will be required. How many levels will depend on the goal set by the specimen x-ray – how many calcifications are being pursued – and the size of the core biopsies. We will cut up to 30 or more levels on a large volume core biopsy to chase a focus of microcalcification and that is justified by a diagnosis rate >95 % and a re-biopsy rate for patients of <10 %. The biopsy procedure may be uncomfortable for the patient, and we as pathologists have a duty to maximize the information gleaned from any tissue sent to us.
6. A further consideration when combining the cutting of further levels and immunohistochemistry is a decision about the sequence of these two approaches. If a lesion has appeared that will benefit from the application of immunohistochemistry, e.g., is the proliferation mixed or a single cell population, it is advisable to ask for the immunohistochemistry to be carried out before the levels. Whether immunohistochemistry is carried out before or after levels is a matter of judgment but should be kept in mind.

Diagnostic and Therapeutic Excision Specimens

The 2005 NHS Breast Screening Guidelines give valuable practical advice about the handling of these specimens and are still very relevant today [2]. Whether an excision specimen is diagnostic or therapeutic but is oriented by the surgeon, e.g., with clips or sutures, it should be handled in the same way. The specimen is inked according to local practice. A specimen x-ray should be available from the surgeon. It is worthwhile looking at the nonoperative core biopsy report(s) at this stage to see if there are any specific issues that need to be resolved. It is better to be forewarned before slicing the specimen, e.g., multisite disease, when one of the lesions has been detected by MRI. The specimen x-ray may show tissue markers which will correlate with sites of previous core biopsies.

Macroscopic examination, of course, has a place in the assessment of these specimens but cannot be relied upon to direct block selection. Excision biopsy specimens for DCIS will often show nothing more than a biopsy site marked by hemorrhage or, if you are lucky, a tissue marker – but even that may be off target or have moved.

There are no hard and fast rules about the use of slice radiography in these excision specimens. Common sense has to be applied here and a balance struck between achieving a satisfactory diagnostic report and managing a large busy breast pathology practice. For smaller specimens of say 25–30 g, I would suggest blocking it in its entirety. For larger excision specimens, generous blocking may suffice, but if possible I would recommend using slice radiography to assist block selection to maximize the yield from the blocks taken (see Chap. 2). The goal with these specimens is to give a confident report on the nature of the disease, its extent, and the status of margins, and well-directed block sampling is the key to this.

Re-excision Specimens

These specimens will normally be oriented with a clip or suture if relating to single margin or with multiple clips/sutures if relating to more than one margin, e.g., superolateral. The new margin is painted in the laboratory, and usually two colors of ink will suffice so that in the example above of the superolateral re-excision I would paint the anterior half red and the posterior black and then serially section the specimen blocking the slices in sequence from the superior extremity to the inferior part of the lateral extremity. Thus the relevant position of each block should be assessable. Normally I block the entire specimen unless it is very large when I sample every other slice retaining the residue which can be blocked later if there is a problem.

Therapeutic Mammoplasties

These procedures are carried out to achieve breast conservation in the face of extensive disease, and the specimens can be very difficult. They normally comprise a generous therapeutic wide local excision, a number of margin re-excisions, and also one or more breast reduction specimens. A sentinel node biopsy is often sent because of the relatively high risk of discovering invasive disease (because of the disease extent). Specimen x-ray(s) will normally be provided for those specimens with calcification.

There will be an expectation that the pathologist will confirm the disease extent as assessed preoperatively, and slice radiography of the therapeutic excision will often be necessary. This will maximize the effectiveness of block-taking and save time and trouble in the long run. I recommend talking to the surgeon before embarking on the cutting of these specimens. He/she will guide you as to which specimens are of particular interest/relevance and which specimens have been taken for purely cosmetic reasons (and therefore only need minimal sampling). It is not always clear which is which from the request form.

Mastectomy Specimens

Mastectomies are usually carried out for extensive disease which is either continuous or apparently multisite and detected following biopsy of widely separated foci of microcalcification. The principles of handling these specimens are no different from therapeutic local excisions aiming to maximize the effectiveness of block-taking. Specimen radiographs will direct the pathologist toward the location and extent of disease, calcifications, and tissue markers. Reference to previous biopsies before cutting the specimen will save time and trouble.

In this laboratory we slice mastectomy specimens in the coronal plane so that our slice x-rays correspond to the two-dimensional specimen x-ray sent from theater. The risk of unsuspected invasive disease is higher in these specimens. With skin-sparing mastectomies, inked blocks should be taken from the anterior (non-skin-covered) margin because a positive margin may require further treatment, e.g., radiotherapy. If the nipple has been conserved, the surgeon will wish to know the status of subareolar ducts, and if the nipple is present in the specimen, it should be blocked in addition to subareolar tissue as disease is often found in these locations.

Disease Extent in Excision Specimens

Extent of disease is not always a straightforward estimation and requires an appreciation of the original imaging abnormality, reassembling sections according to their location in the original excision including three-dimensional reconstructions, relating disease to margins and the original dimensions of the biopsy and where necessary calculating extent from these figures, and finally making additions for any further disease that may be present in re-excision specimens. Disease extent in mastectomies is estimated through a combination of mapping blocks and measuring the separation of different foci on radiographs.

Diagnostic Approaches with Core Biopsies and Excisions

There are subtle but important differences in diagnostic approach depending on whether the specimen is a core biopsy or an excision.

Reporting Diagnostic Core Biopsies (Small and Large Volume)

This is the medium through which the majority of DCIS diagnoses are made. Because of the small size of the specimen and inevitably the limited amount of material, do not attempt to make a diagnosis of ADH. This is a size-based diagnosis, and in a core biopsy, one can have no idea of the extent of such a lesion. Designate it at AIEP and await the excision for the final answer. For non-high-grade DCIS, it is sensible to require more than one duct space or unequivocal lobular cancerization to make the diagnosis. For non-high-grade disease, immunohistochemistry is helpful to support the impression of a single cell proliferation except in the context of a columnar cell proliferation where it is of no help whatsoever. In my practice I use a basal marker such as CK14 and ER. The luminal proliferation should be almost completely devoid of basal phenotype epithelial cells in most cases of non-high-grade DCIS (basal phenotype DCIS does exist and requires a different approach). >90 % of non-high-grade DCIS are ER positive, and the uniform distribution of ER-positive epithelial cells throughout the duct space is a useful counterpoint to the negative CK14 stain.

A diagnosis of high-grade DCIS can be made on a single duct, a cancerized lobule, or even a partial duct profile if the cytology is sufficiently severe. The presence of periductal fibrosis with or without chronic inflammation (Fig. 5.1a), chronic inflammation alone, or distorting sclerosis (Fig. 5.1b, c) should prompt the examination of further levels because of the increased incidence of early invasion in these circumstances [3]. Immunostaining with a pancytokeratin antibody can be very helpful in identifying subtle foci of invasion (Fig. 5.1d).

Reporting Therapeutic Large Core (Vacuum-Assisted) Biopsies

These are carried out increasingly for the therapeutic management of radial scars and papillary lesions diagnosed initially on small volume (14 g) core biopsy. Should an AIEP-type lesion be found in these cores and a diagnosis of DCIS

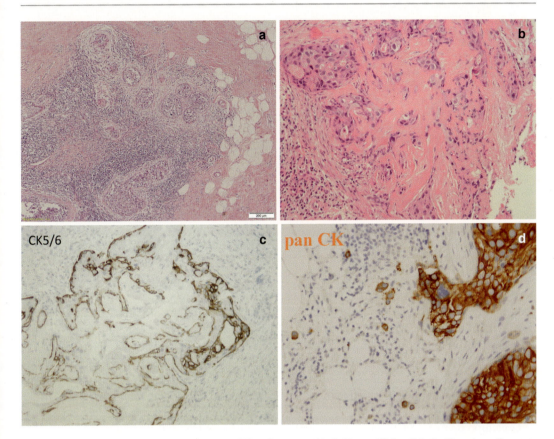

Fig. 5.1 (**a**) Cluster of ducts with high-grade DCIS and surrounding fibrosis and chronic inflammation. (**b**) DCIS with distorting sclerosis (H&E). (**c**) CK5/CK6 immunostain of same area as (**b**) showing preservation of the myoepithelial layer. (**d**) Small foci of invasion adjacent to an area of high-grade DCIS highlighted by pancytokeratin immunostaining

is not possible after exhaustive sectioning, the biopsy should be reported as AIEP and not designated as showing ADH. It is standard practice to follow a large volume excision with atypia by a surgical excision biopsy, and after that all the diagnostic material available should be assessed to make a final diagnosis.

Reporting Excision Biopsies

Two main issues distinguish reporting excision specimen from the core biopsy and both relate to disease extent.

1. Diagnosis of ADH: An excision biopsy is the appropriate medium for diagnosis of ADH.
2. Determining the extent of DCIS as the cytological features ameliorate toward the periphery of

the lesion: In an excision biopsy around the periphery of a zone of DCIS, one may see less severe atypical intraductal proliferations that "tail off" toward the margin (Fig. 5.2). For the purposes of disease extent and margin assessment, these should be regarded as part of the lesion and relevant to discussions about further management including possible re-excision of an involved margin. Obviously such considerations are impossible to apply in core biopsies.

Grading DCIS

The objective of grading DCIS is to provide guidance on prognosis and whether there is a risk of coexistent invasive disease, recurrence after conservation therapy, or a contralateral event. Although this objective is broadly achieved in

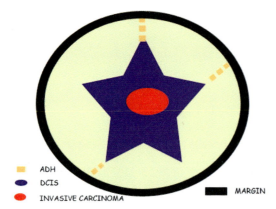

■ ADH
● DCIS
● INVASIVE CARCINOMA
■ MARGIN

Fig. 5.2 Diagrammatic representation of a central carcinoma, peripheral zone of DCIS with ADH extending to the margin of a specimen

populations of patients with DCIS, it has poor applicability for individual patients because of interpretative differences among observers. Data from the Sloane Project [4], for example, showed there was a wide range of recorded high-grade DCIS in different hospitals (30–80 % of cases) that could not be attributed to variation in patient populations [5].

Grading systems for DCIS are primarily based on nuclear morphology with some systems supplementing this information with additional features of comedo necrosis and/or architectural pattern. Both the UK NHS Breast Screening Programme (NHSBSP) and the College of American Pathologists (CAP) currently recommend a system based on nuclear characteristics although there are subtle differences between the two. These two systems are summarized in Tables 5.1a and 5.1b.

It is worth mentioning briefly the Van Nuys grading system which subdivides DCIS on the basis of nuclear grade: high grade and non-high grade, the presence or absence of comedo necrosis, and lesion size [6]. This is attractive because it introduces multiple parameters for assessment, thus reducing reliance on nuclear morphology alone. It also involves binary rather than three-way decisions which usually lead to better consistency among pathologists [7, 8]. The system has never found widespread acceptance or adoption, but its principles are sound and the details could be modified for today's practice. More

recently Pinder and colleagues have identified a subset of DCIS with a very poor outcome which corresponds to the highest Van Nuys grade but requiring >50 % solid architecture and with >50 % of ducts showing comedo necrosis [9].

Interobserver variability and inconsistency in grading undermine the conduct of clinical trials and any progress that might be made in improving the management of this complex disease. The main difficulty lies at the boundary zones between grades (low/intermediate and intermediate/high) with a broad spread of interpretation among pathologists which exceeds substantially the variability of morphology in tissue sections. However, the grading systems in general and pathologists in particular are not wholly to blame for this poor state of affairs. There is enormous variation in clinical practice in the management of DCIS ranging from margin widths, mastectomy rates, management of the axilla, use of radiotherapy, and clinical follow-up to name a few [10, 11, 12]. In the following paragraphs, I will confine my discussion to the NHSBSP system for DCIS grading and discuss the main problems facing pathologists practicing in this area with some suggestions that I hope are helpful.

In the first instance, it is helpful to subdivide DCIS into high grade and non-high grade because, as mentioned above, pathologists are much better at making binary than three-way decisions. This is an exercise in psychology not pathology! Thereafter, if your case is in the non-high-grade group, you will have to make a second subdivision into either low or intermediate grade. However, it has to be mentioned here that from a biological point of view, there is good emerging evidence supporting the division of DCIS into two rather than three prognostic categories [13]. Our difficulty for the future lies in where to draw the line between the two and how to draw it [9].

Low-Grade DCIS

Low-grade DCIS accounts for 5–10 % of DCIS diagnosed in the UK and almost exclusively

Table 5.1a   UK NHSBSP guidelines for grading DCIS

Feature	Low	Intermediate	High
Pleomorphism	Monotonous	Intermediate	Marked
Size	1.0–2×× size of RBC	Intermediate	>3× size of RBC
Chromatin	Diffuse; finely dispersed	Intermediate	Vesicular; irregular distribution
Nucleoli	Only occasional	Intermediate	Prominent; often multiple
Mitoses	Only occasional	Intermediate	*Usually* frequent
Orientation	Polarized toward luminal spaces	Intermediate	*Rarely* polarized

Table 5.1b   College of American Pathologists' guidelines for grading DCIS

Feature	Low	Intermediate	High
Pleomorphism	Monotonous	Intermediate	Marked
Size	1.5–2× size of RBC	Intermediate	>2× size of RBC
Chromatin	Diffuse; finely dispersed	Intermediate	Vesicular; irregular distribution
Nucleoli	Only occasional	Intermediate	Prominent; often multiple
Mitoses	Only occasional	Intermediate	May be frequent
Orientation	Polarized toward luminal spaces	Intermediate	Usually not polarized

through the Breast Screening Programme. There are substantial variations in its incidence among different UK regions with a range of 2–10% in different Scottish regions [14]. The main difficulties encountered by pathologists are in the area of whether the changes seen amount to DCIS at all (rather than an AIEP) and whether minor degrees of nuclear variation consign the lesion to the intermediate grade. Key diagnostic criteria are a small nuclear size, maximum 2× the diameter of a red blood cell (which should be available for comparison within the same tissue section), round nuclei or if ovoid showing some degree of polarization toward any luminal spaces, and inconspicuous nucleoli. Comedo necrosis should be regarded as an absolute exclusion for this diagnosis. Recognizable columnar cells in parts of the duct space usually indicate that the proliferation is incomplete and should be regarded as AIEP. A spectrum of proliferative columnar cell lesions to low-grade DCIS is illustrated in Fig. 5.3.

Intermediate-Grade DCIS

The guidelines are not helpful for this grade of DCIS stating that the features are those in between the low and high grades. Such negative diagnostic criteria "neither low grade nor high grade" do not inspire confidence in the system although one could argue that the pathologist is simply being asked to make two consecutive binary decisions! Having made a decision that the disease is not high grade, the main pathological findings to make a diagnosis of intermediate grade will be nuclear size of 2–3× the diameter of a red blood cell, a degree of nuclear pleomorphism that is not conspicuous, inconspicuous nucleoli, and infrequent mitoses (Fig. 5.4). Nuclear polarization will also be less pronounced than in low-grade disease.

At this point it is worth drilling down on what exactly we mean by "inconspicuous" and "significant" when talking about nuclear pleomorphism and nucleolar prominence. I believe that significant pleomorphism and prominent nucleoli are features that are appreciated easily in an H&E section at ×10 objective magnification (using the ×10 eyepiece) (Fig. 5.5). Comedo necrosis is easily demonstrable at ×4. Again it is worth considering what exactly we mean by comedo necrosis. In my view this is a substantial focus of necrotic debris admixed with polymorphs or their ghosts often with granular,

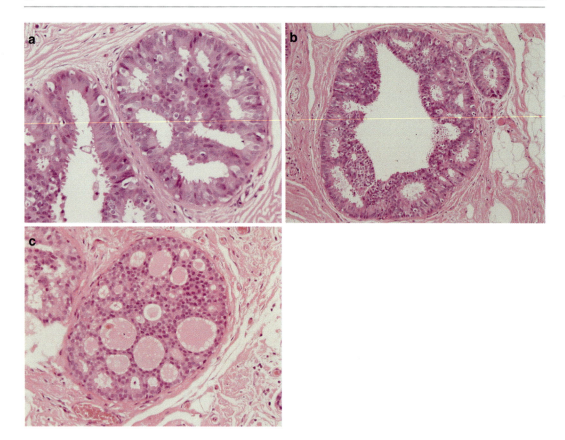

Fig. 5.3 (**a**) Columnar cell hyperplasia (H&E). (**b**) Columnar cell hyperplasia with architectural atypia (H&E). (**c**) Low-grade DCIS (H&E)

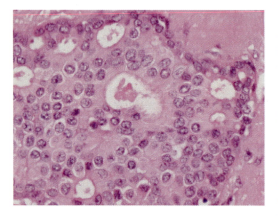

Fig. 5.4 Intermediate-grade DCIS. Note inconspicuous nucleoli and the absence of significant nuclear pleomorphism (H&E)

nearly calcified amphophilic material if not calcified properly. We do not mean the presence of an occasional polymorph admixed with a small amount of degenerate cellular debris that one can see not uncommonly in lower grades of DCIS and occasionally in the lumina of acini showing atypia or even benign proliferations.

High-Grade DCIS

This is more straightforward and is normally a diagnosis made using a low power (×4) objective. Nuclear size is greater than three red blood cell diameters, there is no polarization of cells, and pleomorphism is significant and/or nucleoli conspicuous. Comedo necrosis is often seen but is not exclusive to high grade, and mitoses can be found easily, but in my experience, they are usually at the frequency of one or two mitoses per duct space. I would rank the criteria in descending order of importance as follows: nuclear size, pleomorphism, comedo necrosis, nucleoli, and mitoses.

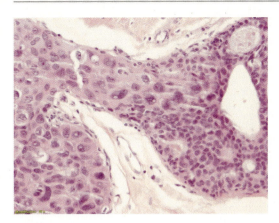

Fig. 5.5 DCIS: a single duct with significant pleomorphism and prominent nucleoli on the left (high-grade area) and insignificant pleomorphism and inconspicuous nucleoli on the right (intermediate-grade area) (H&E)

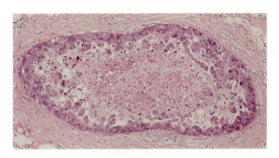

Fig. 5.6 High-grade DCIS showing significant nuclear pleomorphism and prominent nucleoli. There is necrotic debris in the lumen (H&E)

A "full house" is not required to make the diagnosis: nuclear size and pleomorphism are key (Fig. 5.6).

Problems in Grading DCIS

In my practice I would estimate that only 50 % of DCIS cases prove straightforward to grade. This is because many, inevitably, lie on a boundary zone, and in a subset of cases, one grade pattern predominates, but there is a minority population of a higher grade. We should not deviate from the general principle in breast pathology that we grade on the worst area. On occasions this will not be an easy decision because of the sparseness of cells showing higher-grade characteristics.

Table 5.2 Commonly encountered architectural pattern of DCIS in 5000 cases

Architectural pattern	Number	%
Solid alone	1569	31.8
Cribriform alone	925	18.7
Micropapillary alone	164	3.3
Solid and cribriform	1006	20.4
Cribriform and micropapillary	263	5.3

Data source: the Sloane Project

Architectural Patterns and "Special" Types of DCIS

Architectural pattern is not generally helpful in giving prognostic information about the disease. Data from the Sloane Project show that pure histological patterns of DCIS account for 55 % of the total. Of the more commonly reported patterns, Sloane Project data relating to pure and mixed morphology are shown in Table 5.2.

Those forms of DCIS which cause greatest difficulty in either diagnosis or grading are micropapillary and apocrine DCIS and extreme forms of columnar cell atypia/flat epithelial atypia. At the end of this section, there is a brief mention of some rare morphological variants and finally discussion about reporting DCIS following neoadjuvant systemic therapy.

Micropapillary DCIS

In the Sloane Project, a pure micropapillary pattern was identified in 3.3 % of cases. Embedded in the literature based on a study of a total of 140 cases of excised DCIS [15] is an assertion that this pattern of DCIS is frequently multicentric with the implication that it should be treated more aggressively. A review of over 8000 cases from the Sloane Project has failed to substantiate this [5].

Micropapillary DCIS is characterized by the circumferential involvement of one or more duct spaces by small papillary tufts of epithelium with cytological features ranging from the very bland (low grade) to very severe (high grade). The key elements for a firm diagnosis are circumferential involvement, the lack of fibrovascular cores in the tufts, and the presence of cytologically identical epithelium, usually as a single layer, between the tufts. The main area of diagnostic difficulty lies between the usual types, micropapillary pattern epithelial hyperplasia (Fig. 5.7a) and low-grade micropapillary DCIS (Fig. 5.7c).

Apocrine DCIS

The distinction between apocrine metaplasia and atypia DCIS is one of the most difficult areas of breast pathology. Because it is common to make allowances for degrees of cytological variation in apocrine epithelium, it is vital that we agree on what constitutes apocrine change in the first place. Apocrine cells are large, and they have abundant eosinophilic subtly granular cytoplasm giving a ground-glass appearance. The nucleus is centrally placed, and there is a single centrally placed large eosinophilic nucleolus. I believe that "normal" nuclear variation should not be greater than a factor of 2 (Figs. 5.8).

There is a limited literature on what exactly constitutes the diagnostic features of apocrine DCIS. The introduction of a size definition helps pathologists working in this area although the evidence base for such definitions is weak [16, 17]. Taking the best from the available literature, I would suggest the following as guidance in making a diagnosis of apocrine DCIS:

1. The epithelial abnormality is circumferential and in non-high-grade disease involves more than one duct space.
2. There are no specific architectural patterns although solid, papillary, and micropapillary are most common. Architectural abnormalities are the key to diagnosis of intermediate-grade apocrine DCIS.
3. Lesion size of a minimum of 4 mm is a helpful guideline and maintains consistency with (some) working definitions of ADH versus DCIS. A cut-off point of 2 mm has also been promoted as a minimum size for non-high-grade disease [15].

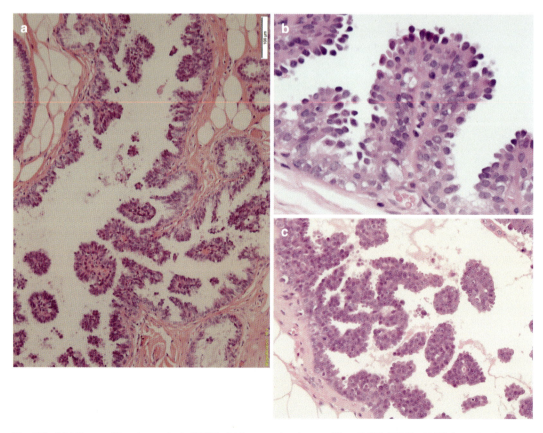

Fig. 5.7 (**a**) Micropapillary hyperplasia (H&E). (**b**) Low grade micropapillary DCIS (H&E). (**c**) High-grade micropapillary DCIS (H&E)

4. Nuclear variation should be >3× but is not a requirement if the architectural pattern is correct.
5. The nuclear membrane may be irregular and the chromatin pattern irregular.
6. Multiple, often small, nucleoli are seen.

Having reached a diagnosis of DCIS, which is hard enough, we should then attempt to grade the lesion. Given the diagnostic criteria above, I think it is very difficult to make a diagnosis of low-grade DCIS in an apocrine lesion. I would suggest a pragmatic approach reserving the high-grade category for those lesions showing gross cytological atypia with or without comedo necrosis. Figure 5.9 illustrates examples of apocrine DCIS of intermediate and high grades.

DCIS Arising in the Context of a Columnar Cell Lesion with Atypia

Columnar cell lesions are described as being with or without hyperplasia and with or without cytological and/or architectural atypia. They may be extensive and drawing the line between atypias and DCIS is often difficult. The spectrum of columnar cell alteration has been dealt with in Chap. 3. In this section I will consider the particular diagnostic challenges relating to DCIS arising in an area of columnar cell proliferation. The first point to appreciate is that when DCIS develops in a columnar cell proliferative lesion, recognizable columnar cell morphology is lost. Partial duct lesions where some of the epithelium is still recognizably columnar should not be

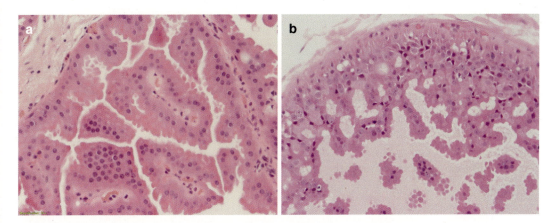

Fig. 5.8 Two examples of apocrine metaplasia with acceptable nuclear variation (H&E)

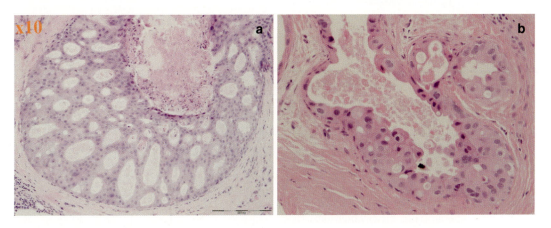

Fig. 5.9 (**a**) Apocrine DCIS, intermediate grade (H&E). (**b**) Apocrine DCIS, high grade (H&E)

diagnosed as DCIS and should be designated AIEP. Thereafter, complete takeover of a duct profile will qualify as DCIS. For *non-high-grade* lesions, I would recommend a minimum of two involved duct spaces to make a diagnosis in a core biopsy. The lesion may be of low, intermediate, or high grade.

Columnar cell hyperplasia (CCH) and CCH-associated DCIS are areas where immunohistochemistry is of no use in helping to support a diagnosis. The proliferations are always monotypic whether hyperplastic or neoplastic, and this is reinforced by negative staining with basal markers and ER. Figure 5.10 shows a partial duct columnar cell lesion which should be designated AIEP.

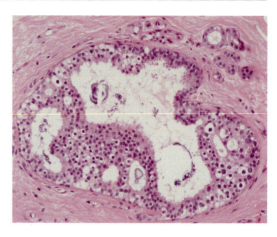

Fig. 5.10 Atypical (partial duct) columnar cell lesion (AIEP) (H&E)

Rare Forms of DCIS

These comprise mucinous, clear cell, small cell, and spindle cell in descending order of frequency. They rarely give rise to diagnostic difficulty and are histological curiosities. Spindle cell forms may show neuroendocrine differentiation staining with markers such as synaptophysin and chromogranin. Normal grading criteria apply to mucinous and clear cell forms. Small cell and spindle cell forms will normally qualify as intermediate grade. Figure 5.11 illustrates the clear cell variant.

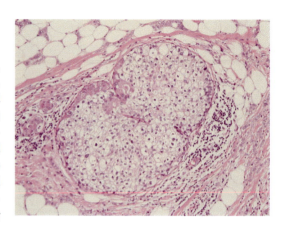

Fig. 5.11 Clear cell DCIS (H&E)

DCIS Following Neoadjuvant Systemic Therapy

Residual DCIS may remain in the breast following neoadjuvant systemic therapy. In the presence of a pathological complete response for invasive disease, its presence is an adverse prognostic indicator [18]. In the ARTemis trial [19], a trial of neoadjuvant chemotherapy with and without the antiangiogenesis agent bevacizumab, residual DCIS was seen in 4% of those cases where a pathological complete response was achieved [20]. Such residual DCIS may be modified by chemotherapy (Fig. 5.12) which can cause difficulties in the assessment of disease extent

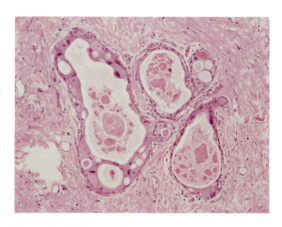

Fig. 5.12 DCIS modified by neoadjuvant systemic chemotherapy (H&E)

and, in conservation cases, margins. There is a limited literature on the use of neoadjuvant systemic therapy for pure DCIS, and at the present time, it is not part of routine practice [21–23].

Microinvasion and Invasion in DCIS

Detection of invasive disease in the presence of widespread DCIS is of critical importance for the effective management of the patient. It has implications for the management of the axilla and for future systemic therapy, e.g., anti-endocrine therapy for ER-positive invasive disease. The distinction between invasion and microinvasion is artificial and is likely to disappear from the UK reporting guidelines [2]. Microinvasion has been defined previously as a focus of invasive disease not more than 1 mm in maximum size extending outside the periductal specialized stroma. This definition originally arose before the days of immunohistochemistry to avoid overdiagnosis of invasive disease. I believe that in both core biopsies and excisions, such minute foci should be referred to simply as small foci of invasion without qualifying them as being microinvasive. Invasive carcinoma in the presence of widespread DCIS is more common in high-grade disease, and there are histological pointers that will alert the pathologist to their potential presence. These are periductal chronic inflammation and fibrosis and also possible so-called distorting sclerosis of ducts [3] (Figs. 5.1a, b).

Identifying small foci of invasion in the presence of widespread DCIS may be difficult, and the pathologist should concentrate his/her effort on those areas with chronic inflammation or fibrosis as these areas are likely to be most fruitful. The most useful stain for identifying such small foci is a pancytokeratin coupled with a CK14 or other basal marker to prove beyond question that the foci are truly invasive. Diagnostic difficulty may arise in cases of DCIS with limited or no stainable myoepithelium, when a judgment will have to be made on the H&E stained section. Difficulties may also arise in those uncommon cases of DCIS showing basal differentiation. In this latter scenario, I usually employ a range of basal markers

such as CK14, smooth muscle myosin, and P63, as the small invasive foci will often express one marker, while the myoepithelium of the in situ component will express a different marker. Examples of small foci of invasion and the use of immunohistochemical markers in their diagnosis are shown in Fig. 5.1d.

Where multiple small foci of invasion are present, they should be reported along the following lines "n foci of invasive carcinoma (grade 1/2/3) ranging in size from x to y mm set in area of DCIS $a \times b$ mm." I would routinely assess ER and PgR in these foci. Usually these patients are not candidates for adjuvant chemotherapy, and HER2 testing may not be feasible, reliable, or necessary.

The Use of Immunohistochemistry in DCIS

The key markers in routine practice include a small panel of basal/myoepithelial markers, a pancytokeratin, and ER. These will be used *in some cases* for the confirmation of a monotypic proliferation in the context of differentiating low-/intermediate-grade DCIS from benign proliferations, distinguishing complex sclerosing processes from invasive disease, confirming the presence of an intact myoepithelial layer in more confluent proliferations which may be in situ or invasive, and detecting small foci of invasion which might be hard to see on an H&E but stand out using a pancytokeratin stain.

Differentiating Low/Intermediate-Grade DCIS from Benign Proliferations

A myoepithelial marker such as CK14 is sensitive and relatively specific and is excellent for detecting myoepithelial cells admixed with luminal epithelial cells in benign proliferations (usual type epithelial hyperplasia). In low- and intermediate-grade DCIS, such admixed cells are uncommon. Occasionally one might see scattered myoepithelial cells in a proliferation that on other grounds is diagnostic of DCIS, and one should not allow these few positive cells to deter one from your diagnosis – but be careful! Myoepithelial markers are of no help whatsoever in sorting out columnar cell lesions. In those cases one has to rely on H&E alone. Figure 5.13 illustrates the difference in staining in usual hyperplasia and low-grade DCIS using CK14 immunostaining.

Distinguishing Complex Sclerosing Processes from Invasive Disease

Normally low power examination of an H&E section will allow these two processes to be distinguished with confidence because of the preservation of architectural features of scleros-

ing lesions and the presence of a preserved myo-epithelial population and bounding basement membrane on higher powered examination. Occasionally the use of a myoepithelial marker such as CK14 or CK5/6 will be helpful in more challenging lesions (Fig. 5.14).

Confluent Proliferations

Occasionally confluent masses of tumor cells, usually high grade, may give rise to difficulties in interpretation as to whether they are invasive or in situ. There may even be some duct profiles showing an unequivocal in situ histological pattern adding to one's doubt. The confluent masses are usually invasive, and the use of a CK14 immunostain can help

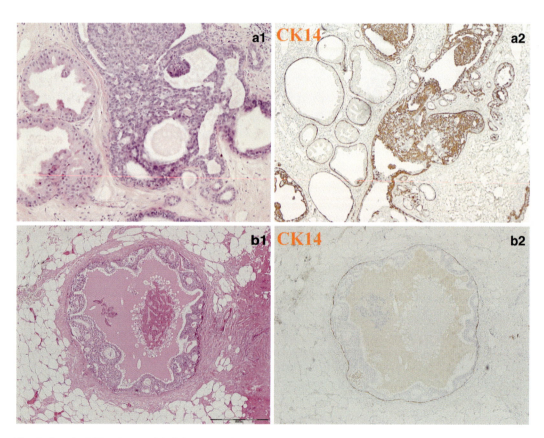

Fig. 5.13 (**a**) (*1*) Usual type epithelial hyperplasia. Note the streaming of a mixed population of epithelial cells within the central duct lumen (H&E). (**a**) (2) Admixed CK14-positive myoepithelial population in usual hyperplasia (H&E). The use of a myoepithelial marker high-lights the mixed population of epithelial cells in usual hyperplasia. (**b**) (*1*) Low-grade DCIS (H&E). (**b**) (2) Low-grade DCIS showing absence of myoepithelial cells in the luminal population with CK14 immunostaining

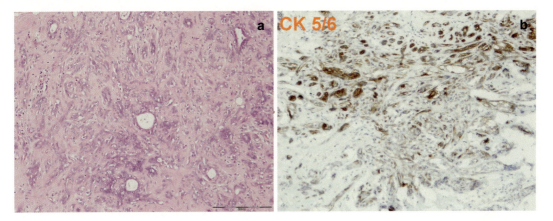

Fig. 5.14 (**a**) Sclerosing adenosis (H&E). (**b**) Sclerosing adenosis: confirmation of preservation of myoepithelial layer by CK5/6 immunostaining

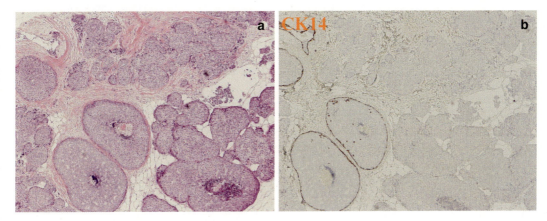

Fig. 5.15 (**a**) Confluent masses of carcinoma with DCIS in the lower part of the section and invasive carcinoma in the upper part (H&E). (**b**) Same area as (**a**) showing absence of myoepithelium in the upper invasive area with immunostaining for CK14

to support this diagnosis (Fig. 5.15), but in case of conflict between your H&E diagnosis and that suggested by immunohistochemistry, it is recommended to follow the direction of the H&E.

References

1. Ellis IO, Humphreys S, Michell M, Pinder SE, Wells CA, Zakhour HD. Guidelines for non-operative diagnostic procedures and reporting in breast cancer screening. NHSBSP Publication No 50, 2001.
2. Ellis IO, Pinder SE, Bobrow L, et al. Pathology reporting of breast disease. NHSBSP Publication No 58. NHS Cancer Screening Programmes and The Royal College of Pathologists 2005.
3. Walters LL, Pang JC, Zhao L, JM Jorns JM. Ductal carcinoma in situ with distorting sclerosis on core biopsy may be predictive of upstaging on excision. Histopathology. 2015;66:565–76.
4. The Sloane Project. www.sloaneproject.co.uk. Accessed 21/03/2015.
5. Thomas J, Hanby AM, Pinder SE, et al. Adverse surgical outcomes in screen-detected ductal carcinoma in situ of the breast. Eur J Cancer. 2014;50:1880–90.
6. Silverstein MJ, Poller D, Craig P, et al. A prognostic index for ductal carcinoma in situ of the breast. Cancer. 1996;77:2267–74.
7. Robertson AJ, Anderson JM, Beck JS, et al. Observer variability in histopathological reporting of cervical biopsy specimens. J Clin Pathol. 1989;42:231–8.
8. Robertson AJ, Beck JS, Burnett RA, et al. Observer variability in histopathological reporting of transitional cell carcinoma and epithelial dysplasia in bladders. J Clin Pathol. 1990;43:17–21.

9. Pinder SE, Duggan C, Ellis IO, et al. A new pathological system for grading DCIS with improved prediction of local recurrence: results from the UKCCCR/ANZ DCIS trial. Br J Cancer. 2010;103:94–100. doi:10.1038/sj.bjc.6605718.

10. Nicholson S, Hanby A, Clements K, et al. Variations in the management of the axilla in screen-detected ductal carcinoma in situ: evidence from the UK NHS Breast Screening Programme audit of screen detected DCIS. Eur J Cancer. 2015;41:86–93.

11. Dodwell D, Clements K, Lawrence G, et al. Radiotherapy following breast-conserving surgery for screen-detected ductal carcinoma in situ: indications and utilisation in the UK. Interim findings from the Sloane Project. Br J Cancer. 2007;97:725–9.

12. Maxwell AJ, Evans A, Carpenter R, et al. Follow-up for screen-detected ductal carcinoma in situ: results of a survey of UK centres participating in the Sloane project. EJSO. 2009;35:1055–9.

13. Meijnen P, Pieterse JL, Antonini N, Rutgers EJ, van der Vijver MJ. Immunohistochemical categorisation of ductal carcinoma in situ of the breast. BJC. 2008;98:137–42.

14. NHS Breast Screening Programme and Association of Breast Surgery an audit of screen detected breast cancers for the year of screening April 2012 to March 2013. Public Health England and The Association of Breast Surgery. PHE publications gateway number: 2013–526 p46.

15. Bellamy CO, McDonald C, Salter DM, Chetty U, Anderson TJ. Noninvasive ductal carcinoma of the breast: the relevance of histologic categorization. Hum Pathol. 1993;24(1):16–23.

16. Tavassoli F, Norris H. Intraductal apocrine carcinoma: a clinicopathologic study of 37 cases. Mod Pathol. 1994;7:813–8.

17. O'Malley FP, Bane A. An update on apocrine lesions of the breast. Histopathology. 2008;52:3–10.

18. von Minckwitz G, Untch M, Blohmer J-U, et al. Definition and impact of pathologic complete response on prognosis after neoadjuvant chemotherapy in various intrinsic breast cancer subtypes. JCO. 2012;30:1796–804.

19. Earl H, Hiller L, Dunn J, et al. Efficacy of neoadjuvant bevacizumab added to docetaxel followed by fluorouracil, epirubicin, and cyclophosphamide, for women with HER2-negative early breast cancer (ARTemis): an open-label, randomised, phase 3 trial. Lancet Oncol. 2015;16:656–66.

20. Thomas J. Lead pathologist for the Artemis Trial. Personal observation.

21. Von Minckwitz G, Darb-Esfahani S, Loibl S, et al. Responsiveness of adjacent ductal carcinoma in situ and changes in HER2 status after neoadjuvant chemotherapy/trastuzumab treatment in early breast cancer—results from the GeparQuattro study (GBG 40). Br Cancer Res Treat. 2012;132:863–70.

22. Keurer HM, Buzdar AU, Mittendorf EA, et al. Biologic and immunologic effects of preoperative trastuzumab for ductal carcinoma in situ of the breast. Cancer. 2011;117:39–47.

23. Chen Y-Y, De Vries S, Anderson J, et al. Pathologic and biologic response to preoperative endocrine therapy in patients with ER-positive ductal carcinoma in situ. BMC Cancer. 2009;9:285.

Abeer Shaaban

Abstract

Lobular neoplasia includes atypical lobular hyperplasia and lobular carcinoma in situ. This chapter details the morphological and immunohistochemical characteristics of in situ lobular neoplasia and its rarer variants with emphasis on diagnostic challenges, significance, and management.

Keywords

Lobular neoplasia • Pleomorphic LCIS • LCIS with necrosis • PALCIS • B3

Abbreviations

ALH	Atypical lobular hyperplasia
DCIS	Ductal carcinoma in situ
ER	Estrogen receptor
FLCIS	Florid lobular carcinoma in situ
HER2	Human epidermal growth factor 2
LCIS	Lobular carcinoma in situ
LOH	Loss of heterozygosity
PALCIS	Pleomorphic apocrine lobular carcinoma in situ
PLCIS	Pleomorphic lobular carcinoma in situ
TDLU	Terminal duct lobular unit
VAE	Vacuum-assisted excision
vs.	Versus

A. Shaaban
Department of Histopathology, Queen Elizabeth Hospital Birmingham and University of Birmingham, Mindelsohn Way, Edgbaston, Birmingham B15 2GW, UK
e-mail: a.shaaban@bham.ac.uk

Introduction

Lobular neoplasia encompasses a spectrum of lesions including atypical lobular hyperplasia (ALH) (at one end of the spectrum) and lobular carcinoma in situ (LCIS) at the other end. Recently, other variants of LCIS have been described including a pleomorphic LCIS (PLCIS), pleomorphic apocrine LCIS (PALCIS), and classical LCIS with comedo necrosis. Lesions showing hybrid features of ductal and lobular carcinoma in situ are also recognized.

Incidence and Significance

The true incidence of LCIS is difficult to ascertain, but it has been reported to represent between 0.5 and 3.8 % of all breast cancers [1, 2]. Classical LCIS is a disease of premenopausal women with

© Springer International Publishing Switzerland 2017
S. Shousha (ed.), *Breast Pathology*, DOI 10.1007/978-3-319-28655-6_6

most lesions diagnosed between the age of 40 and 50. It is often multifocal (in 50 % of cases) and bilateral (up to 30 %). PLCIS may present at an older age (average 55 years) [3], but data available so far is limited.

LCIS has traditionally been regarded as a marker of breast cancer risk [2] with an increased bilateral risk. ALH confers four to five times increased risk for subsequently developing breast cancer compared to the general population. The risk is 8–10× for LCIS. It has subsequently been shown that breast cancer following the diagnosis of ALH is three times more likely to occur in the same breast [4].

The risk of upgrade to invasive malignancy following a core biopsy diagnosis of LCIS varied considerably in studies (0–60 %) with an average of 27 % [5]. Reasons for discrepancy include differences in the cohort population (screening vs. symptomatic, family history vs. sporadic lesions), radiological discordance, lobular neoplasia on top of structured lesions, and variation in the amount of tissue sampled (conventional core vs. mammotome).

More recently, evidence to support the lesion being a direct precursor of invasive lobular carcinoma has emerged such as the coexistence with invasive lobular carcinoma and identification of common loss of heterozygosity (LOH) loci (17q, 17p, 11q) in both LCIS and the adjacent invasive lobular carcinoma [6]. The inactivation of the e-cadherin gene, observed in both LCIS and invasive lobular carcinoma, is a further support of a direct precursor role [7].

Histology

Atypical Lobular Hyperplasia (ALH)

The distinction between ALH and LCIS is quantitative. ALH is diagnosed when less than 50 % of the acini in a given lobule are involved by the lobular cells (Fig. 6.1a). If more than 50 % of acini are filled, distended, and distorted by the characteristic lobular cells, then the proliferation is designated as LCIS (Fig. 6.1b). Both lesions may coexist, and it may be difficult, particularly on a small core biopsy sample, to accurately

separate both, and therefore the term "in situ lobular neoplasia" is favored for those lesions diagnosed on core biopsy.

Classical LCIS

The term "lobular carcinoma in situ" was originally coined by Foote and Stewart in 1941 [8]. Histologically, LCIS is characterized by a solid monomorphic proliferation within a terminal duct lobular unit (TDLU) of discohesive cells with uniform round nuclei, indistinct nucleoli, and scant cytoplasm. Intracytoplasmic lumina are often present, and "pagetoid" spread into the adjacent ducts can be seen (Fig. 6.1c) producing a "cloverleaf" appearance. Calcification may be present (Fig. 6.1b) but is uncommon compared with DCIS and other types of in situ lobular neoplasia.

Classical LCIS can be composed of two types of cells:

- *Type A cells*: small uniform cells with bland nuclei and scant cytoplasm (Fig. 6.1b)
- *Type B cells*: larger cells (up to two times the size of a lymphocyte), with more cytoplasm and some variation in nuclear size and shape (Fig. 6.1d)

Both types may coexist and should be differentiated from the pleomorphic type (PLCIS) in which the lobular cells show nuclear enlargement with marked pleomorphism. LCIS is often e-cadherin negative (Fig. 6.1e).

Pleomorphic LCIS (PLCIS)

PLCIS was first described by Frost et al. in 1996 [9]. It refers to a proliferation of large pleomorphic (grade 3) lobular cells. Prominent nucleoli are commonly seen. Unlike classical LCIS, the lesion is commonly associated with comedo necrosis and luminal calcifications and hence is detected on mammographic screening (Fig. 6.2a). Calcification and comedo necrosis, however, are not a prerequisite for making the histological diagnosis. PLCIS is commonly associated with a background classical LCIS [10].

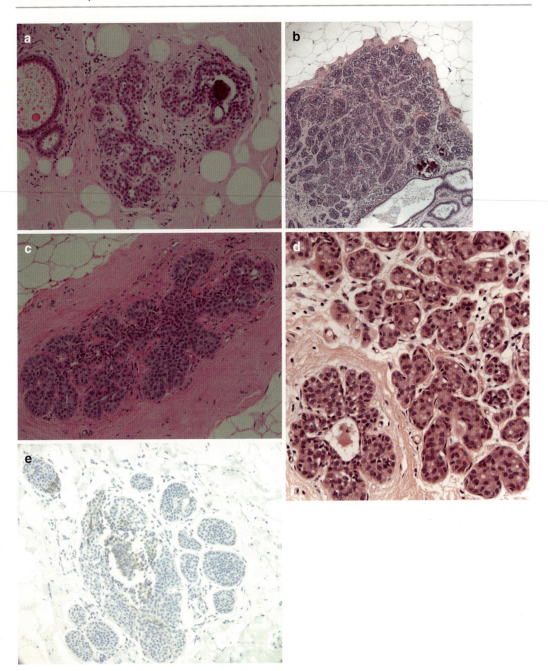

Fig. 6.1 In situ lobular neoplasia. (**a**) ALH showing characteristic lobular cells filling less than 50 % of acini. There is adjacent columnar cell change and calcification in one duct. (**b**) Classical LCIS: a mammary lobule is markedly distended and expanded by discohesive lobular cells of type A. Focal calcification is noted. (**c**) Lobular cells showing "pagetoid" spread along a mammary duct giving a cloverleaf appearance. (**d**) Type B classical LCIS showing larger nuclei with moderate cytoplasm and mild to moderate nuclear pleomorphism. (**e**) LCIS showing negative e-cadherin staining, characteristic of lobular neoplasia

The nuclei of PLCIS are generally large, being three times the size of a lymphocyte or larger, and show marked pleomorphism, similar to the nuclei of a high-grade DCIS. They often have abundant eosinophilic cytoplasm and eccentric nuclei (Fig. 6.2a). Similar to classical LCIS, they show

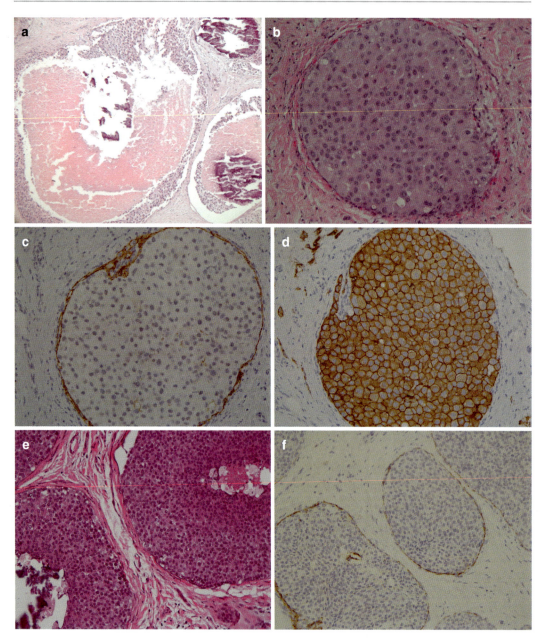

Fig. 6.2 Variants of lobular neoplasia. (**a**) Pleomorphic lobular carcinoma in situ (PLCIS): large ducts with solid proliferation of discohesive cells and associated luminal calcification and comedo necrosis. (**b**) Pleomorphic apocrine LCIS (PALCIS): solid proliferation of lobular cells with abundant eosinophilic cytoplasm. (**c**) E-cadherin immunohistochemistry of the same case. No staining is seen in the lobular cells. Note the positive staining of myoepithelial cells. (**d**) An example of HER2-positive PALCIS. (**e**) Classical LCIS with comedo necrosis: solid proliferation of discohesive lobular cells (types A and B) with luminal calcification and comedo necrosis. Note the absence of large pleomorphic nuclei characteristic of PLCIS. (**f**) The lesion is e-cadherin negative confirming the lobular phenotype

cellular discohesion, pagetoid growth pattern, and intracytoplasmic lumina [10]. Examples composed entirely of signet ring forms have been described [11].

In view of the rarity of the lesion, particularly in its pure form, the natural history of PLCIS remains unclear. Several, albeit small, studies reported a high rate of upgrading to invasive malignancy, predominantly of the lobular type, following a core biopsy diagnosis of PLCIS [12–14]. A recent large meta-analysis has shown an association with invasive carcinoma in 49 % of cases and a recurrence rate of 9.4 % [15]. This data supports managing those lesions as per DCIS.

Pleomorphic Apocrine LCIS (PALCIS)

This is a very rare type of pleomorphic LCIS characterized by striking eosinophilic cells with granular cytoplasm giving the cells an apocrine appearance (Fig. 6.2b). The cells retain the lobular features of being discohesive with intracytoplasmic vacuoles and loss of e-cadherin expression (Fig. 6.2c). Comedo necrosis is commonly present. Chen et al. [16] described ten cases showing myxoid, apocrine, and pleomorphic cytology. The lesion can be positive for HER2 (Fig. 6.2d).

The solid apocrine appearance of PALCIS should be distinguished from apocrine DCIS. Apocrine DCIS does not show cellular discohesion or other cytological features of lobular neoplasia. E-cadherin expression would support the diagnosis of apocrine DCIS.

Classical LCIS with Comedo Necrosis

This is a recently described, rare variant of LCIS characterized by a solid proliferation of classical lobular cells (type A and/or B) with associated comedo necrosis [17] (Fig. 6.2e, f). Fadare et al. [18] described a series of 18 cases, of which 12 were associated with invasive carcinoma. Examples of the same lesion have been included under the term "florid LCIS or FLCIS" by some groups [19, 20]. These lesions are thought to show genetic alterations similar to apocrine LCIS

and therefore may represent an aggressive form of LCIS. Large series of this rare subtype are still needed to illustrate the natural history and define appropriate management.

In Situ Carcinoma of Mixed Ductal and Lobular Features

These are lesions showing features of both ductal and lobular neoplasia and have also been termed "carcinoma in situ with indeterminate features" [21]. These may comprise uniform discohesive cells showing an architecture of DCIS (Fig. 6.3a) or cohesive cells that otherwise show lobular features (Fig. 6.3b). E-cadherin immunohistochemistry in those lesions may show heterogeneous expression (Fig. 6.3c) [21]. If after careful histological and immunohistochemical assessment a lesion cannot be confidently assigned into LCIS or DCIS, then the term "in situ carcinoma with mixed ductal and lobular features" should be used as per the WHO recommendations [17]. The presence of e-cadherin-positive neoplastic cells should be distinguished from residual normal ductal cells involved by lobular neoplasia (Fig. 6.3d). Genuine DCIS and LCIS may coexist in one lesion, sometimes in the same duct (Fig. 6.3e, f).

LCIS with Prominent Basal/ Myoepithelial Proliferation

The association of LCIS with abundant cells showing morphological and immunohistochemical features of myoepithelial cells has been described (Fig. 6.3g). Few case reports showed in situ lobular neoplasia associated with large cohesive cells, with irregular nuclei, eosinophilic to clear cytoplasm, inconspicuous nucleoli, and coarse chromatin [22–24]. These cells were consistently positive for CD10, SMA, CK5, CK14, P63, calponin, and e-cadherin and negative for ER/PR. It is not certain whether these cells represent myoepithelial hyperplasia or neoplastic myoepithelial differentiation. This phenomenon should be distinguished from residual normal ductal epithelial cells and from the mixed DCIS/LCIS examples.

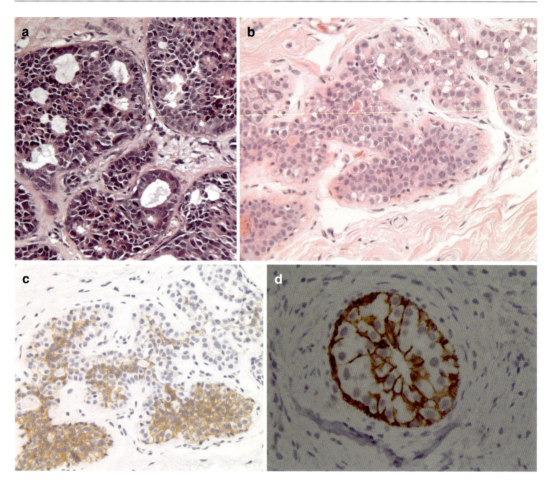

Fig. 6.3 In situ carcinoma with mixed ductal and lobular features. (**a**) Discohesive cells with eccentric nuclei and intracytoplasmic vacuoles (lobular features) arranged in a cribriform pattern (ductal feature). (**b**) Solid atypical intraductal proliferation involving a terminal duct lobular unit. Part of the lesion (right side) shows discohesion, while the remainder is cohesive. (**c**) E-cadherin immuno-histochemistry of the same lesion showing loss of expression in discohesive area with positive staining in the cohesive part. (**d**) LCIS cells (e-cadherin negative) admixed with e-cadherin-positive residual ductal epithe-lial cells. These should not be mistaken for DCIS. (**e**) E-Cadherin immunohistochemistry showing an example of coexistent DCIS (e-cadherin positive) and LCIS (e-cadherin negative) within the same lesion. (**f**) High-grade DCIS (central) comprising large pleomorphic nuclei admixed with small uniform LCIS nuclei (periph-ery) within the same ducts. (**g**) CD10 immunohistochem-istry showing LCIS with prominent CD10-positive myoepithelial cells

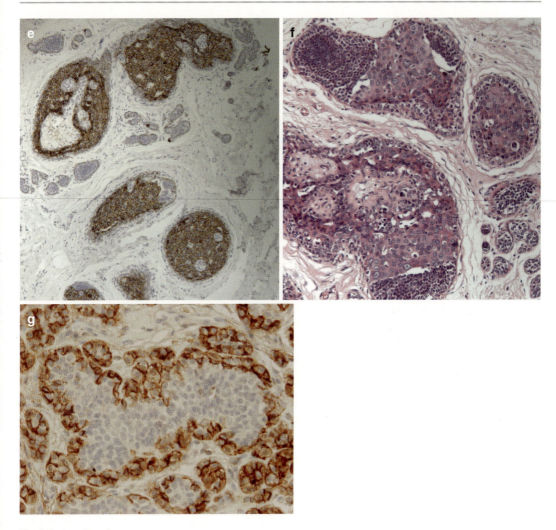

Fig. 6.3 (continued)

Immunoprofile

The majority of classical LCIS lesions are ER positive and HER2 and p53 negative. PLCIS, particularly PALCIS, is more likely to be ER negative and HER2 positive (Fig. 6.2d) and to show higher ki67 proliferation index. Basal cytokeratins (such as cytokeratin 5 and cytokeratin 14) are negative indicating a monomorphous population of cells. This, together with a strong and uniform ER positivity, can be used to confirm the neoplastic nature and differentiate it from florid usual-type ductal hyperplasia.

Classical LCIS and variants are often e-cadherin negative (in up to 90% of cases) (Figs. 6.1e and 6.2c, f) [25]. Aberrant e-cadherin expression may, however, be seen in morphologically typical LCIS cases. It is to be noted that the diagnosis of LCIS is morphological and can be supported by e-cadherin immunohistochemistry. Cases that are histologically lobular should not be reclassified as ductal based on e-cadherin expression. In this context, β-catenin and p120 immunostaining may be helpful since e-cadherin forms complexes with both proteins. β-Catenin is normally lost with e-cadherin, whereas p120 is aberrantly expressed in the cytoplasm of lobular cells. This can be used to confirm the lobular phenotype in difficult cases [26].

Molecular Profile

The hallmark of in situ and invasive lobular neo-plasia is the inactivation of the e-cadherin gene [7]. In situ lobular neoplasia is part of the low-nuclear grade neoplasia family [27] characterized by a loss of chromosome 16q and 17p with gain of 1q. Approximately 50% of lobular carcinomas show mutations of the e-cadherin gene resulting in a nonfunctional protein. Promoter methylation of the e-cadherin gene resulting in transcriptional silencing has also been reported. PLCIS shows all molecular features of classical LCIS but with more marked alterations. These include LOH in 52% of the cases at the p53 locus, 18% at the ESR locus, 19–24% at the HER2 locus, and 27–32% at the BRCA1 locus [28] and amplifica-tions of c-myc and HER2 genes [29]. These changes support the contention that PLCIS is related to classical LCIS, but probably represents an aggressive form of the disease.

There was no specific genomic pattern that distinguished PALCIS from PLCIS and/or classi-cal LCIS. However, some molecular changes occurred or were more prevalent in PALCIS, including amplification of 17q11.2–17q12 (HER2 gene region), amplification of 11q13.3 (cyclin D1 gene region), gain of 16p, and losses of 3q, 11q, 13q, and 17p [3].

Differential Diagnosis

Classical LCIS should be distinguished from low-grade solid DCIS. This may be difficult since DCIS may involve lobules "cancerization of lob-ules" and LCIS can spread into larger ducts.

PLCIS should be distinguished from solid high-grade DCIS. Cellular discohesion is a clue for diagnosing PLCIS. The presence of the typi-cal architecture of DCIS (such as cribriform, micropapillary patterns) in adjacent ducts is a pointer to DCIS. E-cadherin immunohistochem-istry can be helpful. The two lesions may, how-ever, coexist and both should be reported.

The distinction between PLCIS and type B clas-sical LCIS may be difficult, and in many cases a spectrum of changes from classical LCIS to PLCIS is seen. This is of particular importance in core

biopsies (PLCIS is categorized as B5a whereas classical LCIS as B3) and for tumor size measure-ment and margin assessment upon excision.

LCIS may involve other lesions such as fibro-adenoma and sclerosing adenosis. This may give a false impression of invasion. Careful attention to the morphological details of the preexisting lesions and assessment of the surrounding myo-epithelium should help establish the diagnosis. Immunohistochemistry for myoepithelial markers (such as p63 and smooth muscle myosin) should highlight a myoepithelial layer in difficult cases.

Management of LCIS

The management of classical LCIS has been the subject of controversy. Management strategies ranged from surgical excision (ABS/BASO guidelines 2009) to observation [30]. Some authors recommended excision only in the pres-ence of radiological discordance [31], and more recently vacuum-assisted excision (VAE) was proposed for further tissue examination to exclude coexistent invasive carcinoma [32, 33].

Standardization of the management of lesions with uncertain malignant potential on core biopsy (B3 lesions), including lobular neoplasia, is cur-rently underway in the UK. A multidisciplinary group has been commissioned, by the British National Health Service Breast Screening Programme (NHSBSP), to provide guidelines on the management of B3 lesions, and their report is pending publication. The group recommended second-line vacuum-assisted excision (VAE) as the method of choice for sampling, following a core biopsy diagnosis of classical LCIS, whether the lesion was incidental or associated with the mammographic abnormality.

Surgical specimens showing classical LCIS should be sampled well to exclude more advanced disease. The lesion is not included in the mea-surement of whole tumor size. There is no requirement to re-excise margins involved with classical LCIS.

The NHSBSP guidelines (pending publica-tion) recommend coding PLCIS on core biopsy as B5a and treating the disease as per DCIS by excision with clear margin. The European Society for Medical Oncology also recommends managing PLCIS as per DCIS. The size of PLCIS, as for DCIS, is included in the measurement of the whole tumor size. If close/at relevant margin, then re-excision to clear this margin is recommended.

In the current state of knowledge, LCIS with necrosis is best categorized as B4 on core biopsy (pending UK guidelines) and managed by excision for full assessment. Re-excision of involved margins is appropriate.

References

1. Haagensen CD, Lane N, Lattes R, Bodian C. Lobular neoplasia (so-called lobular carcinoma in situ) of the breast. Cancer. 1978;42:737–69.
2. Page DL, Kidd Jr TE, Dupont WD, Simpson JF, Rogers LW. Lobular neoplasia of the breast: higher risk for subsequent invasive cancer predicted by more extensive disease. Hum Pathol. 1991;22:1232–9.
3. Chen YY, Hwang ES, Roy R, et al. Genetic and phenotypic characteristics of pleomorphic lobular carcinoma in situ of the breast. Am J Surg Pathol. 2009;33:1683–94.
4. Page DL, Schuyler PA, Dupont WD, et al. Atypical lobular hyperplasia as a unilateral predictor of breast cancer risk: a retrospective cohort study. Lancet. 2003;361:125–9.
5. Hussain M, Cunnick GH. Management of lobular carcinoma in-situ and atypical lobular hyperplasia of the breast – a review. Eur J Surg Oncol: J Eur Soc Surg Oncol Br Assoc Surg Oncol. 2011;37:279–89.
6. Lakhani SR, Collins N, Sloane JP, Stratton MR. Loss of heterozygosity in lobular carcinoma in situ of the breast. Clin Mol Pathol. 1995;48:M74–8.
7. Berx G, Cleton-Jansen AM, Strumane K, et al. E-cadherin is inactivated in a majority of invasive human lobular breast cancers by truncation mutations throughout its extracellular domain. Oncogene. 1996;13:1919–25.
8. Foote FW, Stewart FW. Lobular carcinoma in situ: a rare form of mammary cancer. Am J Pathol. 1941;17:491–6. 3.
9. Frost AR, Terahata S, Silverberg SG. Pleomorphic lobular carcinoma in situ. Pathol Case Rev. 1996;1:27–30.
10. Carder PJ, shaaban AM. Pleomorphic lobular carcinoma in situ. Diagn Histopathol. 2012;18:119–23.
11. Fadare O. Pleomorphic lobular carcinoma in situ of the breast composed almost entirely of signet ring cells. Pathol Int. 2006;56:683–7.
12. Sneige N, Wang J, Baker BA, Krishnamurthy S, Middleton LP. Clinical, histopathologic, and biologic features of pleomorphic lobular (ductal-lobular) carcinoma in situ of the breast: a report of 24 cases. Mod Pathol Off J U S Can Acad Pathol. 2002;15:1044–50.
13. Chivukula M, Haynik DM, Brufsky A, Carter G, Dabbs DJ. Pleomorphic lobular carcinoma in situ (PLCIS) on breast core needle biopsies: clinical significance and immunoprofile. Am J Surg Pathol. 2008;32:1721–6.
14. Carder PJ, Shaaban A, Alizadeh Y, et al. Screen-detected pleomorphic lobular carcinoma in situ (PLCIS): risk of concurrent invasive malignancy following a core biopsy diagnosis. Histopathology. 2010;57:472–8.
15. Pieri A, Harvey J, Bundred N. Pleomorphic lobular carcinoma in situ of the breast: can the evidence guide practice? World J Clin Oncol. 2014;5:546–53.
16. Chen YY, Fitzgibbons PL, Jacobs TW, Waldman FM. Pleomorphic apocrine lobular carcinoma in situ (PALCIS): phenotypic and genetic study of a distinct variant of lobular carcinoma in situ (LCIS). Mod Pathol: Off J U S Can Acad Pathol. 2005;18 suppl 1:29A.
17. Lakhani SR, Schnitt SJ, O'Malley F, van de Vijver, Simpson PT, Palacois J. Lobular neoplasia. In: Lakhani S, Ellis I, Schnitt S, Tan P, van de Vijver M, editors. WHO classification of tumours of the breast. 4th ed. Lyon: IARC; 2012.
18. Fadare O, Dadmanesh F, Alvarado-Cabrero I, et al. Lobular intraepithelial neoplasia [lobular carcinoma in situ] with comedo-type necrosis: a clinicopathologic study of 18 cases. Am J Surg Pathol. 2006;30: 1445–53.
19. Bagaria SP, Shamonki J, Kinnaird M, Ray PS, Giuliano AE. The florid subtype of lobular carcinoma in situ: marker or precursor for invasive lobular carcinoma? Ann Surg Oncol. 2011;18:1845–51.
20. Shin SJ, Lal A, De Vries S, et al. Florid lobular carcinoma in situ: molecular profiling and comparison to classic lobular carcinoma in situ and pleomorphic lobular carcinoma in situ. Hum Pathol. 2013;44:1998–2009.
21. Jacobs TW, Pliss N, Kouria G, Schnitt SJ. Carcinomas in situ of the breast with indeterminate features: role of E-cadherin staining in categorization. Am J Surg Pathol. 2001;25:229–36.
22. Shousha S, Knee G. In-situ lobular/myoepithelial neoplasia of the breast. Histopathology. 2004;45:93–5.
23. Del Vecchio M, Foschini MP, Peterse JL, Eusebi V. Lobular carcinoma of the breast with hybrid myoepithelial and secretory ("myosecretory") cell differentiation. Am J Surg Pathol. 2005;29:1530–6.
24. Shousha S. In situ lobular neoplasia of the breast with marked myoepithelial proliferation. Histopathology. 2011;58:1081–5.
25. Dabbs DJ, Schnitt SJ, Geyer FC, et al. Lobular neoplasia of the breast revisited with emphasis on the role of E-cadherin immunohistochemistry. Am J Surg Pathol. 2013;37:e1–11.
26. Rakha EA, Patel A, Powe DG, et al. Clinical and biological significance of E-cadherin protein expression in invasive lobular carcinoma of the breast. Am J Surg Pathol. 2010;34:1472–9.

27. Abdel-Fatah TM, Powe DG, Hodi Z, et al. High frequency of coexistence of columnar cell lesions, lobular neoplasia, and low grade ductal carcinoma in situ with invasive tubular carcinoma and invasive lobular carcinoma. Am J Surg Pathol. 2007;31:417–26.

28. Middleton LP, Palacios DM, Bryant BR, et al. Pleomorphic lobular carcinoma: morphology, immunohistochemistry, and molecular analysis. Am J Surg Pathol. 2000;24:1650–6.

29. Reis-Filho JS, Simpson PT, Jones C, et al. Pleomorphic lobular carcinoma of the breast: role of comprehensive molecular pathology in characterization of an entity. J Pathol. 2005;207:1–13.

30. Meroni S, Bozzini AC, Pruneri G, et al. Underestimation rate of lobular intraepithelial neoplasia in vacuum-assisted breast biopsy. Eur Radiol. 2014;24:1651–8.

31. Capobianco G, Simbula L, Soro D, et al. Management of breast lobular carcinoma in situ: radio-pathological correlation, clinical implications, and follow-up. Eur J Gynaecol Oncol. 2014;35:157–62.

32. Parkin CK, Garewal S, Waugh P, Maxwell AJ. Outcomes of patients with lobular in situ neoplasia of the breast: the role of vacuum-assisted biopsy. Breast. 2014;23:651–5.

33. Stratchan C, Horgan K, Millican-Slater R, Shaaban AM, Sharma N. Outcome of a new patient pathway for managing B3 breast lesions by vacuum assisted biopsy – time to change current UK practice? J Clin Pathol, in press 2015.

Emad A. Rakha and Ian O. Ellis

Abstract

Histological grade is a simple and relatively accurate morphological measure of the degree of differentiation of the tumor and provides an overview of its intrinsic biological characteristics. It has a strong correlation with prognosis. This chapter deals with the basic principles of grading, its methodology, and evidence supporting its importance in clinical practice.

Keywords

Breast cancer • Grade • Differentiation • Tubule formation • Mitotic activity • Prognosis • Reproducibility • Methodology

Introduction

Invasive mammary carcinomas are morphologically subdivided according to their growth patterns and degree of differentiation, which reflects how closely they resemble normal breast epithelial cells. This is achieved by assessing histological type and histological grade, respectively. Histological grade is considered as a simple and relatively accurate morphological measure of the degree of differentiation of the tumor and provides an overview of its intrinsic biological characteristics. Although the recognition of the importance of grading of breast cancer goes back to the beginning of the twentieth century [1], the assessment of histological grade has become more objective with modifications of the original Patey and Scarff [2] and Bloom and Richardson [3] methods by Elston and Ellis [4], which is known as the Nottingham grading system (NGS). The NGS refers to the semiquantitative evaluation of three morphological characteristics, tubule formation, nuclear pleomorphism, and mitotic activity, and is a relatively simple and low-cost method, requiring only adequately prepared hematoxylin and eosin (H&E) stained tumor tissue sections to be assessed by an appropriately trained pathologist using a standard protocol.

Following the adoption of NGS criteria, many studies have demonstrated a significant association between histological grade and survival in invasive breast carcinoma [5–11] including the Nottingham group [12] (Fig. 7.1). In multivariate analysis, histological grade has equivalent

E.A. Rakha • I.O. Ellis (✉)
Department of Cellular Pathology, University of Nottingham and Nottingham University Hospitals NHS Trust, City Hospital Campus, Nottingham, UK
e-mail: ian.ellis@nottingham.ac.uk

S. Shousha (ed.), *Breast Pathology*, DOI 10.1007/978-3-319-28655-6_7

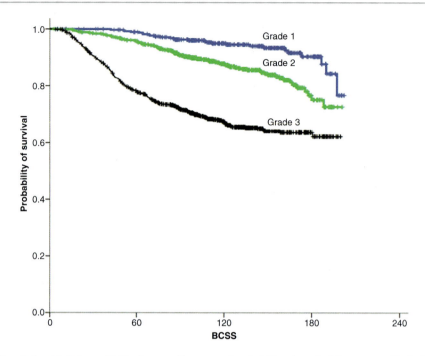

Fig. 7.1 The relationship between Nottingham grading system (grade 1-3) and survival demonstrated in the Nottingham breast cancer series

prognostic value to that of lymph node status [13]. Therefore it was combined with lymph node stage and tumor size to form the Nottingham Prognostic Index [NPI] [14]. NPI has been widely used for the management of patients with breast cancer in the UK [15], its validity has been confirmed in independent studies [16–18], and it has been recognized as the only appropriately validated prognostic index in breast cancer [19]. The NPI grade and lymph node stage have equal weighting. However in another prognostic index (Kalmar Prognostic Index [KPI] [10]), histological grade is given a higher weighting value (1.57), which is less than that for lymph node status (0.79) or tumor size (0.31). NGS is also a key component of other internationally recognized prognostic tools such as Adjuvant! Online and Predict.

In a large study from our group [12] that included 2,219 operable breast cancer cases with a long-term follow-up, grade was combined with lymph node stage and assessed the prognostic significance of the different combinations. The results demonstrated that grade is an important determinant of breast cancer out-come and complementary to lymph node stage. For example, the outcome of patients with grade 2/node-positive tumors (pN1, one to three positive nodes) was better than that of patients with grade 3/node-negative (pN0) tumors. Our results are supported by the study of Henson et al. [20] that included survival rates for 22,616 cases of breast cancer collected from the Surveillance, Epidemiology, and End Results (SEER) program of the National Cancer Institute. Their study showed that patients who were assigned stage II, grade 1, had the same survival as those assigned stage I, grade 3. It was shown that patients with histological grade 1 tumors less than 2 cm in size have excellent prognosis even if they have positive axillary lymph nodes with 99 % 5-year survival. There are also several lines of evidence that demonstrated grade as an independent prognostic factor in unselected series as well as in certain important subgroups, such as small operable breast cancer [6, 12, 21] and estrogen receptor (ER)-positive/HER2-negative cancers [22], and showed strong association between histological grade and prognostic gene signatures [23]. To further emphasize the biological and prognostic significance of breast cancer, several studies have shown an association between higher grade and other poor prognostic biomarkers such as ER negativity [24], HER2, P53, and P-cadherin positivity [25, 26]. Histological grade may also explain the poor prognostic significance of certain classes such as breast cancer in African-American women [27]. Being well recognized is a powerful prognostic factor; NGS is included as a component of the UK Royal College of Pathologists' minimum data set for histological reporting of breast cancer [28] and has been recommended to be provided in routine breast cancer pathology reports by various professional bodies internationally (EU, WHO, and AJCC [29–31]).

This grading system is based on a more objective criteria for assessment of the morphological characteristics of the tumor, including how closely the tumor resembles the normal breast terminal duct lobular unit architecture and cell structure (i.e., the degree of differentiation toward normal breast ducts and lobules), the degree of nuclear pleomorphism, and the number of mitotic figures, a measure of proliferation.

Basic Principles of Grading

Grading Requires High-Quality Tissue Preservation and Section Preparation

A number of studies have shown that delayed fixation can affect assessment of mitotic frequency. Start and colleagues have shown that as little as a 6-h delay may reduce the number of visible mitoses in a given sample by up to 76% [32]. Therefore the first prerequisite for accurate histological grading is good specimen preparation. The fixation step entails three elements: thickness of tissue, type and volume of fixative, and time. Failure to optimize all three elements results in underfixation or overfixation of the tissue. Ideally the tumor should be sliced in the fresh state to allow good penetration of fixative. It is well established that formalin penetrates tissues poorly. Time between removal of tissue and

fixation should be minimized as mitoses may complete their cycle, even after the tissue has been removed from the body, and disappear. Therefore, the specimen should be sent immediately, ideally in the fresh state, to the pathology laboratory. If this is not possible, it should be immediately placed in a fixative after making single or 90° cruciate pair of incisions into the lesion from the posterior aspect, thus preserving the integrity of key margins while allowing immediate penetration of fixative. Good liaison with surgical colleagues is required, and special arrangements may have to be made. Fixation in phosphate-buffered formalin using 10% neutral phosphate-buffered formalin (pH 7) is recommended. This gives perfectly adequate preservation, but the best results are obtained if the tumor is sliced in the fresh state to allow good penetration of fixative. The amount of fixative should be greater than the volume of tissue, and the optimum formalin to tissue ratio is 10:1. Immersing the whole breast unsliced into a specimen pot containing fixative will lead to poor preservation of morphologic details and cannot be endorsed. The length of time a tissue remains in fixative has also become an issue in sample preparation. It has been reported that standard time for complete fixation of tissues is a minimum of 5 h for needle core biopsies (NCB) and 12 or more hours for sections from larger specimens. Adequate fixation is important not only for preservation of mitotic figures but also for accurate assessment of vascular invasion and for retention of proteins such as the estrogen and progesterone receptors.

Careful high-quality tissue processing is important. Sections should be cut at 4–5 mm; if sections are cut too thick, nuclear detail is obscured. Slides of poor quality should not be accepted for assessment. Conventional staining with H&E is sufficient, and special stains are not required for grading. Although the use of immunohistochemistry to assess the proliferative activity of tumors (e.g., Ki-67) may add prognostic information particularly in grade 2 tumors or in the luminal molecular class, the current evidence is still not sufficient for incorporating this into routine practice.

Block Sampling

Blocks should be selected to give good representation of the whole tumor and in particular its periphery and from the optimally fixed areas to provide the best representation of the tumour mitotic activity.

Be Familiar with and Adhere to the Grading Protocol

Histological grading requires commitment and strict adherence to the accepted protocol. See below.

Take Account of Tumor Heterogeneity

Variation in appearance from one part of a tumor to another can occur and is particularly true of tumors of mixed type. Assessment of tubular differentiation is made on the overall appearances of the tumor, and so account is taken of any variation. Nuclear appearances including mitotic frequency are evaluated at the periphery and/or the least differentiated area of the tumor, to obviate differences between the leading edge and the less active center.

Grade All Breast Adenocarcinomas

Grading is carried out in invasive adenocarcinomas; this grading system is not suitable for tumors that are completely or predominantly in situ (see Chap. 5 for grading in situ tumors). It is our policy to grade all histological types of invasive carcinomas. The prognostic value of histological grade has been documented in most tumor types including invasive lobular carcinomas [33].

Audit Grade Distribution

Do not expect equal numbers of cancers to fall in each grade category. Published distribution for grades 1, 2, and 3 is approximately 20%:30%:50% in symptomatic breast carcino-

mas. If an audit of grade distribution shows substantially fewer grade 3 cases, or a majority of grade 2 cases, adherence to the grading protocols should be carefully reviewed and consideration of issues relating to suboptimal fixation considered. Screen-detected carcinoma series are likely to include a smaller proportion of high-grade cases with an approximate ratio of 3:4:3.

Grading Methodology

Three tumor characteristics are evaluated: tubule formation as an expression of glandular differentiation, nuclear pleomorphism, and mitotic counts. A numerical scoring system of 1–3 is used to ensure that each factor is assessed independently (see Table 7.1). Glandular formation is assessed over the whole tumor and is a low-power assessment. Nuclear pleomorphism is evaluated in the worst area. Mitotic counting is done in the most proliferating area. Examples of grades 1, 2, and 3 tumors are shown in Figs. 7.2, 7.3, and 7.4.

When evaluating tubules and glandular structures, only those exhibiting clear central lumina surrounded by polarized neoplastic cells are

Table 7.1 Semiquantitative method for assessing histological grade in breast

Tubule and gland formation
Majority of tumor (>75%) 1
Moderate degree (10–75%) 2
Little or none (<10%) 3
Nuclear pleomorphism
Small, regular uniform cells 1
Moderate increase in size and variability 2
Marked variation 3
Mitotic counts
Dependent on microscope field area 1–3 (see Table 7.2)
Final grading
Add scores for gland formation, nuclear pleomorphism, and mitotic count
Total score 3, 4, or 5 = *grade 1*
Total score 6 or 7 = *grade 2*
Total score 8 or 9 = *grade 3*
From Elston and Ellis [4]

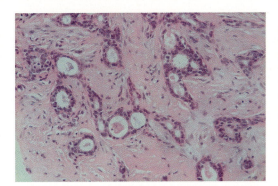

Fig. 7.2 An example of a grade 1 tumor which shows prominent tubule/gland formation throughout (tubule score 1), regular nuclei close to the size of normal breast epithelial cells (nuclear pleomorphism score 1), and no visible mitotic figures (mitotic frequency score 1). Total grade component score = 3 which indicates a grade 1 classification

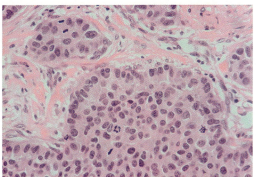

Fig. 7.4 An example of a grade 3 tumor which shows no tubule/gland formation (tubule score 3), and multiple visible mitotic figures (mitotic frequency score 3). Total grade component score = 9 which indicates a grade 3 classification

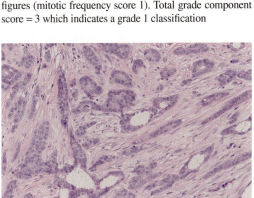

Fig. 7.3 An example of a grade 2 tumor which shows focal tubule/gland formation (tubule score 2), enlarged pleomorphic nuclei when compared with normal breast epithelial cells (nuclear pleomorphism score 3), and no visible mitotic figures (mitotic frequency score 1). Total grade component score = 6 which indicates a grade 2 classification

Table 7.2 Score thresholds for mitotic counts

Field diameter (mm)	Score 1	Score 2	Score 3
0.40	≤4	5–9	≥10
0.41	≤4	5–9	≥10
0.42	≤5	6–10	≥11
0.43	≤5	6–10	≥11
0.44	≤5	6–11	≥12
0.45	≤5	6–11	≥12
0.46	≤6	7–12	≥13
0.47	≤6	7–12	≥13
0.48	≤6	7–13	≥14
0.49	≤6	7–13	≥14
0.50	≤7	8–14	≥15
0.51	≤7	8–14	≥15
0.52	≤7	8–15	≥16
0.53	≤8	9–16	≥17
0.54	≤8	9–16	≥17
0.55	≤8	9–17	≥18
0.56	≤8	9–17	≥18
0.57	≤9	10–18	≥19
0.58	≤9	10–19	≥20
0.59	≤9	10–19	≥20
0.60	≤10	11–20	≥21
0.61	≤10	11–21	≥22
0.62	≤11	12–22	≥23
0.63	≤11	12–22	≥23
0.64	≤11	12–23	≥24
0.65	≤12	13–24	≥25
0.66	≤12	13–24	≥25
0.67	≤12	13–25	≥26
0.68	≤13	14–26	≥27
0.69	≤13	14–27	≥28

counted; cutoff points of 75 and 10 % of glandular/tumor area are used to categorize this variable with >75 % tubule/gland formation = score 1, 10–75 % = score 2, and 10 % = score 3.

Nuclear pleomorphism is assessed by reference to the regularity of nuclear size and shape of normal epithelial cells in adjacent breast tissue. Increasing irregularity of nuclear outlines and the number and size of nucleoli are useful additional features in allocating scores for pleomorphism. Score 1 nuclei are very similar in size (<1.5) to benign preexisting epithelial cells and show minimal pleomorphism and even chromatin pattern, and nucleoli are not visible or very inconspicuous. Score 2 nuclei are larger (1.5–2 × normal area), with mild to moderate pleomorphism and visible but small and inconspicuous nucleoli. Score 3 nuclei are larger in size (>2 × normal area) with vesicular chromatin, vary markedly in size and shape, and show often prominent nucleoli.

Evaluation of mitotic figures requires care and relies on optimal tissue fixation and good section preparation. Observers must count only defined mitotic figures; hyperchromatic and pyknotic nuclei are ignored since they are more likely to represent apoptosis rather than cells in mitosis. Mitotic counts require standardization to a fixed field area. The total number of mitoses per ten high power fields is recorded. Cutoff points for score allocation are dependent on field area. Therefore, for mitotic counting it is essential to calibrate the microscope by measuring the diameter of the high power field (×40 objective, see Table 7.2). Field selection for mitotic scoring should be from the peripheral leading edge of the tumor to find the area with most mitotic activity. If there is heterogeneity, regions exhibiting a higher frequency of mitoses should be chosen. Field selection is by random meander through the chosen area. Only fields with a representative tumor cell burden should be assessed.

The three values are added together to produce scores of 3–9, to which the grade is assigned as follows:

Grade 1 – well differentiated: 3–5 points
Grade 2 – moderately differentiated: 6–7 points
Grade 3 – poorly differentiated: 8–9 points

It is recommended for quality assurance to report the grade giving the individual score components as well as the calculated grade.

Grading of small tissue samples such as needle core biopsy specimens is possible, but it should be recognized that it has limitations, as the small size of the specimens can lead to underestimation of grade components [34].

Reproducibility of Histological Grade

Several studies have reported acceptable levels of inter- and intra-observer concordance of histological grade [4, 6–8, 35–41]. Variation in the proportion of each grade reported in some studies can be explained by the variation in the grading system utilized and the difference in the patient cohorts including age distribution, symptomatic versus screening population, early versus advanced breast cancer groups, and details of tissue fixation. Suboptimal levels of tissue fixation lead to disruption and loss of visibility of mitotic figures which may result in a reduction in the proportion of cases classified as grade 3 [4, 42]. The use of rigorously optimized and standardized methods in Nottingham has provided a high NGS reproducibility in a recently published series [12] and that of an old series published more than two decades ago from the same institution with similar percentage of cases in each grade [42]. Significant improvements in consistency of histological grading have been observed on a national basis in the UK through the publication of guidelines with linked educational activity and associated external quality assurance (EQA) [35]. These guidelines not only provide information on histological grading methodology but also recommendations for application of these methods and guidance on tissue handling.

Misassignments from grade 1 to grade 3 or vice versa are rarely reported. However grade 2 tumors usually show the lowest degree of concordance. This is an expected phenomenon of scoring of a biological variable where scores in the overlap regions are usually most difficult to be categorized. Attempts have been made to improve biological and clinical significance of histological grading by subclassification of grade 2 tumors into two distinct subclasses: a grade 1-like subgroup, which has an excellent outcome and may not require adjuvant chemotherapy, and a grade 3-like subgroup, which comprises tumors that behave in a way similar to high-grade cancers and need more aggressive systemic treatment. Examples of these studies include application of gene expression profiling to subclassify histological grade 2 into two molecular subclasses (G2a and G2b) [43, 44] or using proliferation biomarkers such as Ki-67 expression [45]. However, the clinical usefulness and the cost-benefit ratios of these tests need to be considered.

Some concerns regarding the inaccuracy of assessment of histological grade on needle core biopsy have been raised [46]. Current evidence suggests that histological grading like nodal status can be assessed relatively reliably, whereas other well-established prognostic factors, such as vascular invasion and tumor size, cannot [47–49]. Importantly, selection of patients for neoadjuvant therapy requires prognostic information to be available from nonoperative diagnostic tumor samples.

Molecular Genetics of Histological Grade

Tumors of different histological grades show distinct molecular profiles at the genomic [50–52], transcriptomic [43, 53], and immunohistochemical level [54, 55]. These studies suggest that the majority of high-grade tumors are unlikely to stem from the progression of low-grade cancers and that grades 1 and 3 breast tumors represent different molecular progression pathways with distinct molecular origins, pathogenesis, and behavior [50–52]. Gene expression studies have demonstrated that histological grade better reflects the molecular makeup of breast cancer than lymph node status and tumor size [43, 56, 57]. Importantly, in a number of studies developing molecular signatures, histological grade remained an independent prognostic factor for ER-positive tumors even after the inclusion of gene signatures in the multivariate models [58, 59].

References

1. Greenhough RB. Varying degrees of malignancy in cancer of the breast. J Cancer Res. 1925;9:452–63.
2. Patey DH, Scarff RW. The position of histology in the prognosis of carcinoma of the breast. Lancet. 1928;i:801–4.
3. Bloom HJ, Richardson WW. Histological grading and prognosis in breast cancer; a study of 1,409 cases of which 359 have been followed for 15 years. Br J Cancer. 1957;11:359–77.
4. Elston CW, Ellis IO. Pathological prognostic factors in breast cancer I. The value of histological grade in breast cancer: experience from a large study with long-term follow-up. Histopathology. 1991;19:403–10.
5. Symmers WC. In: Elston CW, Ellis IO, editors. Assessment of histological grade. Edinburgh: Churchill Livingstone; 1998. 381 p.
6. Pereira H, Pinder SE, Sibbering DM, et al. Pathological prognostic factors in breast cancer. IV: should you be a typer or a grader? A comparative study of two histological prognostic features in operable breast carcinoma. Histopathology. 1995;27:219–26.
7. Dalton LW, Page DL, Dupont WD. Histologic grading of breast carcinoma. A reproducibility study. Cancer. 1994;73:2765–70.
8. Frierson Jr HF, Wolber RA, Berean KW, et al. Interobserver reproducibility of the Nottingham modification of the Bloom and Richardson histologic grading scheme for infiltrating ductal carcinoma. Am J Clin Pathol. 1995;103:195–8.
9. Robbins P, Pinder S, de Klerk N, et al. Histological grading of breast carcinomas: a study of interobserver agreement. Hum Pathol. 1995;26:873–9.
10. Sundquist M, Thorstenson S, Brudin L, et al. Applying the Nottingham Prognostic Index to a Swedish breast cancer population. South East Swedish Breast Cancer Study Group. Breast Cancer Res Treat. 1999;53:1–8.
11. Reed W, Hannisdal E, Boehler PJ, et al. The prognostic value of p53 and c-erb B-2 immunostaining is overrated for patients with lymph node negative breast carcinoma: a multivariate analysis of prognostic factors in 613 patients with a follow-up of 14–30 years. Cancer. 2000;88:804–13.
12. Rakha EA, El-Sayed ME, Lee AH, et al. Prognostic significance of Nottingham histologic grade in invasive breast carcinoma. J Clin Oncol. 2008;26:3153–8.
13. Walker RA. Prognostic and predictive factors in breast cancer. 1st ed. New York: Informa Health Care; 2003. p. 10–7.
14. Galea MH, Blamey RW, Elston CE, et al. The Nottingham Prognostic Index in primary breast cancer. Breast Cancer Res Treat. 1992;22:207–19.
15. Elston CW, Ellis IO, Pinder SE. Pathological prognostic factors in breast cancer. Crit Rev Oncol Hematol. 1999;31:209–23.
16. Balslev I, Axelsson CK, Zedeler K, et al. The Nottingham Prognostic Index applied to 9,149 patients from the studies of the Danish Breast Cancer Cooperative Group (DBCG). Breast Cancer Res Treat. 1994;32:281–90.
17. D'Eredita G, Giardina C, Martellotta M, et al. Prognostic factors in breast cancer: the predictive value of the Nottingham Prognostic Index in patients

with a long-term follow-up that were treated in a single institution. Eur J Cancer. 2001;37:591–6.

18. Okugawa H, Yamamoto D, Uemura Y, et al. Prognostic factors in breast cancer: the value of the Nottingham Prognostic Index for patients treated in a single institution. Surg Today. 2005;35:907–11.

19. Clark GM. Do we really need prognostic factors for breast cancer? Breast Cancer Res Treat. 1994;30:117–26.

20. Henson DE, Ries L, Freedman LS, et al. Relationship among outcome, stage of disease, and histologic grade for 22,616 cases of breast cancer. The basis for a prognostic index. Cancer. 1991;68:2142–9.

21. Hanrahan EO, Valero V, Gonzalez-Angulo AM, et al. Prognosis and management of patients with node-negative invasive breast carcinoma that is 1 cm or smaller in size (stage 1; T1a, bN0M0): a review of the literature. J Clin Oncol. 2006;24:2113–22.

22. Desmedt C, Haibe-Kains B, Wirapati P, et al. Biological processes associated with breast cancer clinical outcome depend on the molecular subtypes. Clin Cancer Res. 2008;14:5158–65.

23. Wirapati P, Sotiriou C, Kunkel S, et al. Meta-analysis of gene expression profiles in breast cancer: toward a unified understanding of breast cancer subtyping and prognosis signatures. Breast Cancer Res. 2008;10:R65.

24. Putti TC, El-Rehim DM, Rakha EA, et al. Estrogen receptor-negative breast carcinomas: a review of morphology and immunophenotypical analysis. Mod Pathol. 2005;18:26–35.

25. Domagala W, Harezga B, Szadowska A, et al. Nuclear p53 protein accumulates preferentially in medullary and high-grade ductal but rarely in lobular breast carcinomas. Am J Pathol. 1993;142:669–74.

26. Gamallo C, Moreno-Bueno G, Sarrio D, et al. The prognostic significance of P-cadherin in infiltrating ductal breast carcinoma. Mod Pathol. 2001;14:650–4.

27. Henson DE, Chu KC, Levine PH. Histologic grade, stage, and survival in breast carcinoma: comparison of African American and Caucasian women. Cancer. 2003;98:908–17.

28. Pathology reporting of breast disease. A Joint Document Incorporating the Third Edition of the NHS Breast Screening Programme's Guidelines for Pathology Reporting in Breast Cancer Screening and the Second Edition of The Royal College of Pathologists' Minimum Dataset for Breast Cancer Histopathology. January 2005. NHSBSP Pub. No 58 p.

29. Lakhani SR, Ellis IO, Schnitt SJ, editors. WHO classification of tumours of the breast. 4th ed. Lyon: IARC Press; 2012.

30. Senkus E, Kyriakides S, Ohno S, et al. Primary breast cancer: ESMO Clinical Practice Guidelines for diagnosis, treatment and follow-up. Ann Oncol. 2015;26 Suppl 5:v8–30.

31. Perry NM, Broeders M, de Wolf CJM, editors. European guidelines for quality assurance in breast cancer screening and diagnosis. 4th ed. Luxembourg: Office for Official Publications of the European Communities; 2006.

32. Start RD, Layton CM, Cross SS, Smith JH. Reassessment of the rate of fixative diffusion. J Clin Pathol. 1992;45:1120–1.

33. Rakha EA, El-Sayed ME, Menon S, et al. Histologic grading is an independent prognostic factor in invasive lobular carcinoma of the breast. Breast Cancer Res Treat. 2008;111:121–7.

34. Harris GC, Denley HE, Pinder SE, Lee AH, Ellis IO, Elston CW, Evans A. Correlation of histologic prognostic factors in core biopsies and therapeutic excisions of invasive breast carcinoma. Am J Surg Pathol. 2003;27:11–5.

35. Ellis IO, Coleman D, Wells C, et al. Impact of a national external quality assessment scheme for breast pathology in the UK. J Clin Pathol. 2006;59:138–45.

36. Theissig F, Kunze KD, Haroske G, et al. Histological grading of breast cancer. Interobserver, reproducibility and prognostic significance. Pathol Res Pract. 1990;186:732–6.

37. Jacquemier J, Charpin C. Reproducibility of histoprognostic grades of invasive breast cancer. Ann Pathol. 1998;18:385–90.

38. Chowdhury N, Pai MR, Lobo FD, et al. Interobserver variation in breast cancer grading: a statistical modeling approach. Anal Quant Cytol Histol. 2006;28:213–8.

39. Page DL, Gray R, Allred DC, et al. Prediction of node-negative breast cancer outcome by histologic grading and S-phase analysis by flow cytometry: an Eastern Cooperative Oncology Group Study (2192). Am J Clin Oncol. 2001;24:10–8.

40. Third Edition of the NHS Breast Screening Programme's Guidelines for Pathology Reporting in Breast Cancer Screening and the Second Edition of The Royal College of Pathologists' Minimum Dataset for Breast Cancer Histopathology. SheffieldJanuary 2005. NHSBSP Pub. No 58 p.

41. European Commission. European guidelines for quality assurance in mammography screening. Luxembourg: Office for Official Publications of the European Communities; 1996.

42. Elston CW. The assessment of histological differentiation in breast cancer. Aust N Z J Surg. 1984;54:11–5.

43. Sotiriou C, Wirapati P, Loi S, et al. Gene expression profiling in breast cancer: understanding the molecular basis of histologic grade to improve prognosis. J Natl Cancer Inst. 2006;98:262–72.

44. Ivshina AV, George J, Senko O, et al. Genetic reclassification of histologic grade delineates new clinical subtypes of breast cancer. Cancer Res. 2006;66:10292–301.

45. Aleskandarany MA, Rakha EA, Macmillan RD, et al. MIB1/Ki-67 labelling index can classify grade 2 breast cancer into two clinically distinct subgroups. Breast Cancer Res Treat. 2011;127:591–9.

46. Fitzgibbons PL, Page DL, Weaver D, et al. Prognostic factors in breast cancer. College of American

Pathologists Consensus Statement 1999. Arch Pathol Lab Med. 2000;124:966–78.

47. Damera A, Evans AJ, Cornford EJ, et al. Diagnosis of axillary nodal metastases by ultrasound-guided core biopsy in primary operable breast cancer. Br J Cancer. 2003;89:1310–3.

48. Denley H, Pinder SE, Elston CW, et al. Preoperative assessment of prognostic factors in breast cancer. J Clin Pathol. 2001;54:20–4.

49. Rakha EA, Ellis IO. An overview of assessment of prognostic and predictive factors in breast cancer needle core biopsy specimens. J Clin Pathol. 2007;60:1300–6.

50. Roylance R, Gorman P, Hanby A, et al. Allelic imbalance analysis of chromosome 16q shows that grade I and grade III invasive ductal breast cancers follow different genetic pathways. J Pathol. 2002; 196:32–6.

51. Buerger H, Mommers EC, Littmann R, et al. Ductal invasive G2 and G3 carcinomas of the breast are the end stages of at least two different lines of genetic evolution. J Pathol. 2001;194:165–70.

52. Natrajan R, Lambros MB, Rodriguez-Pinilla SM, et al. Tiling path genomic profiling of grade 3 invasive ductal breast cancers. Clin Cancer Res. 2009;15:2711–22.

53. Rhodes DR, Yu J, Shanker K, et al. Large-scale meta-analysis of cancer microarray data identifies common transcriptional profiles of neoplastic transformation and progression. Proc Natl Acad Sci U S A. 2004;101:9309–14.

54. Abd El-Rehim DM, Ball G, Pinder SE, et al. High-throughput protein expression analysis using tissue microarray technology of a large well-characterised series identifies biologically distinct classes of breast cancer confirming recent cDNA expression analyses. Int J Cancer. 2005;116:340–50.

55. Malamou-Mitsi VD, Syrrou M, Georgiou I, et al. Analysis of chromosomal aberrations in breast cancer by comparative genomic hybridization (CGH). Correlation with histoprognostic variables and c-erbB-2 immunoexpression. J Exp Clin Cancer Res. 1999;18:357–61.

56. Yu K, Lee CH, Tan PH, et al. A molecular signature of the Nottingham prognostic index in breast cancer. Cancer Res. 2004;64:2962–8.

57. Lu X, Lu X, Wang ZC, et al. Predicting features of breast cancer with gene expression patterns. Breast Cancer Res Treat. 2008;108:191–201.

58. Dunkler D, Michiels S, Schemper M. Gene expression profiling: does it add predictive accuracy to clinical characteristics in cancer prognosis? Eur J Cancer. 2007;43:745–51.

59. Weigelt B, Baehner FL, Reis-Filho JS. The contribution of gene expression profiling to breast cancer classification, prognostication and prediction: a retrospective of the last decade. J Pathol. 2010;220:263–80.

Fibroepithelial Lesions

8

Andrew H.S. Lee

Abstract

This chapter deals mainly with fibroadenomas and phyllodes tumor and concentrates on the histological distinction of benign phyllodes tumor from fibroadenoma and distinction of malignant phyllodes from breast sarcomas and spindle cell carcinoma in both surgical specimens and needle core biopsy. The genetics of both lesions and prognostic factors of phyllodes tumor are also discussed.

Keywords

Fibroadenoma • Phyllodes tumor • Needle core biopsy • Genetics • Prognostic factors • CD34

Introduction

As the name implies, fibroepithelial lesions have stromal and epithelial components. Luminal epithelial cells are surrounded by a layer of myoepithelium, and the stromal component is thought to be derived from the specialized intralobular stroma. This chapter will concentrate on the histological distinction of benign phyllodes tumor from fibroadenoma and distinction of malignant phyllodes from spindle cell carcinoma in both surgical specimens and needle core biopsy. The genetic changes and prognostic factors in phyl-

lodes tumor will also be discussed. Azzopardi said of the phyllodes tumor that "This is one of the most difficult tumours of the breast on which to make pronouncements" [1]; both making the diagnosis and giving accurate prognostic information can be difficult.

Fibroadenoma

Fibroadenoma is much the commonest fibroepithelial lesion in the breast. Although seen most frequently in young adult women, fibroadenomas can occur at almost any age. Macroscopically, the lesion is circumscribed and rounded or lobulated with a white or gray, rubbery or firm cut section. The circumscription is also apparent histologically. Two growth patterns are recognized. In the pericanalicular pattern, round or oval glands are surrounded by

A.H.S. Lee
Histopathology Department, City Hospital Campus,
Nottingham University Hospitals,
Hucknall Rd, Nottingham NG5 1PB, UK
e-mail: andrew.lee@nuh.nhs.uk

© Springer International Publishing Switzerland 2017
S. Shousha (ed.), *Breast Pathology*, DOI 10.1007/978-3-319-28655-6_8

stroma. In the intracanalicular pattern, the glands are elongated and may form leaflike areas with clefts. Often, the surrounding stroma will show myxoid change, which can be very marked in Carney's syndrome. Hyalinization of the stroma is common in older women. In most cases, the above features are present and the diagnosis is straightforward (Fig. 8.1a). Typically, the stromal cells show minimal atypia, but plumper forms are not uncommon (Fig. 8.1b). Bizarre multinucleate giant cells occasionally occur in the stroma and, like those seen in otherwise normal breast tissue, have no clinical significance. Occasional stromal mitoses may be present especially in younger women. Epithelial hyperplasia of usual type is common, as is fibrocystic change, including apocrine change and sclerosing adenosis. Pseudoangiomatous stromal hyperplasia can be present in fibroadenomas and phyllodes tumors as well as hamartomas. Smooth muscle can be seen, and if prominent, the term muscular hamartoma may be used. Adipose tissue occurs uncommonly in the stroma, typically near the edge of the lesion. Carcinoma may rarely be present within a fibroadenoma – lobular carcinoma in situ and ductal carcinoma in situ are less rare than invasive carcinoma [2].

Juvenile fibroadenoma is most often seen in adolescents or young adults and may grow rapidly or to a large size. It has a more cellular stroma than a typical fibroadenoma. The proportions of stroma and epithelium are usually similar throughout the lesion – this is a useful feature when trying to distinguish juvenile or cellular fibroadenoma from phyllodes tumor. Occasional stromal mitoses may be present [3]. Typically there is a pericanalicular architecture with usual type hyperplasia of the epithelium often with a micropapillary pattern resembling gynecomastia [4].

Fibroadenomas are multiple in about 10 % of patients. Recurrences are described as common, but some of these may be new tumors rather than true recurrences. One study estimated the true recurrence rate at 17 % [5].

Phyllodes Tumor

Macroscopically phyllodes tumor may resemble a fibroadenoma, but sometimes leaflike clefts will be apparent. The name phyllodes comes from the Greek word φύλλο (phyllos) meaning leaf. Most phyllodes tumors are circumscribed, but malignant phyllodes tumors may have an irregular edge. Phyllodes tumors tend to occur at an older age than fibroadenomas, but this is of little practical help as both lesions can be seen in a wide range of ages.

Malignant and borderline phyllodes tumors are usually straightforward to recognize if there is an epithelial component with a leaflike architecture. Malignant phyllodes tumors often have an invasive border and typically show nuclear pleomorphism, mitoses (Fig. 8.2a–c), and overgrowth of the stromal component (defined as a ×4 objective field of stroma with no epithelium). If

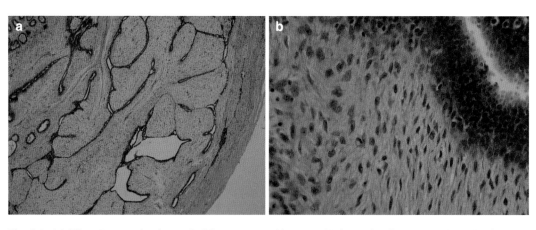

Fig. 8.1 (**a**) Fibroadenoma showing typical low-power architecture. (**b**) Stromal cells are normal on the right and plumper on the left

there is no glandular component in the initial sections, the differential diagnosis includes spindle cell carcinoma and sarcomas.

Differentiating Malignant Phyllodes Tumor from Sarcomas and Spindle Cell Carcinoma

Primary mammary sarcomas and sarcomas metastatic to the breast are rare, and spindle cell carcinoma is the commonest (or least uncommon) malignant spindle cell lesion of the breast. It is important to sample the lesion thoroughly looking for evidence of a benign glandular component, which supports the diagnosis of phyllodes tumor. Features supporting spindle cell carcinoma are associated conventional invasive carcinoma, usually of no special type, or ductal carcinoma in situ, cohesive foci often with a

squamoid appearance or cytokeratin expression by the spindle cells. It is important to use a range of antibodies including antibodies to both basal and luminal cytokeratins as no antibody stains all spindle cell carcinomas. A pitfall is that phyllodes tumors can show cytokeratin expression in the stromal component, but this is typically focal [6]. p63 has been suggested as a marker of spindle cell carcinoma, but it can also be expressed by malignant phyllodes tumors [7]. CD34 is expressed by most phyllodes tumors (Fig. 8.2d) [6, 8]. Although CD34 is less frequently expressed by malignant phyllodes tumors, it is still a useful marker when it is positive as spindle cell carcinoma is negative. An important pitfall is that CD34 is expressed in the normal stroma around ducts and lobules, so if there are entrapped benign glands in a spindle cell carcinoma (typically near the edge of the tumor), the staining needs to be assessed away from the glands. CD34 can also be

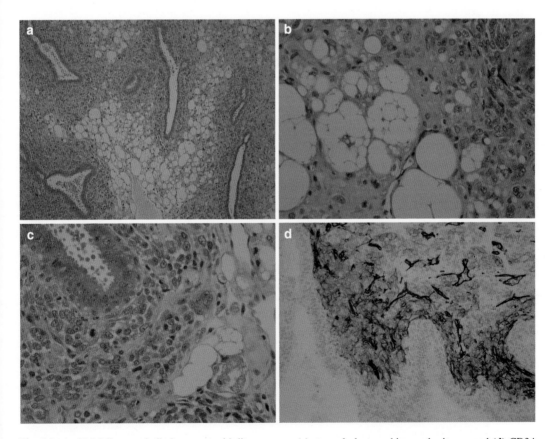

Fig. 8.2 (**a**, **b**) Malignant phyllodes tumor with liposarcoma, (**c**) stromal pleomorphism and mitoses, and (**d**) CD34 expression

expressed in some primary sarcomas such as dermatofibrosarcoma protuberans.

Malignant heterologous elements are present in a minority of malignant phyllodes tumors, and the most common is liposarcoma (Fig. 8.2a, b) [9, 10]. Chondrosarcoma and osteosarcoma can be seen in both phyllodes tumors and spindle cell carcinomas [11, 12]. Very rarely, rhabdomyosarcoma, leiomyosarcoma, or angiosarcoma may be present. Benign adipose tissue and cartilaginous and osseous areas can also be components of phyllodes tumors [10].

Differentiating Benign Phyllodes Tumor from Fibroadenoma

The main differential diagnosis of benign phyllodes tumor is fibroadenoma. A key feature in the diagnosis of benign phyllodes tumor is increased stromal cellularity compared with a typical fibroadenoma (Figs. 8.3, 8.4, and 8.5). Sometimes this increase is patchy, and a phyllodes tumor may contain areas resembling a fibroadenoma. Both lesions usually have a circumscribed margin. A leaflike architecture is almost always present in benign phyllodes, but can also be seen in a fibroadenoma (Fig. 8.5a, b). Most phyllodes tumors arise de novo, but progression from a fibroadenoma is described. Stromal overgrowth is more frequent in phyllodes tumors but can occur in fibroadenomas. The presence of stromal mitoses favors phyllodes tumor, but occasional mitoses can be present in fibroadenoma, particularly in younger women. Stromal atypia is usually not a feature of either diagnosis, although some plumpness of the stromal cells can be seen in both lesions. No single feature can be relied on to separate the two, and the more features that are present, the more likely is the diagnosis of

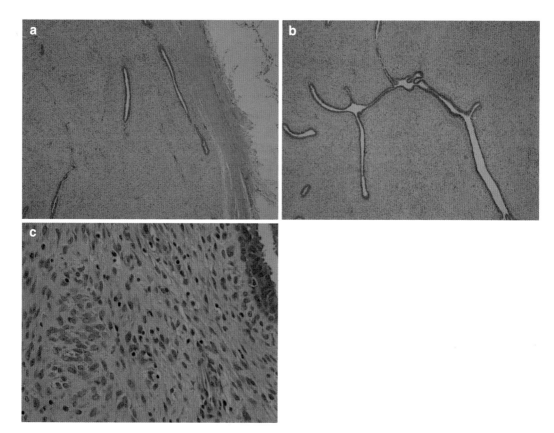

Fig. 8.3 (a) Benign phyllodes tumor with (a) circumscribed edge and stromal expansion, (b) leaflike architecture, and (c) increased stromal cellularity

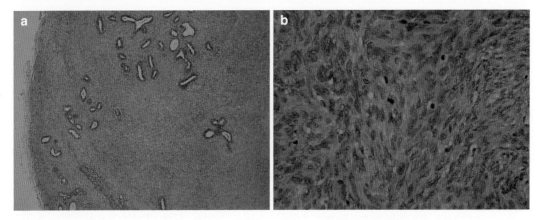

Fig. 8.4 (**a**) Fibroepithelial lesion with stromal expansion, but no leaflike architecture. (**b**) The stroma shows a clear increase in cellularity and mitoses so this lesion is best regarded as a phyllodes tumor

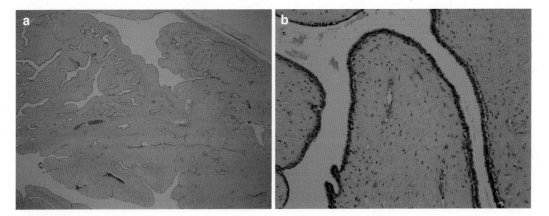

Fig. 8.5 (**a**) This fibroepithelial lesion has a leaflike architecture, (**b**) but stromal cellularity is low favoring a fibroadenoma

phyllodes tumor. Phyllodes tumors can contain epithelial hyperplasia of the usual type as in fibroadenomas, but apocrine change is less frequent. Tumors at the margin between fibroadenoma and phyllodes tumor can be difficult to categorize with poor reproducibility between pathologists [13]. Immunohistochemistry is not of value in separating phyllodes tumors and fibroadenomas in routine practice. For example, although the percentage of Ki67-positive stromal cells is higher on average in phyllodes tumors, there is a large overlap with fibroadenoma. CD34 is typically positive in both. When there is histological ambiguity, the WHO working group recommends a diagnosis of fibroadenoma rather than benign phyllodes tumor in order to avoid overtreatment [14]. Prospective studies are needed to look at the behavior of such lesions at the margin between cellular fibroadenoma and benign phyllodes tumor.

Core Biopsy Diagnosis

Accurate preoperative diagnosis of fibroepithelial lesions is helpful for the management of these lesions. Most fibroadenomas and hamartomas do not need surgery, whereas phyllodes tumors should be excised.

Needle core biopsy of the breast is very good at establishing certain diagnoses such as invasive carcinoma. As discussed above, the diagnosis of fibroepithelial lesions can be challenging in surgical specimens, so it is not surprising that distinction of fibroadenomas and phyllodes tumors in core biopsy cannot always be made. There is clearly a wide variation in diagnostic practices. The proportion of phyllodes tumors with a definite diagnosis of phyllodes tumor in the preceding core biopsy varies between 9 and 65 % in the literature [15–17]. Similarly, there is a wide variation in the proportion of lesions categorized as cellular fibroepithelial lesion on core biopsy that turn out to be a phyllodes tumor in the subsequent excision specimen: 16–76 % in the larger studies [18–21]. No study discusses the frequency of false-positive diagnosis of phyllodes tumor, but it is likely that this occurs occasionally.

There are two groups of studies looking at histological features useful for distinguishing phyllodes tumors and fibroadenomas in core biopsy. One group started with core biopsies with a cellu-

lar fibroepithelial lesion and correlated the features in the core biopsy with the subsequent excision diagnosis [21–24]. The other studies started from the excision diagnosis and looked at features in the preceding core biopsy [17, 20, 25]. The results from these two approaches are similar.

An intracanalicular growth pattern and a leaf-like architecture are seen at a similar frequency in both fibroadenomas and phyllodes tumors in core biopsy, so these are not useful discriminatory features. Increased stromal cellularity, defined as cellularity more than that in a typical fibroadenoma, favors a phyllodes tumor (Fig. 8.6a). Stromal overgrowth, defined as a ×10 or ×20 field containing stroma with no glands, is more frequent in phyllodes tumor (Fig. 8.6b). The presence of stromal mitoses favors phyllodes tumor, particularly if there are three or more mitoses per ten high-power fields. Marked stromal atypia strongly favors phyllodes tumor, but when this is

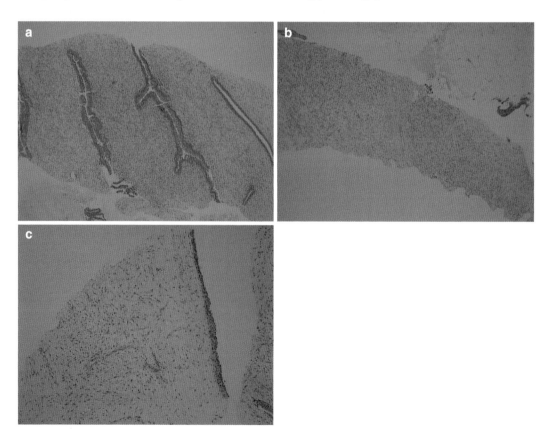

Fig. 8.6 Core biopsy of cellular fibroepithelial lesion showing (**a**) increased stromal cellularity, (**b**) stromal overgrowth, and (**c**) fragmentation

present, the biopsy usually shows other features of phyllodes tumor. Some plumpness of the stromal nuclei is quite common in fibroadenoma. Fragmentation, defined as a fragment of stroma with epithelium at one or both ends, is more frequent in phyllodes tumor (Fig. 8.6c).

There are some features that favor phyllodes tumor in some but not all studies: an irregular margin, an increased stromal cellularity adjacent to the epithelium, the absence of epithelial hyperplasia, and the presence of adipose tissue within the stroma.

No individual feature is completely specific for fibroadenoma or phyllodes tumor. The more features that are present, the more likely is the diagnosis of phyllodes tumor [20]. Morgan et al. created a model using logistic regression which included age and mitoses [25]. I think age is of limited value as although phyllodes tumors occur on average at an older age, fibroadenoma is still more common in all ages. Yasir et al. found a mitotic count of three or more per ten high-power fields; stromal overgrowth, stromal fragmentation, adipose tissue infiltration, stromal heterogeneity, subepithelial condensation, and stromal atypia were useful for distinguishing phyllodes tumor from cellular fibroadenoma [21]. Three or more of these features were present in 85 % of phyllodes tumors and 11 % of cellular fibroadenomas. Further studies looking at the best way to combine histological features would be useful, ideally with separate hypothesis generating and validation series. Sometimes, it is possible to

make a definite diagnosis of phyllodes tumor, but often this is not possible and a phrase like "phyllodes tumor cannot be excluded" needs to be used. In our experience, repeating a core biopsy is not helpful if a definite diagnosis is not possible in the first biopsy [20].

It is important to be aware that it is not possible to detect all phyllodes tumors with a core biopsy: between 7 and 39 % of phyllodes tumors have a false-negative core biopsy [15–17, 20]. The most frequent reason is tumor heterogeneity with the core biopsy appropriately reported as a fibroadenoma. I suspect that some of the false-negative cases in the literature are the result of the core biopsy missing the lesion. Occasionally, diagnostic error is the cause.

Almost all core biopsy diagnoses of fibroadenoma are accurate. We found that of 1,757 core diagnoses of fibroadenoma, only 11 (0.6 %) were later found to be phyllodes tumor during a study period of 7.5 years [20]. Similarly, Van Osdol et al. found that 3 (1 %) of 261 lesions diagnosed as fibroadenoma on core biopsy followed up for a median of 8 years were later found to be benign phyllodes tumors [26]. Abdulcadir et al. identified 41 phyllodes tumors (2 %) among 2,255 fibroadenomas diagnosed on core biopsy after an unspecified duration of follow-up [19].

As with surgical specimens, the diagnosis of malignant phyllodes tumors in core biopsies is usually straightforward if the epithelial component is present (Fig. 8.7a, b). If no epithelial component is present, then the differential diagnosis

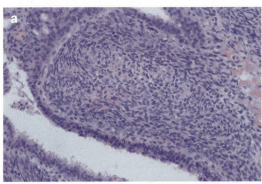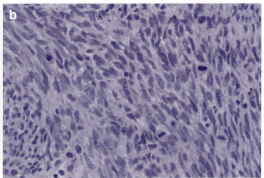

Fig. 8.7 Core biopsy of malignant phyllodes showing (**a**) biphasic lesion with increased stromal cellularity with (**b**) stromal atypia and mitoses

includes spindle cell carcinoma and sarcomas and the approach described above for surgical specimens is appropriate.

When making a diagnosis of a fibroepithelial lesion on a core biopsy, one should have a balance between trying to identify features suggesting a phyllodes tumor and avoiding overinterpreting minor changes and therefore excising too many fibroadenomas. As discussed above, some false-negative diagnoses of phyllodes tumours are unavoidable on core biopsy. The multidisciplinary meeting has a useful role in trying to reduce the frequency of missing phyllodes tumors. It is reasonable to excise lesions diagnosed on core biopsy as fibroadenoma that are larger than 30 mm or are growing or the occasional lesion with septa shown on ultrasound [15, 20].

A study of vacuum-assisted excision of phyllodes tumor found that 15 of 27 (56%) had residual tumor in subsequent surgical excision, and 2 of 23 (9%) phyllodes tumors classified as benign in the vacuum-assisted excision were malignant in the surgical excision [27]. None of 14 patients who were followed up by ultrasound after the vacuum-assisted excision had residual disease – but in view of the fact that 56% had residual disease detected by surgical excision, it is likely that ultrasound is poor at detecting small areas of residual tumor. This study suggests that surgical excision is the appropriate management of a cellular fibroepithelial lesion in which phyllodes tumor cannot be excluded on core biopsy.

Genetics

Older studies found that fibroadenomas have polyclonal stromal and epithelial components, whereas phyllodes tumors typically have a clonal stromal component and polyclonal epithelial component [28, 29]. However, a clonal stromal component has been described in occasional fibroadenomas, for example, in areas of stromal overgrowth or in fibroadenomas that had a phyllodes tumor develop later at the same site [29, 30]. Also allelic imbalance and monoclonality have been described in the epithelium

as well as the stroma of phyllodes tumors [29, 31]. Estrogen receptor and progesterone receptor expression in the epithelium is more frequently seen in benign than malignant phyllodes tumors, suggesting interaction between the stromal and epithelial components [32]. Usually, only the stromal component is present in metastases of phyllodes tumors, but a pulmonary metastasis with epithelium and myoepithelium as well as stroma raises interesting questions about the relationship between the different components [33]. For example, could the two components arise from a common progenitor? However, genetic abnormalities confined to the epithelium have been described in some phyllodes tumors [31].

A study using comparative genomic hybridization found recurrent chromosomal imbalances in 55, 91 and 100% of benign, borderline, and malignant phyllodes tumors [34]. The mean number of chromosomal changes was 1, 6, and 6, respectively. Another study found aneuploidy in 0% of benign, 25% of borderline, and 43% of malignant phyllodes tumors. Intratumoral heterogeneity was detected even between areas that histologically were similar [35].

Recent studies have shown that mutations in MED12 are present in about 70–80% of phyllodes tumors [36, 37]. Some studies show a similar frequency in all grades, but others found a lower frequency in malignant phyllodes tumors. MED12 mutations are also common in fibroadenomas, particularly those with an intracanalicular growth pattern. The MED12 mutations in both lesions are most often missense mutations affecting codon 44. This suggests a biological continuum between these lesions similar to the histological continuum. Mutations in the TERT promotor are present in 50–60% of phyllodes tumors and are much less common in fibroadenomas (0–7%) [38, 39]. The MED12 and TERT mutations are present in the stroma of these lesions and not in the adjacent breast tissue, so they are somatic mutations of the stroma. Mutations in known cancer driver genes such as TP53, RB1, NF1, ERBB4, and EGFR appear to be restricted to malignant and borderline phyllodes tumors [40].

Prognostic Factors of Phyllodes Tumors

Several different grading systems have been proposed for phyllodes tumors, and there is no international consensus on which system to use. Most systems use similar histological features. The World Health Organization classification proposes a three-tiered classification with benign, borderline, and malignant categories [14]. According to this system, benign phyllodes tumors have a well-defined border, usually mild stromal cellularity, mild or no stromal atypia, fewer than five mitoses per ten high-power fields ($0.196 \, mm^2$), and no stromal overgrowth. The majority of phyllodes tumors are benign. Borderline phyllodes tumors have a well-defined border, which may be focally permeative, usually moderate stromal cellularity, mild or moderate stromal atypia, usually five to nine mitoses per ten high-power fields, and absent or very focal stromal overgrowth (Fig. 8.8). Malignant phyllodes tumors have a permeative border, usually marked stromal cellularity, marked stromal atypia, and more than ten mitoses per ten high-power fields, and stromal overgrowth is often present. If there are malignant heterologous elements, the tumor is classified as malignant.

A weakness of this and other classifications is the lack of objective criteria for defining mild, moderate, and marked stromal cellularity and atypia. Tumor heterogeneity is quite common: it is best to grade the tumor in the more atypical areas. Furthermore, not all tumors fall neatly into one of these three categories. One approach is to use some judgment for such cases. Alternatively, more flexible criteria can be used. A system proposed in Nottingham uses the same five histological features as the WHO [41]. Five criteria are defined for benign tumors, and if four are

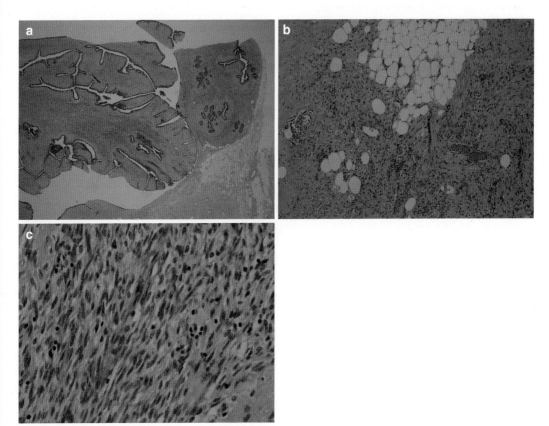

Fig. 8.8 Borderline phyllodes with (**a**) leaflike architecture, (**b**) focally invasive edge, and (**c**) clear increase in stromal cellularity. There were also several mitoses per ten high-power fields (not shown)

present, the tumor is categorized as benign. A similar approach is used for malignant tumors and tumors that do not satisfy the criteria for benign or malignant are called borderline. Furthermore, there are few data on whether different degrees of importance should be attached to each criterion. There is some evidence that stromal overgrowth is a particularly important feature suggesting malignant behavior. With the different definitions and lack of objective criteria, it is not surprising that there is a wide variation of the proportion of benign, borderline, and malignant phyllodes tumors in different series. Numerous biological markers have been shown to correlate with histological grade, but they are not of use in routine practice [42].

Distant metastases occur most often to the lungs and bone, but metastases to many other sites are described. Almost all distant metastases are from malignant phyllodes tumors. In a recent analysis of series published since 2000 including 2,350 tumors, metastases occurred in 0.1 % of benign, 1.6 % of borderline, and 17 % of malignant phyllodes tumors [43]. Metastases to axillary nodes are rare, so routine axillary surgery is not recommended.

The majority of local recurrences are of the same grade, but in a recent large series, 32 % were of higher grade and 5 % were of lower grade [44]. This is consistent with molecular data showing the acquisition of new genetic changes in some recurrences [35]. There is evidence of a relationship between grade and risk of local recurrence, but this is much weaker than the association with distant recurrence. The most powerful predictor of local recurrence is the completeness of excision, but it is a far from perfect marker [41, 43]. There is a clear increase in risk if the tumor reaches the margin [45], but local recurrence is not inevitable in this situation and it can occur in apparently widely excised tumors. Also, it is not clear if a larger margin reduces the risk as very few studies have investigated this: this question is particularly important for borderline and malignant tumors. The standard approach in the past was to aim for a 1 cm clear margin. A review of the literature found that the local recurrence rate is lower after wide local excision than after local excision [46]. Detailed studies of large series of patients looking at the distance to the margin and risk of recurrence in the three grades of tumors are needed.

As discussed above, many phyllodes tumors are not diagnosed preoperatively. As a result, the initial surgical procedure often results in incomplete excision. A wait-and-see policy has been proposed for incompletely excised benign phyllodes tumors [47]. For such tumors, local recurrence is not inevitable and most recurrences are benign, so this is a reasonable option to discuss with the patient. However, if local recurrence does occur, the surgeon should aim to completely excise it. The potential for aggressive behavior is higher for borderline and malignant tumors, so it is prudent to re-excise any involved margins after the initial excision. It is important to be aware that patients rarely die from phyllodes tumor (2–4 % in recent series) [44, 48, 49]: distant recurrences are largely only seen in malignant tumors, which represent a small proportion of phyllodes tumors.

References

1. Azzopardi JG. Sarcomas of the breast. In: Problems in breast pathology. WB Saunders, London 1979 p. 346–78.
2. Kuijper A, Mommers EC, van der Wall E, van Diest PJ. Histopathology of fibroadenoma of the breast. Am J Clin Pathol. 2001;115:736–42.
3. Tay TK, Chang KT, Thike AA, Tan PH. Paediatric fibroepithelial lesions revisited: pathological insights. J Clin Pathol. 2015;68(8):633–41. doi:10.1136/jclinpath-2015-202956.
4. Pike AM, Oberman HA. Juvenile (cellular) adenofibromas. A clinicopathologic study. Am J Surg Pathol. 1985;9:730–6.
5. Organ CH, Organ BC. Fibroadenoma of the female breast: a critical clinical assessment. J Natl Med Assoc. 1983;75:701–4.
6. Chia Y, Thike AA, Cheok PY, Chong LYZ, Tse GMK, Tan PH. Stromal keratin expression in phyllodes tumours of the breast: a comparison with other spindle cell breast lesions. J Clin Pathol. 2012;65:339–47. doi:10.1136/jclinpath-2011-200377.
7. Cimino-Mathews A, Sharma R, Illei PB, Vang R, Argani P. A subset of malignant phyllodes tumors express p63 and p40: a diagnostic pitfall in breast core needle biopsies. Am J Surg Pathol. 2014;38:1689–96. doi:10.1097/PAS.0000000000000301.

8. Lee AHS. Recent developments in the histological diagnosis of spindle cell carcinoma, fibromatosis and phyllodes tumour of the breast. Histopathology. 2008;52:45–57. doi:10.1111/j.1365-2559.2007.02893.x.

9. Powell CM, Rosen PP. Adipose differentiation in cystosarcoma phyllodes. A study of 14 cases. Am J Surg Pathol. 1994;18:720–7.

10. Tan PH, Jayabaskar T, Chuah KL, Lee HY, Tan Y, Hilmy M, et al. Phyllodes tumors of the breast: the role of pathologic parameters. Am J Clin Pathol. 2005;123:529–40.

11. Silver SA, Tavassoli FA. Osteosarcomatous differentiation in phyllodes tumors. Am J Surg Pathol. 1999;23:815–21.

12. Rakha EA, Tan PH, Shaaban A, Tse GM, Esteller FC, van Deurzen CH, et al. Do primary mammary osteosarcoma and chondrosarcoma exist? A review of a large multi-institutional series of malignant matrix-producing breast tumours. Breast. 2013;22:13–8. doi:10.1016/j.breast.2012.09.010.

13. Lawton TJ, Acs G, Argani P, Farshid G, Gilcrease M, Goldstein N, Koerner F, Rowe JJ, Sanders M, Shah SS, Reynolds C. Interobserver variability by pathologists in the distinction between cellular fibroadenomas and phyllodes tumors. Int J Surg Pathol. 2014;22:695–8. doi:10.1177/1066896914548763.

14. Tan PH, Tse G, Lee A, Simpson JF, Hanby AM. Fibroepithelial tumours. In: Lakhani SR, Ellis IO, Schnitt SJ, Tan PH, van de Vijver MJ, editors. WHO classification of tumours of the breast. 4th ed. Lyon: International agency for research on cancer; 2012. p. 141–7.

15. Dillon MF, Quinn CM, McDermott EW, O'Doherty A, O'Higgins N, Hill AD. Needle core biopsy in the diagnosis of phyllodes neoplasm. Surgery. 2006;140:779–84.

16. Foxcroft LM, Evans EB, Porter AJ. Difficulties in the pre-operative diagnosis of phyllodes tumours of the breast: a study of 84 cases. Breast. 2007;16:27–37.

17. Tsang AK, Chan SK, Lam CC, Lui PC, Chau HH, Tan PH, et al. Phyllodes tumours of the breast – differentiating features in core needle biopsy. Histopathology. 2011;59:600–8. doi:10.1111/j.1365-2559.2011.03939.x.

18. El-Sayed ME, Rakha EA, Reed J, Lee AHS, Evans AJ, Ellis IO. Predictive value of needle core biopsy diagnoses of lesions of uncertain malignant potential (B3) in abnormalities detected by mammographic screening. Histopathology. 2008;53:650–7. doi:10.1111/j.1365-2559.2008.03158.x.

19. Abdulcadir D, Nori J, Meattini I, Giannotti E, Boeri C, Vanzi E, et al. Phyllodes tumours of the breast diagnosed as B3 category on image-guided 14-gauge core biopsy: analysis of 51 cases from a single institution and review of the literature. Eur J Surg Oncol. 2014;40:859–64. doi:10.1016/j.ejso.2014.02.222.

20. Lee AHS, Hodi Z, Ellis IO, Elston CW. Histological features useful in the distinction of phyllodes tumour and fibroadenoma on needle core biopsy of the breast. Histopathology. 2007;51:336–44.

21. Yasir S, Gamez R, Jenkins S, Visscher DW, Nassar A. Significant histologic features differentiating cellular fibroadenoma from phyllodes tumor on core needle biopsy specimens. Am J Clin Pathol. 2014;142:362–9. doi:10.1309/AJCPZUZ96RESGPUP.

22. Jacobs TW, Chen YY, Guinee DG, Holden JA, Cha I, Bauermeister DE, et al. Fibroepithelial lesions with cellular stroma on breast core needle biopsy: are there predictors of outcome on surgical excision? Am J Clin Pathol. 2005;124:342–54.

23. Resetkova E, Khazai L, Albarracin CT, Arribas E. Clinical and radiologic data and core needle biopsy findings should dictate management of cellular fibroepithelial tumors of the breast. Breast J. 2010;16:573–80. doi:10.1111/j.1524-4741.2010.01013.x.

24. Jara-Lazaro AR, Akhilesh M, Thike AA, Lui PC, Tse GM, Tan PH. Predictors of phyllodes tumours on core biopsy specimens of fibroepithelial neoplasms. Histopathology. 2010;57:220–32. doi:10.1111/j.1365-2559.2010.03607.x.

25. Morgan JM, Douglas-Jones AG, Gupta SK. Analysis of histological features in needle core biopsy of breast useful in preoperative distinction between fibroadenoma and phyllodes tumour. Histopathology. 2010;56:489–500. doi:10.1111/j.1365-2559.2010.03514.x.

26. Van Osdol AD, Landercasper J, Andersen JJ, Ellis RL, Gensch EM, Johnson JM, et al. Determining whether excision of all fibroepithelial lesions of the breast is needed to exclude phyllodes tumor: upgrade rate of fibroepithelial lesions of the breast to phyllodes tumor. JAMA Surg. 2014;149:1081–5. doi:10.1001/jamasurg.2014.73.

27. Youk JH, Kim H, Kim EK, Son EJ, Kim MJ, Kim JA. Phyllodes tumor diagnosed after ultrasound-guided vacuum-assisted excision: should it be followed by surgical excision? Ultrasound Med Biol. 2015;41:741–7. doi:10.1016/j.ultrasmedbio.2014.11.004.

28. Noguchi S, Motomura K, Inaji H, Imaoka S, Koyama H. Clonal analysis of fibroadenoma and phyllodes tumor of the breast. Cancer Res. 1993;53:4071–4.

29. Kuijper A, Buerger H, Simon R, Schaefer KL, Croonen A, Boecker W, et al. Analysis of the progression of fibroepithelial tumours of the breast by PCR-based clonality assay. J Pathol. 2002;197:575–81.

30. Noguchi S, Yokouchi H, Aihara T, Motomura K, Inaji H, Imaoka S, et al. Progression of fibroadenoma to phyllodes tumor demonstrated by clonal analysis. Cancer. 1995;76:1779–85.

31. Sawyer EJ, Hanby AM, Ellis P, Lakhani SR, Ellis IO, Boyle S, Tomlinson IPM. Molecular analysis of phyllodes tumors reveals distinct changes in the epithelial and stromal components. Am J Pathol. 2000;156:1093–8.

32. Tse GMK, Lee CS, Kung FYL, Scolyer RA, Law BKB, Lau T, Putti TC. Hormonal receptors expression in epithelial cells of mammary phyllodes tumors correlates with pathologic grade of the tumor: a multicenter study of 143 cases. Am J Clin Pathol. 2002;118:522–6.

33. Kracht J, Sapino A, Bussolati G. Malignant phyllodes tumor of breast with lung metastases mimicking the primary. Am J Surg Pathol. 1998;22:1284–90.

34. Laé M, Vincent-Salomon A, Savignoni A, Huon I, Fréneaux P, Sigal-Zafrani B, et al. Phyllodes tumors of the breast segregate in two groups according to genetic criteria. Mod Pathol. 2007;20:435–44.

35. Jones AM, Mitter R, Springall R, Graham T, Winter E, Gillett C, et al. A comprehensive genetic profile of phyllodes tumours of the breast detects important mutations, intra-tumoral genetic heterogeneity and new genetic changes on recurrence. J Pathol. 2008;214:533–44. doi:10.1002/path.2320.

36. Yoshida M, et al. Frequent MED12 mutations in phyllodes tumours of the breast. Br J Cancer. 2015;112:1703–8. doi:10.1038/bjc.2015.116.

37. Piscuoglio S, et al. MED12 somatic mutations in fibroadenomas and phyllodes tumours of the breast. Histopathology. 2015;67:719–29. doi:10.1111/his.12712.

38. Yoshida M, et al. TERT promoter mutations are frequent and show association with MED12 mutations in phyllodes tumors of the breast. Br J Cancer. 2015;113:1244–8. doi:10.1038/bjc.2015.326.

39. Piscuoglio S, Ng CKY, Murray M, Burke KA, Edelweiss M, Geyer FC, et al. Massively parallel sequencing of Phyllodes tumours of the breast reveals actionable mutations, and *TERT* promoter hotspot mutations and *TERT* gene amplification as likely drivers of progression. J Pathol 2016;238:508–18. doi:10.1002/path.4672.

40. Tan J, Ong CK, Lim WK, Ng CC, Thike AA, Ng LM, et al. Genomic landscapes of breast fibroepithelial tumors. Nat Genet. 2015;47:1341–5. doi:10.1038/ng.3409.

41. Moffat CJ, Pinder SE, Dixon AR, Elston CW, Blamey RW, Ellis IO. Phyllodes tumours of the breast: a clinicopathological review of thirty-two cases. Histopathology. 1995;27:205–18.

42. Karim RZ, O'Toole SA, Scolyer RA, Cooper CL, Chan B, Selinger C, et al. Recent insights into the molecular pathogenesis of mammary phyllodes tumours. J Clin Pathol. 2013;66:496–505. doi:10.1136/jclinpath-2012-201082.

43. Tan BY, Acs G, Apple SK, Badve S, Bleiweiss IJ, Brogi E, et al. Phyllodes tumours of the breast: a consensus review. Histopathology. 2016;68:5–21. doi:10.1111/his.12876.

44. Tan PH, Thike AA, Tan WJ, Thu MM, Busmanis I, Li H, et al. Predicting clinical behaviour of breast phyllodes tumours: a nomogram based on histological criteria and surgical margins. J Clin Pathol. 2012;65:69–76. doi:10.1136/jclinpath-2011-200368.

45. Jang JH, Choi MY, Lee SK, Kim S, Kim J, Lee J, et al. Clinicopathologic risk factors for the local recurrence of phyllodes tumors of the breast. Ann Surg Oncol. 2012;19:2612–7. doi:10.1245/s10434-012-2307-5.

46. Barth RJ. Histologic features predict local recurrence after breast conserving therapy of phyllodes tumors. Breast Cancer Res Treat. 1999;57:291–5.

47. Zurrida S, Bartoli C, Galimberti V, Squicciarini P, Delledonne V, Veronesi P, Bono A, de Palo G, Salvadori B. Which therapy for unexpected phyllode tumour of the breast? Eur J Cancer. 1992;28:654–7.

48. Barrio AV, Clark BD, Goldberg JI, Hoque LW, Bernik SF, Flynn LW, et al. Clinicopathologic features and long-term outcomes of 293 phyllodes tumors of the breast. Ann Surg Oncol. 2007;14:2961–70.

49. Belkacémi Y, Bousquet G, Marsiglia H, Ray-Coquard I, Magné N, Malard Y, et al. Phyllodes tumor of the breast. Int J Radiat Oncol Biol Phys. 2008;70:492–500.

Sami Shousha

Abstract

This chapter deals with the spectrum of mucinous lesions of the breast which extend from simple mucinous cysts at one end to invasive mucinous carcinoma at the other end and include mucocele-like lesions and mucinous DCIS. All lesions are characterized by the presence of abundant, usually acidic, mucin, and the majority express WT1. There is also a discussion of reporting mucocele-like lesions in core biopsies and a brief account of signet ring cell carcinoma.

Keywords

Mucocele-like lesions • Mucinous DCIS • Invasive mucinous carcinoma • Signet ring cell carcinoma • WT1

Introduction

In 1993, Weaver et al. suggested that mucinous lesions of the breast form a pathological continuum [1]. This was based on the morphological study of 23 consecutive cases of invasive mucinous carcinomas where intermediate mucinous lesions were commonly found in association with the invasive tumor. These lesions included simple mucous cysts and cysts lined by hyperplastic, atypical, or malignant epithelium, present singly or in combinations. Similar cysts were only rarely found in association with non-mucinous carcinomas of the breast. In another study, Kim et al. found that both mucocele-like lesions and type A invasive mucinous carcinoma express the same type of MUC, namely, MUC1 but not MUC5B [2]. MUC2 has also been shown to be expressed in mucocele-like lesions and mucinous carcinoma [3].

On the other hand, 65 % of pure mucinous carcinomas of the breast are known to express the Wilms' tumor gene (WT1) [4, 5], and we have shown that 85 % of mucocele-like lesions as well as simple mucinous cysts and mucinous ductal carcinoma in situ (DCIS) express WT1 [6]. This in our opinion has completed the circle, providing further evidence supporting Weaver's original idea of the presence of a pathological continuum of mucinous lesions of the breast, which is also

S. Shousha
Department of Histopathology, Charing Cross Hospital & Imperial College,
Fulham Palace Road, London W6 8RF, UK
e-mail: s.shousha@imperial.ac.uk

probably a specific pathway for the development of mucinous carcinoma of the breast.

Simple Mucinous Cysts

These are intact simple cysts distended with mucin and lined by simple flattened (Fig. 9.1a) or cuboidal (Fig. 9.1b) epithelium that may occur singly or in small groups. In H&E-stained sections, they appear to contain basophilic secretion that stains blue with Alcian Blue/PAS stain indicating the presence of acidic mucin (Fig. 9.1c). Luminal calcification may be present (Fig. 9.1b). The lining epithelium usually expresses WT1 (Fig. 9.1d). This is in contrast to other benign breast cysts which might contain eosinophilic secretion (Fig. 9.1e, f) or are lined by apocrine-type epithelium (Fig. 9.1g) which is WT1 negative.

The true incidence of these simple mucinous cysts in the breast is not known. They are occasionally seen, singly or in small groups, in association with fibrocystic change, but are more commonly seen as part of a mucocele-like lesion or in association with in situ or invasive mucinous carcinoma. The occasionally seen WT1-positive small normal-looking acini could be the early precursors of the mucinous continuum (Fig. 9.1h).

Mucocele-Like Lesions

Mucocele-like lesions of the breast were first described by Rosen in 1986 as "benign breast lesions composed of multiple cysts lined by flat, cuboidal or columnar epithelium with only focal hyperplasia" [7]. The cysts may rupture and discharge mucus and epithelium into the surrounding tissue which may then lead to confusion with mucinous carcinoma [7]. Later on, it was realized

that the lining epithelium of these cysts can sometimes show atypia or in situ malignant change [1, 8–13] and several cases were described in association with invasive mucinous carcinoma [1, 3, 9–12].

Currently, mucocele-like lesions are mostly diagnosed by mammographic screening, because of the common presence of microcalcification in the cysts. A core biopsy might show a closely packed group of mucin-containing cysts of variable sizes (Fig. 9.2a), intact and ruptured cysts (Fig. 9.2b, c), or even a single large ruptured cyst (Fig. 9.2d–f). The appearance of all these lesions in an H&E-stained section may be bland, but careful attention to the cyst will recognize the presence of faintly stained mucin in the lumen, and in many cases luminal calcifications will be also present. The latter may be in the form of a relatively large calcific focus (Fig. 9.2g) or very fine calcium "sands" floating in the n mucin. An AB/PAS will confirm the diagnosis by detecting the blue-stained mucin (Fig. 9.2c, e). The epithelium lining of most of these lesions expresses WT1 (Fig. 9.2f, g).

Once the diagnosis of a mucocele-like lesion is made, attention must be then directed to the lining epithelium. This can widely vary from a single layer of flattened (Fig. 9.1a), cuboidal (Fig. 9.1b), or columnar (Fig. 9.3a, b) epithelium to epithelium with variable degrees of hyperplasia or atypia. These may include cysts lined by cells showing columnar cell hyperplasia (Fig. 9.3c, d), papillary hyperplasia (Fig. 9.3e), or flat epithelial atypia (Fig. 9.3f, g). All will contain acidic mucin (Fig. 9.3c) and most will express WT1 (Fig. 9.3b, d, g).

Difficulties sometime arise in deciding whether the lining epithelium is atypical or even malignant or not. In these cases, strict criteria have to be applied. If the lining is of the atypical flat epithelial type but shows areas with abnormal

---

Fig. 9.1 (**a**) Simple mucinous cysts lined by flattened epithelium (H&E). (**b**) Simple mucinous cysts lined by cuboidal epithelium (H&E). (**c**) Simple mucinous cysts lined by flattened epithelium and containing acidic mucin (AB/PAS). (**d**) WT1 expression in a simple mucinous cysts lined by cuboidal epithelium (immunoperoxidase).

(**e**) Cystic pseudolactational change with psammoma bodies in a 48-year-old woman. (**f**) Same lesion in e stained with AB/PAS. (**g**) Apocrine cysts (H&E). (**h**) A few WT1-positive small acini seen adjacent to a normal breast lobule (immunoperoxidase)

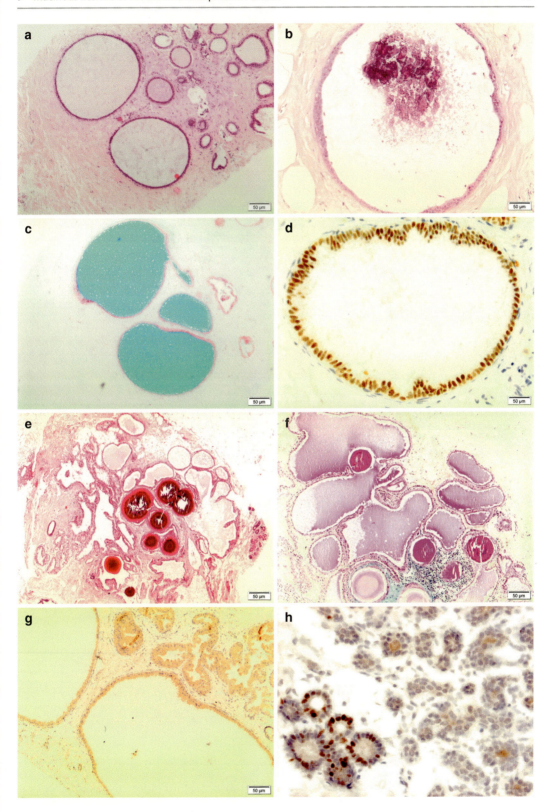

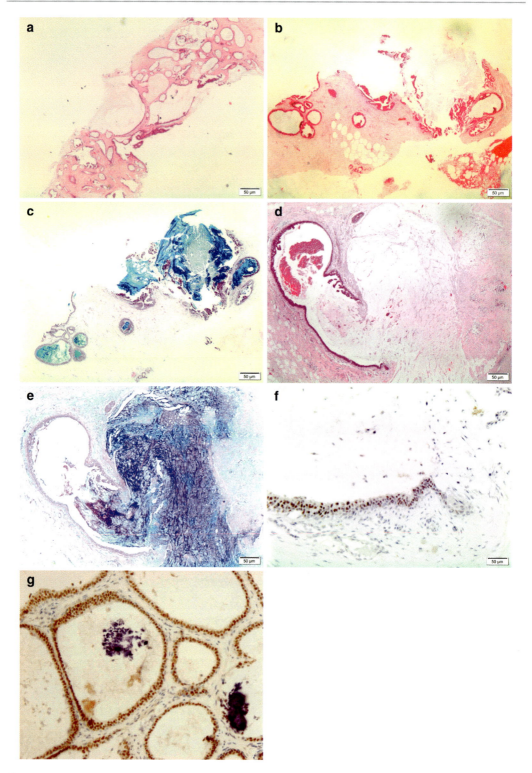

Fig. 9.2 (**a**) Mucocele-like lesion in a core biopsy (H&E). (**b**) Mucocele-like lesion in a core biopsy showing a ruptured cyst (H&E). (**c**) Same as in b stained with AB/PAS. (**d**) Mucocele-like lesion in a core biopsy showing a single ruptured cyst (H&E). (**e**) Same lesion as in d stained with AB/PAS. (**f**) Same core biopsy seen in d stained for WT1 (immunoperoxidase). (**g**) The same core biopsy seen in a stained for WT1 (immunoperoxidase)

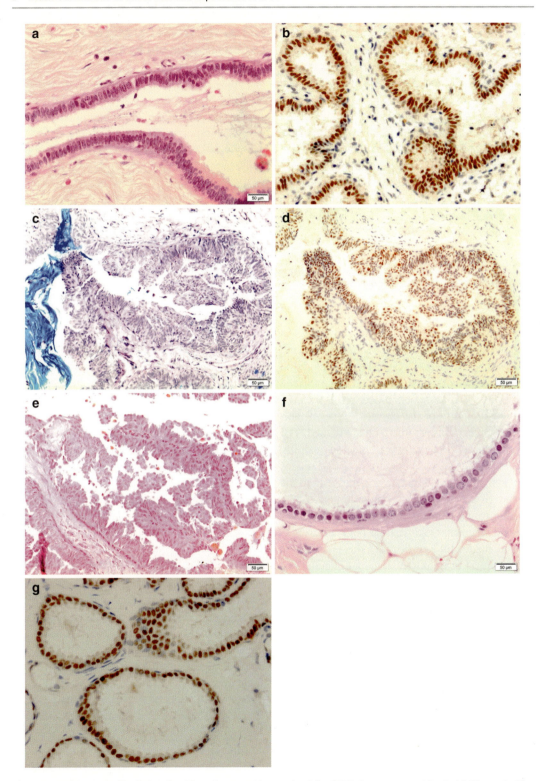

Fig. 9.3 (**a**) Mucocele-like lesion lined by columnar epithelium (H&E). (**b**) Mucocele-like lesion lined by WT1-positive columnar cells (immunoperoxidase). (**c**) Mucocele-like lesion showing florid columnar cell hyperplasia stained with AB/PAS. (**d**) Same biopsy seen in c stained for WT1 (immunoperoxidase). (**e**) Mucocele-like lesion lined by epithelium showing papillary hyperplasia (H&E). (**f**) Mucocele-like lesion lined by epithelium showing flat atypia (H&E). (**g**) Cysts lined by WT1-positive flat epithelial atypia

architectural patterns like papillae or Roman bridges, the case has to be classified as having atypical epithelial proliferation (ADH) as long as the atypia is of a low grade (Fig. 9.4a–c). If the atypia is of a higher grade in part of the lesion, the case would be labeled as mucocele-like lesion with focal in situ malignant change (Fig. 9.4d). If there are atypical changes involving more than two adjacent ducts in a wider lesion, the case would be diagnosed as mucocele-like lesion with foci of DCIS (Fig. 9.4e–g). By definition, acidic mucin will be present (Fig. 9.4f) and WT1 is commonly expressed (Fig. 9.4g).

Ruptured and Unruptured Mucous Cysts

It is obvious from Rosen's original publications that the lesion he described included ruptured and unruptured cysts [7, 12]. The demonstration of WT1 reactivity in both intact and ruptured mucinous cysts, as demonstrated in this chapter, and the similarity of the chemical type of their mucus content indicate that both are related. The differences between the two seem to be quantitative as regards their size and amount of mucus they contain, which ultimately would lead to the rupture of the larger ones. A more important distinction would be the type of their epithelial lining and whether it is of regular or atypical type. Indeed, many of the cystic mucinous lesions seen with atypical or frankly malignant epithelial lining are unruptured (Figs. 9.3g, 9.4a–e).

Scoring Core Biopsies

Cases of mucocele-like lesions diagnosed at core biopsies are usually given a B3 regardless of the presence or absence of atypia which would indicate the need for a further excision. However, in the absence of atypia, maybe this can be carried out by a vacuum-assisted biopsy rather than a surgical excision. A surgical excision will be needed if there is atypia because of a higher possibility of upgrading to malignancy (see below). Cases with focal malignant change are given B5a.

Follow-Up Studies of Mucocele-Like Lesions Diagnosed by Core Biopsy

In a study of 57 patients, varying in age between 38 and 72 years, 35 (61%) had excision biopsies at our institution. These included 18 cases with no atypia in whom no atypia or malignancy was seen on excision, and 16 had atypia in the core of whom 4 (25%) showed low-grade DCIS on excision. The remaining patient had focal in situ malignant change in the core biopsy and more extensive DCIS on excision. These findings are similar to those of several other studies [14–17] and suggest that cases with no atypia in the core are unlikely to show malignancy on excision.

However, there are two published studies indicating and upgrading of mucocele-like lesions with no atypia to DCIS. In one study, 1 (2%) out of 45 cases was upgraded to DCIS and was thought to be the result of radiological-pathological discordance [18]. In another multi-institutional study, in which the diagnosis was reviewed by the local pathologist only, upgrading to DCIS was made in 2 (4%) out of 54 cases [19]. As a compromise, vacuum-assisted, rather than surgical, excision may be adequate for treating cases with no atypia, as long as the lesions have been thoroughly sampled and there is strict radiological-pathological concordance.

Mucinous DCIS

Pure mucinous ductal carcinoma in situ of the breast is rare. In a study of 44 cases of malignant mucinous breast lesions, only 4 (9%) were pure mucinous DCIS [20]. On the other hand, mucinous DCIS is seen in 68–92% of cases of invasive mucinous carcinoma [20, 21] and as discussed above is now also encountered occasionally as part of a mucocele-like lesion. According to "Stanford Medicine," the diagnostic criteria include the presence of extracellular mucin within a duct involved by DCIS and that epithelium must surround all the mucin-containing spaces (Fig. 9.5a). Like other types of DCIS, the lesions are classified as low,

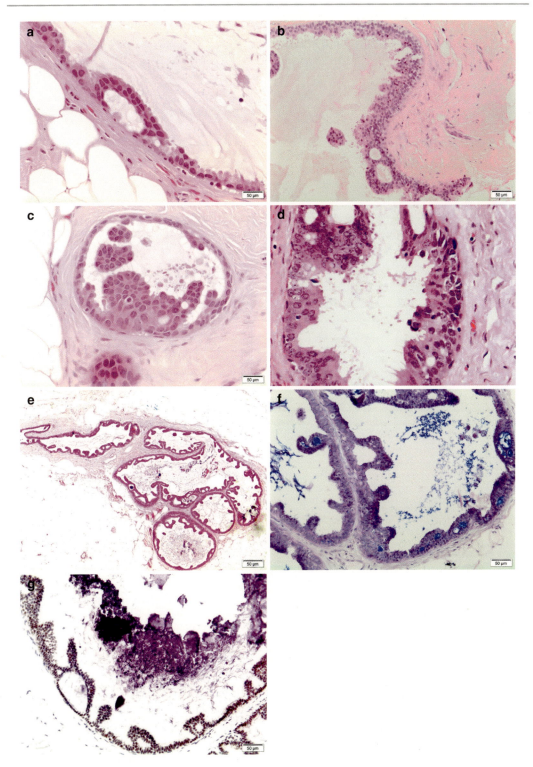

Fig. 9.4 (a) Mucocele-like lesion showing atypical epithelial proliferation in the form of a Roman bridge (H&E). (b) Mucocele-like lesion showing atypical epithelial proliferation in the form of a Roman bridge and short papillae (H&E). (c) Part of a mucocele-like lesion with atypical epithelial proliferation (H&E). (d) Part of a mucocele-like lesion showing in situ malignant change (H&E). (e) Mucocele-like lesion including a focus of low-grade micropapillary mucinous DCIS (H&E). (f) Same case seen in e stained with AB/PAS. (g) Same case as in e stained for WT1 (immunoperoxidase)

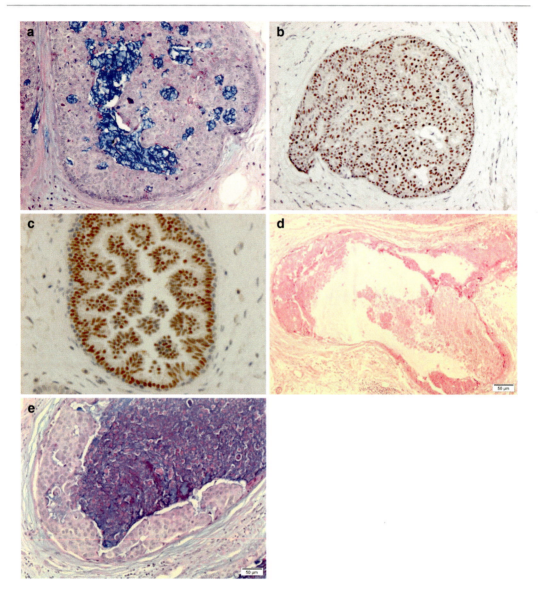

Fig. 9.5 (**a**) Low-grade cribriform mucinous DCIS stained with AB/PAS. (**b**) WT1-positive cribriform mucinous DCIS (immunoperoxidase). (**c**) WT1-positive micro-papillary mucinous DCIS (immunoperoxidase). (**d**) High-grade mucinous DCIS with comedo necrosis (H&E). (**e**) Same case as in d stained with AB/PAS

intermediate, or high grade according to the nuclear morphology (see Chap. 5). The architectural pattern can be cribriform (Fig. 9.5a, b), micropapillary (Figs. 9.4e–g and 9.5c), or flat. Comedo necrosis may be present and mixed with mucin in high-grade lesions (Fig. 9.5d, e). Most mucinous DCIS express WT1 (Fig. 9.5b, c).

Mucinous DCIS has to be differentiated from cystic hypersecretory DCIS [22] where the luminal secretion is eosinophilic "colloid-like" and the lining neoplastic cells are usually high grade (Fig. 9.6). There is no information available about WT1 expression in cystic hypersecretory DCIS.

Invasive Mucinous Carcinoma

These are tumors characterized by the presence of extracellular mucin in which the tumor cells float (Fig. 9.7a–c). They can occur in male as well as female patients [23]. The ratio of tumor cells to mucin is variable, and accordingly

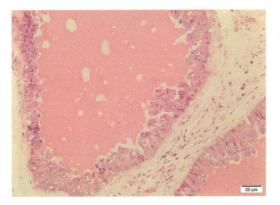

Fig. 9.6 Cystic hypersecretory DCIS

mucinous carcinomas have been subclassified into two types. Type A has more mucin than tumor cells, and type B has more tumor cells than mucin. Neuroendocrine granules are more commonly encountered in type B than type A [24, 25]. Most mucinous carcinomas are grade 1 or 2, ER positive, and HER2 negative. Axillary lymph node metastasis has been reported in 12–18 % of cases [25, 26] and distal metastasis in 2 % [25], but in general, the prognosis of the pure type, where more than 90 % of the tumor is mucinous, is favorable when compared with other more common types of breast carcinoma [26]. Mixed mucinous and other types, usually ductal, have less favorable prognosis [27]. WT1 is expressed in around 65 % of the tumors [4] (Fig. 9.7c).

Mucinous carcinomas of the breast are usually CK7 positive, CK20 negative, and p63 negative. This helps to differentiate them from mucinous carcinomas of the colorectum (CK20 positive,

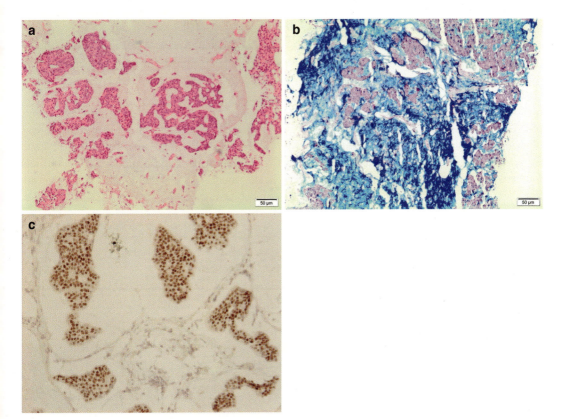

Fig. 9.7 (**a**) Invasive mucinous carcinoma (H&E). (**b**) Invasive mucinous carcinoma stained with AB/PAS. (**c**) WT1-positive invasive mucinous carcinoma (immunoperoxidase)

CK7 negative) and mucinous carcinoma of the skin (p63 positive).

As mucinous carcinomas of the breast are thought to be genomically distinct from other types of breast carcinomas [5, 28, 29], it would be interesting to find out if mucocele-like lesions share any genetic abnormalities with mucinous carcinomas and at which stage of the mucinous continuum these genetic abnormalities start to appear.. This, if proved, would confirm the presence of a unique, morphologically distinct, pathway along which mucinous carcinomas of the breast develop. It may be worth mentioning here that MUC1 and MUC2 expression were found to be similar in mucocele-like lesions and type A mucinous carcinoma of the breast [2].

Differentiating Detached Epithelial Fragments in a Ruptured Mucoceles from Invasive Mucinous Carcinoma

When a mucocele ruptures, usually only mucin escapes into the adjacent stroma (Fig. 9.2a, d). However, sometimes fragments of the lining epithelium may escape with the mucin (Fig. 9.8a) [13]. The presence of these small epithelial fragments floating in the escaped mucin can cause problems with interpretation particularly in core biopsies and when the lining epithelium is atypical or malignant. The possibility of invasive mucinous carcinoma might arise and has to be ruled out. In most cases, the clue is in the presence of a relatively large part of the intact wall of the ruptured mucocele in continuity with the escaped mucin and its floating epithelium (Fig. 9.8a). Also, the amount of epithelium is usually small and may be seen in the form of short strips or small groups rather than larger clumps as is usually seen in mucinous carcinoma. Myoepithelial markers are not useful in these circumstances as the epithelium is usually detached without its underlying myoepithelium (Fig. 9.8b).

Signet Ring Cell Carcinoma

These are mucin-producing carcinomas in which most of the mucin produced is kept inside the cell rather than secreted outside. The accumulated intracellular mucin sometimes pushes the nucleus to one side producing a "signet ring" appearance. Most of these tumors are E-cadherin negative and are considered to be a variant of invasive lobular carcinoma (Fig. 9.9a, b). However, in a study of 19 cases of signet ring cell carcinomas of the breast, 7 (37 %) proved to be E-cadherin positive [30] and thus can be considered of ductal phenotype (Fig. 9.9c–e).

Signet ring cell tumors are mostly ER positive (Fig. 9.9f), and the single case we tested was GATA3 and CA125 positive (Fig. 9.9g, h) and WT1 negative and had a mixture of neutral and acidic mucin (Fig. 9.9d, e). These tumors are almost always CK7 positive, CK20 negative,

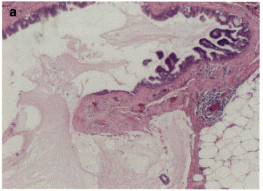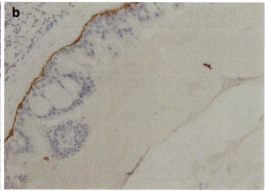

Fig. 9.8 (**a**) Mucocele-like lesion with detached atypical epithelium floating in the mucin (H&E). (**b**) The detached epithelium is devoid of myoepithelial cells as demonstrated by CK5 immunostaining

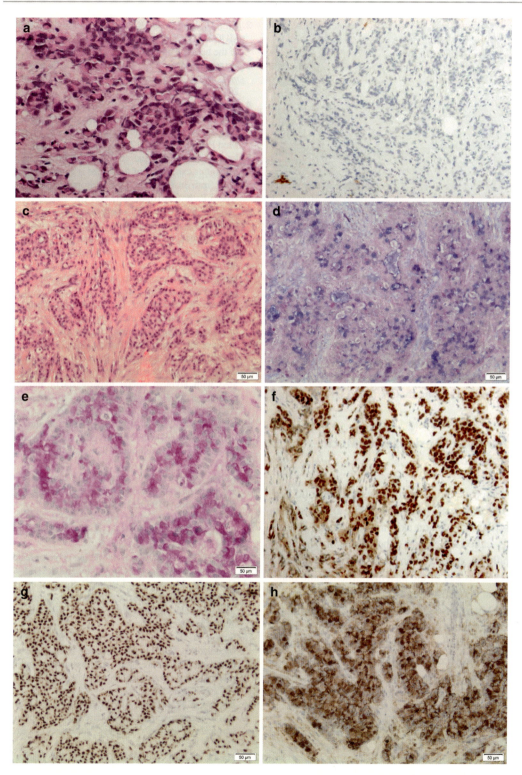

Fig. 9.9 (**a**) Signet ring cell carcinoma (H&E). (**b**) Same tumor seen in a stained for E-cadherin (immunoperoxidase). (**c**) Signet ring cell carcinoma with ductal phenotype (H&E) stained with diastase AB/PAS in (**d**) and diastase PAS in (**e**). (**f**) Same tumor seen in c stained for estrogen receptors, (**g**) GATA3, (**h**) CA125, and (**i**) WT1 (immunoperoxidase)

Spindle Cell Lesions

10

Sami Shousha

Abstract

This chapter deals with benign and malignant spindle cell lesions of the breast other than spindle cell carcinoma and fibroepithelial lesions which are dealt with in Chaps. 12 and 8, respectively. It starts with outlining the scheme that should be followed for diagnosing spindle cell lesions in core biopsies. Important benign and malignant lesions are then discussed individually.

Keywords

Fibromatosis • Myofibroblastoma • Diabetic mastopathy • Stromal sarcoma • Fibrosarcoma • CD10-expressing sarcoma

Introduction

Although spindle cell lesions of the breast are not common, they can cause problems in their diagnosis particularly on core biopsies. This is because there is a wide range of lesions that have a spindle architecture. These vary from simple bland bundles of fibrous tissue that are the result of a previous surgery or even a previous core biopsy, to the more aggressive-looking bundles of a sarcoma or high-grade spindle cell carcinoma. As usual, it is the lesions that lie in the middle of this spectrum that cause most diagnostic problems.

Spindle Cell Lesions in Core Biopsies

All spindle cell lesions in core biopsies are given a B3 (lesions of uncertain malignant potential) to start with, which can go up in some cases to B5 (malignant) on further analysis. The first step in the analysis should be a cytokeratin (CK) stain to exclude (CK negative), or prove (CK positive), the possibility of spindle cell carcinoma. It is usually advised to use at least two cytokeratin stains as there is no single antibody that can stain all spindle cell carcinomas. Studies have shown that MNF116 is the best cytokeratin stain in this

S. Shousha
Department of Histopathology, Charing Cross Hospital & Imperial College,
Fulham Palace Road, London W6 8RF, UK
e-mail: s.shousha@imperial.ac.uk

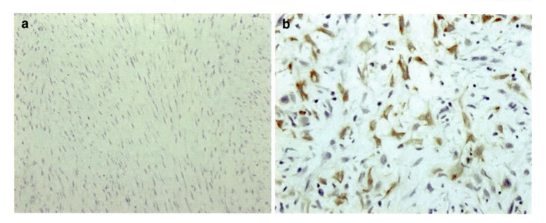

Fig. 10.1 Spindle cell lesions stained for a pan-cytokeratin (AE1/AE3). (**a**) *Negative*; indicating a "soft tissue" lesion. (**b**) *Positive*; indicating a spindle cell carcinoma

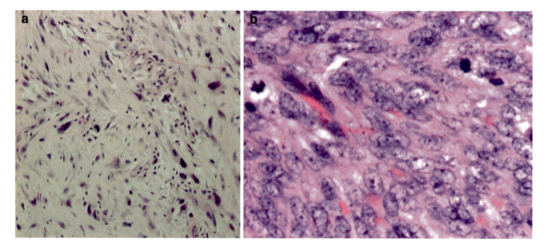

Fig. 10.2 Spindle cell lesion showing evidence of malignancy on H&E-stained sections. (**a**) "Fibrosarcoma." (**b**) Part of a malignant phyllodes tumor

respect as it stains up to 93%, followed by Ck14 (90%), EMA (43%), AE1/AE3 (41%), and Cam 5.2 (40%) [1] (Fig. 10.1a, b). If spindle cell carcinoma is excluded, the second step would be to try to decide whether the lesion is benign or malignant. This is determined by examination of the H&E-stained sections, looking for signs of malignancy. The presence of marked nuclear pleomorphism and prominent mitotic activity indicates malignancy, and a score of B5b (invasive malignant tumor) can be safely given (Fig. 10.2a, b). But even in the absence of such clear signs, a malignant potential cannot be excluded, and a score of B3 is given. Whether the spindle cell lesion is malignant or not, the next step would be to try and give it a "name."

Benign Spindle Cell Lesions

Fibromatosis

This is a nonencapsulated, infiltrative, and well-differentiated fibroblastic growth arising within the mammary gland [2]. The lesion recurs in up to 27% of patients, but does not metastasize [3]. Age incidence is 14–80°years. There may be a history of trauma, including previous surgical operations for benign or malignant breast lesions. Several cases have been reported in association with breast implants, also possibly as a result of surgical trauma [4].

Microscopically, the lesion consists of bland spindle-shaped cells with oval or tapering nuclei, arranged in long sweeping fascicles (Fig. 10.3a). The degree of cellularity is variable. Mitotic figures are infrequent, but may be numerous focally [5]. The lesion is usually stellate shaped with irregular extensions into adjacent tissue that may entrap ducts and acini (Fig. 10.3b). Immunohistochemically, the cells usually stain positive for muscle-specific and smooth muscle actin, and an occasional cell may be positive for desmin and S100 [5]. The lesion typically shows positive nuclear staining for β-catenin [6] and is usually negative for CD34, CKs, and p63. It has to be noted here that β-catenin is not specific for fibromatosis

as originally thought as it can be seen in many other spindle cell lesions (Fig. 10.3c) and focal weak nuclear staining has been detected in some spindle cell carcinomas [6].

A similar condition is now more frequently seen after local surgical excision and radiotherapy for breast carcinoma (intramammary postoperative scar), which can be confused radiologically with a recurrent carcinoma. A core biopsy of such a lesion and a cytokeratin stain would establish the diagnosis. A more limited area of fibroblastic proliferation may also be seen after core biopsies or fine needle aspirations. A more extensive form, which has been called "reactive spindle cell nodules," has been described in patients with papillary or complex sclerosing lesions [7].

The differential diagnosis includes nodular fasciitis, myofibroblastoma, fibrosarcoma, malignant fibrous histiocytoma, and spindle cell (metaplastic) carcinoma.

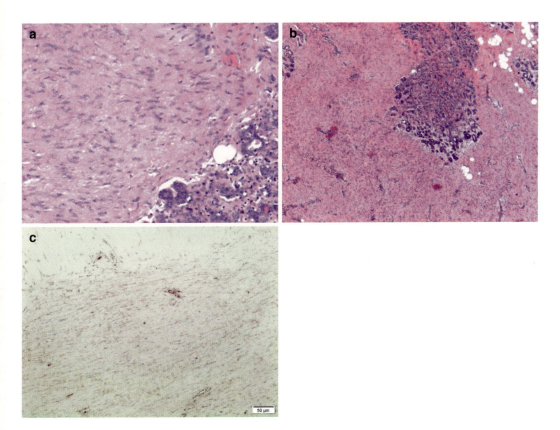

Fig. 10.3 Fibromatosis. (**a**) The cells are bland and are arranged in fascicles (**b**) that insinuate themselves between normal glandular structures (H&E). (**c**) A fibrous needle tract showing positive staining for β-catenin

Myofibroblastoma

This is an uncommon benign and nonrecurring stromal tumor. Originally thought to occur mainly in elderly men, it is now recognized to arise with equal frequency in women of all ages (reported range 25–84 years [5]. Grossly, the tumors are rubbery and can vary in size between 0.9 and 10 cm, the average size being 2 cm. Microscopically, the tumors are usually well circumscribed and consist of spindle cells arranged in short fascicles and clusters, as well as dispersed bundles of collagen fibers. No epithelial elements are present within the lesion. Mitotic figures are infrequent. Multinucleated giant cells, fat cells, cartilage, and myxoid areas may be present.

Several variants have been described including collagenous, epithelioid, cellular, lipomatous, and deciduoid [8–10]. In the collagenous variant, collagen bundles predominate. In the epithelioid variant, 50 % of the tumor consists of polygonal or epithelioid cells arranged in alveolar patterns. The cellular variant consists of dense proliferation of myofibroblasts, which may show a degree of atypia, peripheral infiltrative margin, and focal absence of collagen bundles.

Cases of myofibroblastoma admixed with spindle cell lipoma have been described [11] (Fig. 10.4a, b), and it has been suggested that myofibroblastoma, spindle cell lipoma, and solitary fibrous tumor of the breast may be interrelated [12].

Immunohistochemically, myofibroblastomas are negative for cytokeratins, and the majority are positive for actin, desmin, vimentin, and CD34 as well as androgen and estrogen receptors (Fig. 10.4c).

The differential diagnosis includes fibromatosis, nodular fasciitis, fibrosarcoma, and spindle cell carcinoma.

Nodular Fasciitis

These are well-circumscribed, nonencapsulated, rapidly growing, but self-limiting, mass-forming lesions that may be tender or painful. Adjacent breast ducts and acini may be pushed aside by the lesion, but are not infiltrated [5]. Lymphoid aggregates may be seen at the periphery. The degree of cellularity is variable, and focal collagenization may occur in older lesions. Myxoid change is common, and extravasated red blood cells may be present. CD68-positive osteoclast-like giant cells are occasionally seen. In early lesions, plump cells with prominent mitosis are seen arranged in short fascicles and whorls in a loose myxoid matrix, resembling fibroblasts in tissue culture. Nuclear atypia, abnormal mitosis, and necrosis are absent. The central zone may be markedly hypocellular or even cystic. The spindle cells, presumably myofibroblasts, are positive for muscle-specific and smooth muscle actin. Rarely, focal positivity for desmin may be present [5].

Pseudoangiomatous Stromal Hyperplasia (PASH)

This is a benign proliferation of keloid-like fibrous tissue within which there are slit-like pseudovascular spaces. Its main importance is in its similarity to low-grade angiosarcoma and spindle cell carcinoma [13]. PASH often presents as a component of other breast lesions, particularly fibroadenomas and hamartomas, but may rarely present as a pure circumscribed nodular mass. Microscopically, the lesion consists of a collagenous stroma separated by slit-like, interanastomosing spaces lined by spindle cells resembling endothelial cells (Fig. 10.5a, b). The cells can be positive for CD34 but are negative for other endothelial markers and show variable degrees of positivity for smooth muscle actin and desmin. Because of the difficulty in distinguishing the pure form of these lesions from angiosarcoma in a core biopsy, the UK Royal College of Pathologists guidelines recommend categorizing them as B3, indicating the need for a further diagnostic/excision biopsy for the definitive diagnosis.

Diabetic Mastopathy

These are fibrotic lumps presenting in patients with long-standing diabetes mellitus, particularly the insulin-dependent variety. Clinically, the lesions are hard on palpation, raising a concern about malignancy. Patients may have other diabetic complications or hypertension

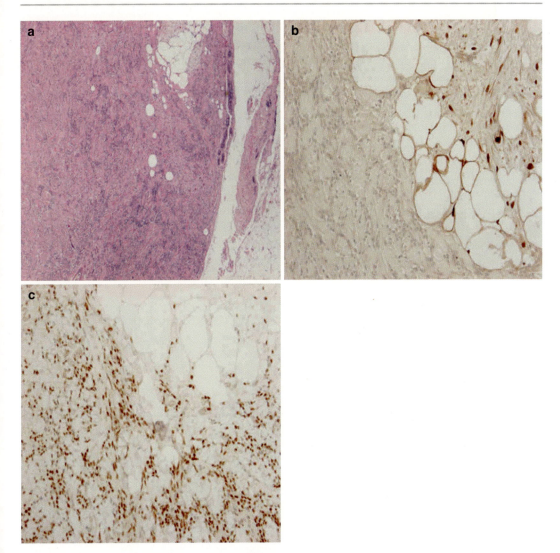

Fig. 10.4 Myofibroblastoma containing fat and spindle cell lipomatous elements. (**a**) H&E, note the well-circumscribed border. (**b**) S100 staining. Note negative myofibroblasts and positive spindle cell lipomatous elements, on the right-hand side. (**c**) Same case showing strong positive staining for androgen receptors

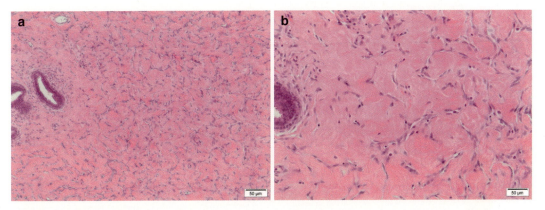

Fig. 10.5 Pseudoangiomatous stromal hyperplasia (PASH) in a fibroadenoma. (**a**) Low power. (**b**) High power showing the lesion's intercommunicating spaces lined by spindle-shaped cells (H&E)

[14, 15]. The lesions can vary in size between 2 and 6 cm and are bilateral in 50 % of patients. Microscopically, there is dense keloid-like fibrosis and heavy lobular and perivascular lymphocytic infiltrate. Lymphocytic aggregates may be present (Fig. 10.6a). Worrying 'epithelioid' fibroblasts, sometimes multi-nucleated are commonly seen scattered in the stroma (Fig. 10.6b). These atypical fibroblasts are usually positive for CD10, suggesting a myofibroblastic origin [16] (Fig. 10.6c). Cysts are typically absent. The disease is self-limiting, but can recur after surgical excision [17]. It has been described in men as well as in women [16, 18], and rare cases have been described in non-diabetic patients [17].

Leiomyoma, Myoid Hamartoma, Schwannoma, and Inflammatory Myofibroblastic Tumor

These are some of the more rare benign spindle cell lesions that can be encountered in the breast. Many are detected via screening. In spite of their benign nature, they are given a score of B3 on a core biopsy with a recommendation for excision because of their uncertain clinical behavior in the breast.

Leiomyoma usually develops in the nipple and subareolar region and presents as a painful, ill-defined mass [19]. Occasionally, they develop deeper in the breast and are detected by mammography as an ill-defined mass "possibly a

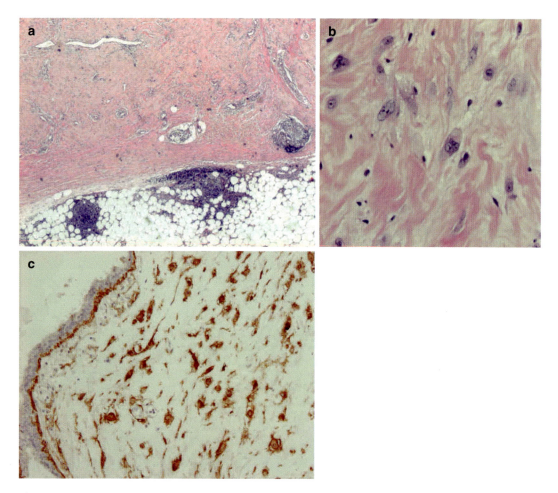

Fig. 10.6 Diabetic mastopathy. (**a**) Low-power view showing a well-circumscribed fibrotic lesion with heavy lymphocytic infiltrate. (**b**) Scattered atypical fibroblasts (**c**) which are CD10 positive

fibroadenoma." Microscopically, the lesion consists of interlacing bundles of smooth muscle fibers with no or minimal intervening fibrous tissue. No glandular elements are present within the lesion, and there is no mitosis, nuclear atypia, or necrosis (Fig. 10.7a, b). Like normal subareolar smooth muscle fibers, they are estrogen and progesterone receptor positive [20], in addition to being positive for smooth muscle actin, desmin, and vimentin and negative for cytokeratin and S100. Complete excision is usually curative although recurrences can occur [19].

Myoid hamartoma is a well-defined lesion that is usually detected radiologically with features suggestive of fibroadenoma. Microscopically, it is a well-circumscribed lesion composed of irregularly arranged bundles of bland spindle-shaped cells that are smooth muscle actin positive and a variable number of scattered small normal-looking ducts (Fig. 10.8). Areas of sclerosing adenosis may be seen at its periphery.

Schwannoma consists of spindle-shaped cells that are positive for S100 and negative for cytokeratins and smooth muscle markers. The cells are usually arranged in the classical biphasic pattern of Antoni A and Antoni B, with the cells in the latter being more loosely arranged. We have recently seen a case that was β-catenin, as well as S100, strongly positive (Fig. 10.9a–d). Another case also seen recently was picked up by mammography as a 7 mm well-defined calcified lesion that microscopically showed marked degenerative changes with coarse calcification (Fig. 10.9e, f). Judging by other anatomical sites, excision of these lesions should be curative.

Inflammatory myofibroblastic tumor is an extremely rare lesion in the breast, usually presenting as a painless circumscribed firm mass. Microscopically, the lesion consists of fascicles of bland spindle-shaped cells heavily infiltrated with chronic inflammatory cells including abun-

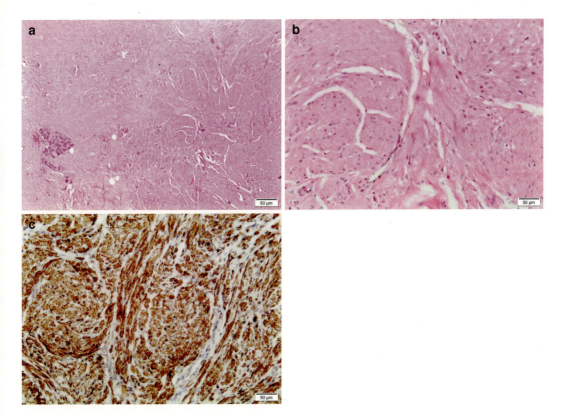

Fig. 10.7 Leiomyoma of the breast detected by mammography. (**a**) H&E low-power view. (**b**) High-power view. (**c**) Strongly positive desmin immunostaining

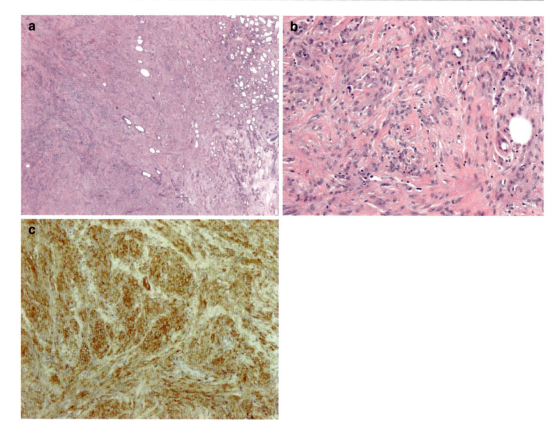

Fig. 10.8 Myoid hamartoma. (**a**) Low-power view of an H&E-stained section showing the lesion composed mainly of bundles of spindle-shaped cells with scattered small glands. (**b**) High-power view of the spindle-shaped cells. (**c**) Strong positive staining for smooth muscle actin

dant plasma cells. Immunohistochemically, the tumor cells are positive for smooth muscle actin and occasionally desmin or keratin. Fifty percent of cases are positive for anaplastic lymphoma kinase (ALK) [21].

Malignant, Non-epithelial, Spindle Cell Lesions

Pure primary sarcomas of the breast, with no associated epithelial elements, comprise less than 1 % of all malignant mammary tumors [22–27]. Male patients can be rarely affected. The tumor can arise de novo or after radiotherapy to the breast. All types of soft tissue sarcomas have been described in the breast with the most common being fibrosarcoma-malignant fibrous histiocytoma [28] and angiosarcoma. Several cases of leiomyosarcoma, rhabdomyosarcoma, liposarcoma, synovial sarcoma, and spindle cell melanoma have also been reported. More recently, mammary sarcoma with CD10 expression has been described [29], and it has been suggested that up to one-third of breast sarcomas may belong to that group.

Fibrosarcoma-Malignant Fibrous Histiocytoma [28]

These can be divided into low- and high-grade lesions according to the degree of nuclear atypia and frequency of mitosis. Low-grade lesions consist of spindle cells arranged in uniform fascicular patterns. There is mild nuclear pleomorphism and low mitotic activity, usually less than 5/10 high-power fields. High-grade

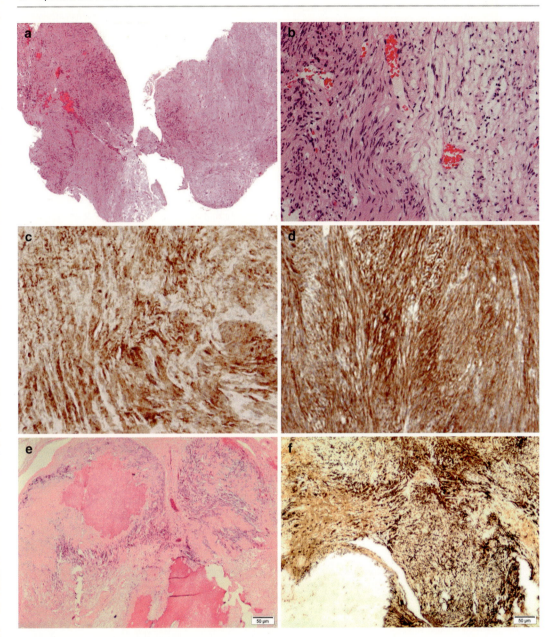

Fig. 10.9 Schwannoma. (**a**) Low-power view of a core biopsy. Note the presence of dark and pale areas reflecting the biphasic Antoni A and Antoni B patterns. (**b**) High-power view showing the two patterns. (**c**) Strong immunostaining for S100. (**d**) Also strong positive staining for β-catenin. (**e**) H&E-stained section of a degenerative focally calcified schwannoma (Courtesy of Dr. Desai, London). (**f**) Same lesion in e showing strong S100 positive staining

lesions consist of larger spindle cells with marked nuclear pleomorphism and high mitotic rate (more than 5/10 high-power field). Multinucleated tumor giant cells and lymphocytic infiltration may be present (Fig. 10.10). The cells are arranged in fascicles or storiform patterns. The cells in both grades can be positive for vimentin and smooth muscle actin, but are negative for cytokeratins, desmin, S100, and endothelial markers. Low-grade lesions are slow growing, show less tendency to recur, and do not usually metastasize, in contrast to high-grade lesions which metastasized in 25 % of patients [28].

Stromal Sarcoma

This term should be reserved to the rare cases of breast sarcomas that can be traced to the specialized periductal and peri-lobular stroma of the breast [22]. This can be confirmed by the presence of prominent stromal proliferation in intact lobules adjacent to the tumor (Fig. 10.11a, b). It is proba-

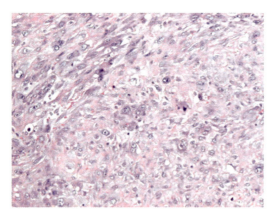

Fig. 10.10 High-grade fibrosarcoma-malignant fibrous histiocytoma of the breast developing after mammary radiotherapy (H&E)

bly equivalent to phyllodes tumor except for the absence of epithelial elements. The tumor grows rapidly, reaching large sizes, and tends to recur.

CD10-Expressing Breast Sarcoma

This is a breast sarcoma showing strong CD10 expression. In a report of seven cases, in addition to CD10 and vimentin positivity, there was EGFR expression in five, SMA in three, and p63 and calponin in two. All seven cases were negative for CK 5/6, 34BE12, CK14, CK17, ER, PgR, CD34, desmin, and h-caldesmon [29]. According to that report, the absence of CD34 expression differentiates these tumors from many other sarcomas including malignant phyllodes and stromal sarcoma. We have recently seen two cases in our hospital. One recurred 6 months after initial excision (Fig. 10.12a–e). The second was associated with an adjacent tubular carcinoma.

Angiosarcoma

These are classified into low, intermediate, and high grade, and it is the latter that can be difficult to diagnose sometimes in a breast core or a skin punch biopsy, as the biopsy may consist entirely of neoplastic spindle-shaped cells with no easily identifiable neoplastic vascular channels

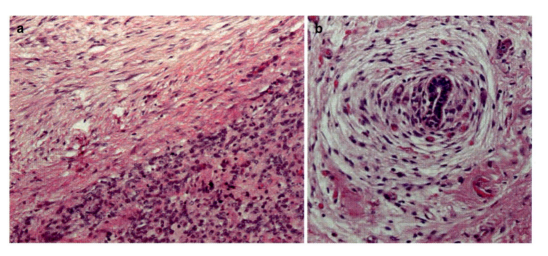

Fig. 10.11 (**a**) Stromal sarcoma. (**b**) Adjacent breast tissue showing prominent periductal stromal proliferation

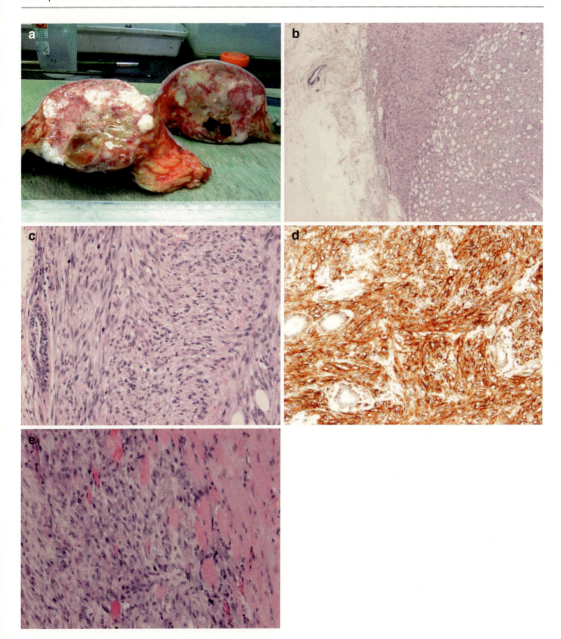

Fig. 10.12 Mammary sarcoma with CD10 expression. (**a**) Gross specimen. (**b**) Low-power view of the tumor infiltrating fat. (**c**) High-power view showing the fascicu- lar arrangement of the spindle-shaped tumor cells. (**d**) Strong CD10 expression. (**e**) Same tumor recurring after 6 month with infiltration of the chest wall

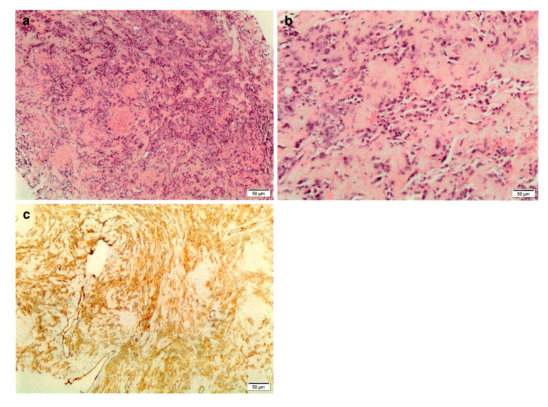

Fig. 10.13 High-grade angiosarcoma in a skin punch biopsy from a patient who had breast carcinoma 8 years earlier treated by wide local excision and radiotherapy. (**a**) Most of the biopsy consisted of solid proliferation of spindle-shaped cells. (**b**) Careful examination identified ill-formed neoplastic vascular channels which pointed to the possibility of angiosarcoma. (**c**) The diagnosis is confirmed by CD31-positive staining

(Fig. 10.13a, b). The presence of a history of previous breast carcinoma treated by radiotherapy and the clinical presentation as red skin patches in the irradiated field usually help in suggesting the diagnosis. This can then be confirmed by immunohistochemistry for endothelial markers like CD31 (Fig. 10.13c).

Sarcomas Developing After Breast Radiotherapy

These can develop within the skin, breast tissue, or chest wall. Angiosarcoma seems to be the most commonly reported, but many other types can occur including fibrosarcoma-malignant fibrous histiocytoma, leiomyosarcoma, rhabdomyosarcoma, liposarcoma, and osteosarcoma [30, 31]. The latency period between radiotherapy and the development of sarcoma varies between 3 and 20 years [30], and the prognosis seems to be worse than sarcomas developing with no prior history of irradiation [31].

Chest Wall Sarcomas Presenting as Breast Lumps

Rare cases of sarcomas developing in the chest wall and presenting as breast lumps have been described. There are two such cases in our files, one was an osteosarcoma and the other a giant cell tumor of soft tissue (Fig. 10.14a) [32]. In both cases, no normal or neoplastic breast tissue was seen in the lesions, and origin from chest wall was confirmed radiologically (Fig. 10.14b).

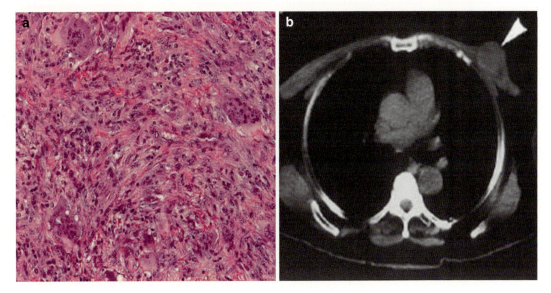

Fig. 10.14 Giant cell tumor of soft tissue presenting as a breast lump. (**a**) H&E-stained section. (**b**) CT scan showing origin of tumor from chest wall

References

1. Carter MR, Hornick JL, Lester S, Fletcher CDM. Spindle cell (sarcomatoid) carcinoma of the breast. A clinicopathologic and immunohistochemical analysis of 29 cases. Am J Surg Pathol. 2006;30:300–9.
2. Wargotz ES, Norris HJ, Austin RM, Enzinger FM. Fibromatosis of the breast. A clinical and pathological study of 28 cases. Am J Surg Pathol. 1987;11:38–45.
3. Rosen PP, Ernsberger D. Mammary fibromatosis. A benign spindle-cell tumor with significant risk for local recurrence. Cancer. 1989;63:1363–9.
4. Balzer BL, Weiss SW. Do biomaterials cause implant-associated mesenchymal tumors of the breast? Analysis of eight new cases and review of the literature. Hum Pathol. 2009;40:15564–1570.
5. McMenamin ME, DeSchryver K, Fletcher CDM. Fibrous lesions of the breast. Int J Surg Pathol. 2000;8:99–108.
6. Lacroix-Triki M, Geyer FC, Lambros MB, et al. beta-catenin/Wnt signalling pathway in fibromatosis, metaplastic carcinomas and phyllodes tumours of the breast. Mod Pathol. 2010;23:1438–48.
7. Gobbi H, Tse G, Page DL, Olson SJ, Jensen RA, Simpson JF. Reactive spindle cell nodules of the breast after core biopsy or fine needle aspiration. Am J Clin Pathol. 2000;113:288–94.
8. Wargotz ES, Weeiss SW, Norris HJ. Myofibroblastoma of the breast. Sixteen cases of a distinctive benign mesenchymal tumor. Am J Surg Pathol. 1987;11: 493–502.
9. Margo G. Epithelioid myofibroblastoma of the breast: expanding the morphologic spectrum. Am J Surg Pathol. 2009;33:1085–92.
10. Wahbah MM, Gilcrease MZ, Wu Y. Lipomatous variant of myofibroblastoma with epithelioid features: a rare and diagnostically challenging breast lesion. Ann Diag Pathol. 2011;15:454–8.
11. Ibrahim HAH, Shousha S. Myofibroblastoma of the female breast with admixed but distinct foci of spindle cell lipoma: a case report. Case Reports in Pathology 2013; Article ID 7380b14
12. Margo G, Bisceglia M, Michal M, Eusebi V. Spindle cell lipoma-like tumor, solitary fibrous tumor and myofibroblastoma of the breast: a clinico-pathological analysis of 13 cases in favor of a unifying histogenetic concept. Virchows Arch. 2002; 440:249–60.
13. Brahim RE, Sciotto CG, Weidner N. Pseudoangiomatous hyperplasia of mammary stroma. Some observations regarding its clinicopathologic spectrum. Cancer. 1989;63:1154–60.
14. Tomaszewski JE, Brooks JSJ, Hicks D, Livolsi VA. Diabetic mastopathy: a distinctive clinicopathologic entity. Hum Pathol. 1992;23:780–6.
15. Seidman JD, Schnaper LA, Phillips LE. Mastopathy in insulin-requiring diabetes mellitus. Hum Pathol. 1994;25:817–24.
16. Shousha S. Diabetic mastopathy: strong CD10+ immunoreactivity of the atypical stromal cells. Histopathology. 2008;52:648–50.

17. Ely KA, Tse G, Simpson JF, Clarfeld R, Page DL. Diabetic mastopathy. A clinicopathologic review. Am J Clin Pathol. 2000;113:541–5.

18. Weinstein SP, Canant EF, Orel SG, Lawton TJ, Acs G. Diabetic mastopathy in men: imaging findings in two patients. Radiology. 2001;219:797–9.

19. Nascimento AG, Rosen PP, Karas M, Caron AG. Leiomyoma of the nipple. Am J Surg Pathol. 1979;3:151–4.

20. Chaudhary KS, Shousha S. Leiomyoma of the nipple, and normal subareolar, muscle fibres, are oestrogen and progesterone receptor positive. Histopathology. 2004;44:626–8.

21. Fletcher CDM. Inflammatory myofibroblastic tumour. In: Lakhani SR, Ellis IO, Schnitt SJ, Tan PH, van de Vijver, editors. WHO classification of tumours of the breast. Lyon: IARC; 2012. p. 133.

22. Callery CD, Rosen PP, Kinne DW. Sarcoma of the breast. A study of 32 patients with reappraisal of classification and therapy. Ann Surgery. 1985;201:527–32.

23. Blanchard DK, Reynolds CA, Grant CS, Donohue JH. Primary nonphylloides breast sarcomas. Am J Surgery. 2003;186:359–61.

24. Zelek L, Liombart-Cusssac A, Terrier P, Pivot X, Guinebretiere JM, Le Pechoux C, et al. Prognostic factors in primary breast sarcomas: a series of patients with long-term follow-up. J Clin Oncol. 2003;21:2583–8.

25. Adem C, Reynolds C, Ingle JN, Nascimento AG. Primary breast sarcoma: clinicopathologic series from the mayo clinic and review of the literature. Brit J Caner. 2004;91:237–41.

26. Al-Benna S, Poggeman K, Steinau H-U, Steinstraesser L. Diagnosis and management of primary breast sarcoma. Breast Cancer Res Treat. 2010;122:619–26.

27. Voutsadakis IA, Zaman K, Leyvraz S. Breast sarcomas: current and future perspectives. Breast. 2011;20:199–204.

28. Jones MW, Norris HJ, Wargotz ES, Weiss SW. Fibrosarcoma-malignant fibrous histiocytoma of the breast. A clinicopathological study of 32 cases. Am J Surg Pathol. 1992;16:667–74.

29. Leibl S, Moinfar F. Mammary NOS-type sarcoma with CD10 expression. A rare entity with features of myoepithelial differentiation. Am J Surg Pathol. 2006;30:450–6.

30. Kirova YM, Vilcoq JR, Asselian B, Sastre-Garau X, Fourquet A. Radiation-induced sarcomas after radiotherapy for breast carcinoma. Cancer. 2005;104:856–63.

31. Gladdy RA, Qin L-X, Moraco N, Edger MA, Antoneecu CR, Alektiar KM, et al. Do radiation-associated soft tissue sarcomas have the same prognosis as sporadic soft tissue sarcomas? J Clin Oncol. 2010;28:2064–9.

32. Shousha S, Sinnett HD. Chest wall tumors presenting as breast lumps. Breast J. 2004;10:150–3.

Papillary Carcinomas

11

Emad Rakha

Abstract

Papillary lesions of the breast comprise a heterogeneous group of diseases with overlapping features and varied clinical behavior. The differential diagnosis includes benign, atypical, and malignant noninvasive and invasive disease. Pathologists should be aware of the different entities and the differential diagnosis of each entity and should follow the updated guideline recommendation for their diagnosis and management. Recognition of papillary carcinomas as a malignant entity (in situ or invasive) by pathologists is high, but concordance of its classification into in situ and invasive disease is sometimes problematic. These rare lesions that usually require additional diagnostic work-up and difficult cases should trigger consensus opinion or expert referral.

Keywords

Breast cancer • Papillary carcinoma • Encapsulated • Solid • In situ • Invasive • Diagnosis • Management

Introduction

Papillary lesions of the breast are a heterogeneous group of diseases characterized by the presence of epithelial proliferation supported by fibrovascular stalks. The majority of papillary lesions arise within the ducto-lobular system of the breast and show a cystic structure with intracystic finger-like projections containing fibrovascular cores covered by epithelium. Typical examples include intraductal papilloma, intraductal papillary DCIS, encapsulated and solid papillary carcinoma, and invasive papillary carcinoma [1–5]. Some papillary lesions show florid epithelial proliferation resulting in a solid appearance. Although this solid pattern of growth is usually focal in intraductal papilloma and encapsulated papillary carcinoma (EPC), it is the predominant growth pattern in solid papillary carcinoma (SPC) [1–6]. Defining these solid lesions as papillary is

E. Rakha
Department of Cellular Pathology,
Division of Cancer and Stem Cells,
The University of Nottingham and Nottingham University Hospitals NHS Trust, Nottingham City Hospital, University of Nottingham, City Hospital Campus, Hucknall Road, Nottingham NG5 1PB, UK
e-mail: Emad.Rakha@nottingham.ac.uk;
Emad.Rakha@nuh.nhs.uk

© Springer International Publishing Switzerland 2017
S. Shousha (ed.), *Breast Pathology*, DOI 10.1007/978-3-319-28655-6_11

based on demonstration of fibrovascular cores within the proliferating epithelial cell population. The presence of these fibrovascular cores is generally accepted as the hallmark of papillary lesions in the breast whether they are cystic or solid, well circumscribed or show irregular margins or are frankly invasive [2–5]. Malignant breast lesions featuring small papillary-like clusters lacking fibrovascular cores are designated as micropapillary carcinomas. Clinical evidence indicates that breast carcinomas featuring predominant papillary morphology are associated with better outcome compared to the non-papillary counterparts including grade-matched cases [5–9]. However, invasive micropapillary carcinomas are associated with aggressive behavior despite being estrogen receptor positive [10].

Papillary morphogenesis is not a feature of normal breast tissue, and its development during the neoplastic process is not completely understood. Apart from papillary apocrine metaplasia, papillary architecture is seen in neoplastic lesions, and it appears to involve a complex process of tissue remodeling and epithelial-mesenchymal interaction resulting from an early alteration of yet undefined genes. The presence of central fibrovascular cores seems to reflect an active process that represents a complex genetic program leading to cell-matrix interaction with growth and budding of stromal tissue accompanied by proliferation of covering cells and acquisition of branching morphogenesis. Further growth and interconnection of these branching structures will eventually result in the arborizing papillary pattern characteristic of papillary lesions [11–13]. Several genes have been proposed to be implicated in the process of papillary morphogenesis during normal and neoplastic tissue development including the hepatocyte growth factor receptor c-Met (also known as Met), RET/PTC, $\alpha3\beta1$ integrin, Sonic hedgehog (Shh), and bone morphogenetic protein (BMP) [11, 13–15]. Phenotypic evidence indicates that papillary morphogenesis is a dynamic process during oncogenesis [16]. We and others have demonstrated that breast in situ tumors with typical papillary carcinoma morphology often lose their papillary configuration during the process of invasion producing conventional non-papillary-type carcinomas such as no special type (NST), mucinous, or micropapillary [4–7]. Papillary morphology is not only observed in the in situ and invasive stage but also in the metastatic sites with different degrees of temporal and spatial papillary differentiation [16]. Although papillary morphology is coined with ductal phenotype, rare in situ and invasive carcinomas may acquire lobular morphology with arborizing growth pattern [16].

Papillary lesions of the breast can present with nipple discharge or as palpable masses when centrally located or located near the skin surface and are relatively large. Peripheral, deeper, and multiple small lesions can be detected by imaging or can be identified incidentally in breast biopsies obtained for other reasons. Ultrasound with color Doppler is the most sensitive methodology for the evaluation of papillary breast lesions. Ultrasound may suggest the presence of a frond-like mass within a dilated duct, a complex intracystic lesion, or a homogeneous solid lesion.

Papillary lesions of the breast can be classified into several types based on the following:

(i) Location in the duct system: Papillary lesions can arise from large ducts including solitary papilloma, EPC and SPC, or small ducts (terminal duct lobular units) including multiple papillomas and papillary DCIS.
(ii) Nature of the proliferating epithelial cells and the presence or absence of myoepithelial cells: This distinguishes benign from malignant papillary lesions.
(iii) Location of myoepithelial cells when present: This not only distinguishes benign from malignant papillary lesions but also can differentiate specific subtypes of malignant papillary lesions (see below).

The most common papillary lesion in the breast is benign intraductal papilloma, also called solitary papilloma. However, other entities, despite being rare, attract more attention due to their unique nature and behavior particularly

EPC and SPC. Invasive papillary carcinoma is very rare and poorly defined making extraction of reliable data on its behavior a challenging task. Multiple papillomas also cause some confusion regarding their risk of malignancy due to the frequent association with epithelial atypia and the diffuse nature of some lesions. Even papillary DCIS, which is a histological variant of DCIS, can cause some diagnostic confusion due to the presence of some overlap with other papillary lesions.

So, the differential diagnosis of papillary lesions includes a spectrum of diseases with typical benign intraductal papilloma at one end and invasive papillary carcinoma at the other. It is in the middle of the spectrum that some of the most challenging diagnostic entities exist. The challenges stem from the following:

(i) Overlapping morphological and immunohistochemical features among benign, atypical, and malignant papillary lesions

(ii) Lack of reliable and reproducible criteria for the diagnosis and classification of atypia within a papilloma, including flat epithelial atypia (FEA)-like epithelial changes and atypical ductal hyperplasia (ADH)

(iii) How to report the presence of low- or high-grade DCIS or lobular neoplasia within an otherwise benign papillary lesion

(iv) Lack of clear criteria to differentiate EPC from SPC and papillary DCIS

(v) Absence of clear criteria to what constitutes invasion or microinvasion particularly as regards SPC and EPC to guide classifying the lesion as in situ or invasive

(vi) Difficulties that may arise in differentiating true/frank invasion from mimics, such as benign glandular entrapment and mechanical dislodgment during a previous biopsy

(vii) How to assess prognostic and predictive parameters in invasive disease associated with noninvasive papillary carcinomas

(viii) Difficulty in linking specific pathological entities to their clinical behavior to guide management decision

Differentiating Benign from Malignant Papillary Lesions

(i) In malignant papillary lesions, the papillae are usually more delicate and less fibrotic than those of benign intraductal papilloma. This generally results in a basophilic (blue) appearance of the papillae in the malignant and an eosinophilic (pink) appearance of the papillae in the benign lesions on low magnification.

(ii) The epithelium in malignant lesions is usually composed of a single cell population with a uniform appearance compared to the heterogeneous variable appearances of the component cells in benign lesions resulting from the presence of a mixture of epithelial, myoepithelial, and basal cells in benign papillomas. In malignant lesions, the epithelium may consist of one to several layers of columnar cells with varying degrees of stratification or may show more pronounced proliferation of uniform cells in solid or cribriform growth patterns (Table 11.1). Florid epithelial proliferation and contiguous growth of the epithelium may partially or completely obliterate the spaces between papillae, obscuring the underlying papillary architecture, but this feature may be seen in both benign and malignant entities.

(iii) The nuclei of the malignant epithelial cells are most often of low or intermediate grade.

(iv) Myoepithelial cells are maintained throughout at the epithelial/stromal interface within the cores and at the periphery of the benign papillary lesion and typically absent in the cores of malignant lesions. They are frequently absent at the periphery of encapsulated and solid papillary carcinomas and always absent in invasive papillary carcinomas (Tables 11.2 and 11.3).

(v) Other important findings that may help are the presence of apocrine metaplasia in benign and mitotic figures in malignant papillary lesions.

(vi) The last but may be the most important clue to differentiate benign from malignant

Table 11.1 Differentiation between benign and malignant papillary lesions

Variables	Papilloma	Papillary carcinoma
Age	30–50 years	60–70 years
Appearance	Eosinophilic (pink)	Basophilic (blue)
Fibrovascular core	Usually broad and frequently sclerotic	Usually fine and less fibrotic
Cell types	Biphasic (epithelial and myoepithelial)	Single (epithelial)
Nuclei	Normochromatic and variable in size and shape	Hyperchromatic and usually uniform with increased nuclear/cytoplasmic ratio
Cell orientation	Haphazard	Orderly, solid or cribriform
	May show hyperplasia of usual type (HUT)	May show mucinous secretion, spindle, columnar or transitional epithelium
Mitosis	Infrequent/absent	More frequent (>1/10hpf) ± abnormal forms
Apocrine metaplasia	Frequent (~36%) benign	Absent (<15%)/atypical
Adjacent ducts	Benign changes	May be DCIS

Table 11.2 Differentiation between encapsulated (EPC) and solid (SPC) papillary carcinomas

Variables	EPC	SPC
Anatomy	Usually solitary and central	Usually central and more often multinodular but may involve peripheral areas
Appearances	Typically cystic but may show solid areas focally	Typically solid
Peripheral capsule	Usually well developed and continuous	Usually not well developed and focal
Papillary cores	Smaller than in papilloma but obvious	Rudimentary, inconspicuous
Cells	Similar to those of DCIS but may be columnar	Frequently show neuroendocrine and mucinous differentiation and may show spindle cell morphology
Nuclear palisading	Absent or only focal	Focal or diffuse and obvious
Associated invasion	Less frequent. When present, it is usually of no special type (NST), but other types may occur	More frequent. When present, it is usually mucinous but may be NST or invasive solid papillary type

Table 11.3 Role of myoepithelial (ME) cells in the diagnosis of papillary lesions

	ME cells in papillae (epithelial/fibrous core interface)	ME cells at periphery (tumor/adjacent stromal interface)
Papilloma	Present	Present
Papilloma with atypia/DCIS	Present but absent/reduced in atypical areas	Present
Papillary DCIS	Absent	Present
Encapsulated PC	Absent	Frequently absent (>85%)
Solid PC	Absent	Usually absent (>70%)
Invasive PC	Absent	Absent

papillary lesions is immunohistochemistry using a panel of markers to assess the presence of myoepithelial cells, tumor cell clonality, and other markers such as those used for detecting neuroendocrine and mucinous differentiation that are typically absent in benign papillary lesions (see below).

Noninvasive Papillary Carcinomas

General Considerations

Papillary carcinomas of the breast account for 0.5–1 % of breast cancers [2, 3, 5–7, 17–23]. They can be either localized and form an expansile mass corresponding to encapsulated and solid variants or diffuse within terminal duct lobular units and correspond to papillary variant of ductal carcinoma in situ (papillary DCIS) [2, 3, 5, 24–26]. Compared to EPC, SPC is typically solid, characterized by mucin production and neuroendocrine features, and is more often multinodular [6, 26–28], while papillary DCIS is typically surrounded by a peripheral layer of myoepithelial cells [5, 7, 25, 29]. The term encapsulated papillary carcinoma (EPC) has recently been introduced to define papillary carcinomas that are typically circumscribed and often encapsulated (separated from surrounding mammary stroma by a fibrous capsule) and lacking myoepithelial cells at their periphery [6, 7]. Although we and others have included SPC in the term EPC [7, 26, 27], the current view is to consider them as separate entities but with acknowledgment that some cases show overlapping features and are difficult to be distinguished from each other [6].

Papillary carcinomas can be present as an isolated lesion or associated with conventional non-papillary in situ or invasive carcinoma. The term papillary carcinoma is used in the literature to describe a heterogeneous group of malignant neoplasms including noninvasive (in situ) and invasive carcinomas, and its classification remains extremely varied [2, 3, 6, 9, 17, 25, 28–31]. Although categorization of papillary DCIS and invasive papillary carcinoma as in situ and invasive disease, respectively, is easy and straightforward, categorization of EPC and SPC into an in situ (noninvasive) or invasive disease created a great deal of debate and controversy due to the mismatch between histological features and behavior [6, 7, 28, 29, 32, 33]. They have long been regarded as a form of in situ carcinoma, but the observation of the absence of myoepithelial cells at the tumor-stromal interface

[34–39] has led to the proposal that these lesions are, in fact, invasive carcinomas with an expansile growth pattern [6, 7, 17, 33–35]. The adoption of this concept was supported by the results of some studies which reported cases with axillary nodal [6, 7, 36, 40] or distant metastases [20, 21, 41] developing in patients after a diagnosis of EPC lacking conventional morphological forms of invasion. In addition, we have seen cases of encysted papillary carcinoma showing failure of multiple attempts of local control with a subsequent local infiltration of the surrounding fat and muscles of the chest wall.

What constitutes invasion in papillary carcinomas is not well defined, and different authorities use different definitions; the majority of these are not based on clinical behavior. As a consequence of these observations and the difficulty in distinguishing in situ from invasive papillary carcinomas, a proportion of these cases will be potentially called invasive and grouped with the more aggressive conventional-type invasive carcinomas, but may not benefit from adjuvant treatment. This concern is supported by the varied proportion of cases termed as invasive papillary carcinoma (from 13 % [21, 42] to 59 % [43] of papillary carcinomas in these series were invasive). However, the current opinion is to consider EPC and SPC as a noninvasive form of breast cancer (Tis) for management purpose despite the fact that they show some biological features of invasive disease [6, 28]. The frequency of clinical events is considered too low and insufficient for diagnosing these tumors as invasive. We have proposed a new terminology for these lesions as malignant tumors with limited metastatic potential to reflect the presence of a degree of uncertainty regarding their clinical behavior [44].

In a previous study of 302 cases of papillary carcinoma (EPC and SPC) [7], 247 cases were identified as pure papillary carcinoma without coexisting conventional-type invasive carcinomas. Of the 247 cases, 208 (84 %) were diagnosed as EPC, 30 (12 %) were diagnosed as SPC, and 9 (4 %) cases were diagnosed as papillary DCIS. The median size of the lesions was 18 mm (range 2.5–100 mm). Seventy-five percent of the patients were treated with local excision and 18 % with mastectomy, while 6 % had no data on further surgery (of whom four patients were treated with hormone therapy alone). Seventy-one percent of cases were associated with DCIS in the surrounding tissue. Lymphovascular invasion (LVI) was reported in five cases. Two cases were recurrences. Of 70 patients who had node sampling, 4 had positive nodes. Stromal/fat invasion was seen in seven cases, including five who showed skeletal muscle invasion while maintaining their cystic papillary morphology with the absence of surrounding myoepithelial cells. Follow-up data were available in 108 cases with a median of 53 months; 7 patients developed local recurrences. Distant metastasis occurred only in patients who developed subsequent invasive carcinoma following papillary carcinoma diagnosis.

Many papillary carcinomas are bounded by zones of fibrosis, chronic inflammation, and recent or resolved hemorrhage. Papillary or tubular structures are routinely found within these areas, parallel to the layer of reactive stroma, and these do not constitute invasion but rather entrapped epithelium. Diagnosis of minimally invasive papillary carcinoma can be difficult. Frank invasion is recognized by the presence of neoplastic cells with infiltrative appearances beyond the zone of reactive stroma into mammary parenchyma and fat. Invasive areas, in general, do not display papillary features (frond-forming), but rather exhibit the morphology of an invasive ductal NST or other types such as mucinous and invasive cribriform carcinoma. Cytological appearances are varied, and nuclear pleomorphism and increased numbers of mitoses may be seen. Mucin secretion is frequently seen in papillary carcinomas particularly the solid variant, and in such cases, it should be distinguished from mucinous carcinoma. In most cases, micropapillary or cribriform ductal carcinoma in situ is present in adjacent ducts.

Intraductal Papillary Carcinoma (Papillary DCIS)

This is a rare type of breast cancer. Although intraductal papillary carcinoma is the term endorsed by the World Health Organization

(WHO) working group and is used to describe this lesion in the relevant chapter of the fourth edition of WHO blue book [29], here we refer to it using the most frequent term that we use in routine practice (papillary DCIS) to avoid confusion with other noninvasive papillary carcinomas, namely, EPC and SPC. Our view is also supported by adopting this terminology (papillary DCIS) in the table included in page "104" of the intraductal papillary carcinoma chapter of the WHO book to describe it when compared to other types of papillary lesions [29]. Papillary DCIS is basically a variant of the classic DCIS because it originates in the terminal duct lobular unit and is distributed in the same manner and, therefore, requires similar management. It is typically multifocal and peripheral in location and usually coexists with other variants of DCIS particularly cribriform DCIS. It is therefore important to distinguish solitary, central papillary carcinomas from papillary DCIS, as the latter may require a wider excision because of its more extensive distribution. Papillary DCIS often present, as other variants of DCIS, with mammographic microcalcification. Rarely papillary DCIS presents as a nipple discharge or a mass lesion which are the most common presentation of EPC and SPC. No specific macroscopic features for papillary DCIS have been recognized.

Papillary DCIS is a subtype of DCIS that show a papillary growth pattern, characterized by fibrovascular cores covered by neoplastic epithelium (Fig. 11.1). Unlike DCIS involving papilloma, papillary DCIS lacks evidence of residual preexisting benign papillary lesion. The absence of myoepithelial cells within the intraluminal papillary fronds with their preservation at the peripheral epithelial-stromal interface throughout the lesion is one of the most important distinguishing features of papillary DCIS. The epithelial cells supported by the fibrovascular stalks can display a variety of proliferative patterns in addition to the typical papillary pattern even with the same ducts including cribriform, solid, micropapillary, or stratified spindle cell patterns. Other rare cell types which can be seen in papillary DCIS include tall hyperchromatic cell with tall cells covering thin fibrous stalks with or without nuclear clearing similar to

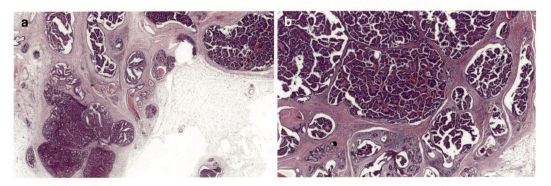

Fig. 11.1 (**a**) Papillary DCIS showing multiple ducts with malignant papillary growth of low-grade neoplastic cells. Myoepithelial cells are maintained at the periphery of the ducts. (**b**) High-power view of the same case

the tall cell variant of papillary thyroid carcinoma. This variant is also observed in EPC. Malignant cells of papillary DCIS can rarely present as compact uniform columns or as transitional cell, which resembles transitional cell carcinoma of the bladder. The neoplastic cells often appear bland and are categorized as low or intermediate grade. High-grade papillary DCIS does occur, albeit with lower frequency. Localized apocrine metaplasia is generally absent, although rarely, complete apocrine differentiation may be present leading to what is called apocrine papillary intraductal carcinoma. These apocrine papillary DCIS often displays abundant epithelial proliferation in solid or cribriform pattern, with well-defined epithelial atypia.

We have noted the presence of myoepithelial cells within the papillae of papillary DCIS, albeit in reduced numbers when compared with benign intraductal papillomas. In our view, these probably represent preexisting benign intraductal papillomas that have become extensively involved by DCIS rather than de novo papillary DCIS.

It should be noted that although most papillary DCIS, EPC, and SPC have a single, uniform cell population, some feature a dimorphic cell population, in which the second population consists of cells with abundant, pale cytoplasm that are most often in a basal location, the so-called globoid cells. These cells should not be mistaken for myoepithelial cells and can be distinguished from them with immunohistochemical markers for epithelial cells such as low-molecular-weight CKs and GCDFP-15 and myoepithelial cells, if necessary. In addition, they show nuclear features and chromatin pattern similar to that of the neoplastic epithelial population. The prognosis and predictive factors for papillary DCIS are the same as those for DCIS in general [29].

Encapsulated Papillary Carcinoma (EPC)

EPC was traditionally termed "encysted" or "intracystic" papillary carcinoma to reflect their cystic circumscribed nature. The incidence of EPC is difficult to determine but comprises <1 % of breast cancers. These lesions usually present as a subareolar mass and/or with nipple discharge, most frequently in elderly women with an average age of 65 years (range 34–92 years [6, 7]. Presentation of EPC may be indistinguishable from that of solitary papilloma apart from the tendency of EPC to affect elderly patients and being larger in size.

On gross examination, these lesions appear as a friable or bosselated mass within a cystic space. Microscopically, they are characterized by one or occasionally multiple nodules of papillary carcinomas with well-defined margins surrounded by a thick fibrous capsule which can be appreciated at low-power examination (Fig. 11.2). Other diagnostic features include dark basophilic (blue) color of the lesions which reflects the increase nucleocytoplasmic ratio of the component neoplastic cells, nuclear hyperchromasia, and lack of apocrine metaplasia or myoepithelial cells. Neoplastic cells, like papillary DCIS, are often monomorphic and bland looking and typically

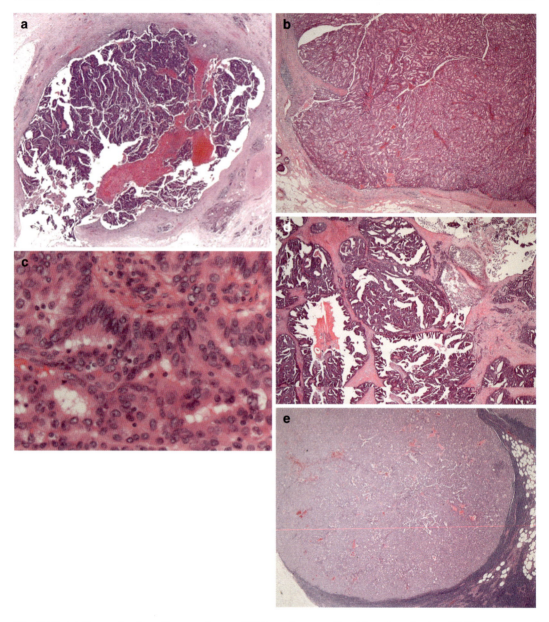

Fig. 11.2 (**a**) Encapsulated papillary carcinoma (EPC) features cystic lesion with thick peripheral fibrous tissue capsule. Focal pushing of the tumor cells in the capsule may be seen, (**b**) but no infiltration beyond the capsule should be seen in pure EPC. (**c**) Shows high-power view of case 11.2B featuring nuclear appearances reminiscent of the nuclei of tall cell papillary thyroid carcinoma with tall columnar cells with nuclear clearing. (**d**) Shows a case of invasive EPC with a mixture of typical EPC clusters lacking peripheral myoepithelial cells and showing some irregularity of the outlines and admixed with frank invasive foci that maintain papillary pattern; the whole tumor in such cases should be considered as an invasive disease. (**e**) Shows a case of invasive EPC like pattern in a lymph node

graded as low or intermediate. High-grade lesions are extremely rare and should be classified as an invasive disease [23]. Focal spindling of the neoplastic cells may be observed in some cases. Tumors are typically cystic with intracystic papillary projections, but cribriform and solid areas may be identified focally, unlike SPC which shows a predominant solid growth pattern.

The surrounding fibrous capsule is thick, often complete, and may show some inflammatory cell infiltration. It is clear that this capsule is not a native layer akin to the basement membrane surrounding DCIS but a reactive process that has also been observed in EPC seen outside the breast, in muscles and lymph node [7]. In addition, it is not uncommon to find entrapped neoplastic epithelial cells within the fibrous capsule, a feature that may be interpreted as microinvasion/frankly invasive carcinoma. However, this phenomenon appears to have no or insignificant clinical impact [7].

Myoepithelial cells are not present in the papillae of EPC. However, in contrast to papillary DCIS, in which there are myoepithelial cells at the periphery of the involved spaces, no myoepithelial cells are present at the periphery of the tumor nodules of EPC in the majority of cases (>80 % [7]). This observation supported the view that these lesions may be in fact a form of low-grade invasive carcinoma with an expansile growth pattern or part of a spectrum of progression from in situ to invasive disease [6, 7, 33]. The finding of metastases in patients with EPC that do not show evidence of frank invasive carcinoma but lack myoepithelial cells provided further support for this concept. EPC showing peripheral myoepithelial cells is biologically and clinically in situ disease and can be considered as a variant of DCIS with no expected invasive behavior.

Regardless of whether these lesions are biologically in situ or invasive in nature, outcome studies have demonstrated that they are associated with an excellent prognosis with adequate local therapy alone [6, 7]. Therefore, it is most prudent to continue to manage patients with EPC and SPC as they are currently managed (i.e., similar to DCIS).

EPC may occur alone, but more often, the surrounding breast tissue contains foci of low- or intermediate-grade DCIS, usually with a cribriform or micropapillary pattern. Typical EPC may also be associated with focal conventional-type non-papillary invasive carcinoma such as ductal NST or mucinous carcinoma. These can range from microinvasive to larger foci. These foci

should be differentiated from entrapped epithelium; the putative invasion should be clearly present beyond the fibrous capsule of the lesion.

Another challenge in the diagnosis of EPC, but is more problematic in SPC, is when they show multiple nodules of variable size and irregular outlines. This creates the problem of trying to differentiate typical SPC and EPC, which are considered noninvasive disease, from invasive forms of SPC and EPC. In an attempt to differentiate in situ from invasive SPC and EPC, some authors defined invasion as nests showing papillary architecture (blunt invasion) and displaying a pattern inconsistent with that of branching ducts or terminal duct lobular units located within nonspecialized stroma [2, 17, 36], while others define stromal invasion by the presence of clusters of papillary carcinoma 10 mm or more beyond the capsule [41]. However, the latter authors did not ascribe any clinical value to this form of stromal invasion [41], and this definition has also been criticized by others [38]. In fact this diagnostic challenge is mainly observed with SPC, while in EPC the main challenge is to identify invasive tumor that is typically non-papillary and seen beyond the capsule. The details of the definition of invasive SPC are described in details below.

EPC are positive for estrogen and progesterone receptors and negative for HER2. Rare case may show triple-negative or HER2-positive phenotype, but these cases are typically high grade and should be considered as invasive tumors [23]. Molecular studies of EPC have reported alterations similar to those observed in other low-grade estrogen receptor-positive breast cancers with frequent LOH at 16q and 1q, low gene copy number aberrations, and frequent PIK3CA mutations [44]. It was also reported that the papillary histologic pattern is unlikely to be underpinned by a highly recurrent expressed fusion gene or a highly recurrent expressed mutation [45].

The consensus of the WHO working group is to manage EPC lacking evidence of conventional invasive carcinoma as in situ disease (stage Tis) [6]. When frankly invasive carcinoma is present in association with an EPC, the size type and grade of the invasive component only should be

of pure invasive SPC as defined above without conventional-type carcinoma is unknown, but it is prudent to report tumors showing such features as invasive disease in routine practice, and sufficient data on their outcome may emerge in the future.

Complete excision of the lesion or total/partial mastectomy is the treatment of choice for SPC. As these cases are staged as Tis disease, sentinel lymph node may not be indicated. However, the high frequency of coexistent invasive conventional-type carcinoma and the possibility of changing the diagnosis to an invasive SPC on excision specimen make recommendation for sentinel node biopsy advisable or subject to further discussion.

The role of postoperative radiation and endocrine therapy in EPC and SPC remains controversial. However, most of these malignant tumors show large size and are likely to be treated using breast-conserving surgery procedures, so there is a likely possibility that the patients will be candidate for local radiotherapy. Also, the majority of these tumors are estrogen receptor strongly positive making those patients candidate for hormone therapy especially when surgery is not possible [7].

Diagnosing Invasion in Encapsulated/ Solid Papillary Carcinoma

Current evidence supports the concept that papillary carcinomas unless associated with frank invasion behave as an intraductal in situ lesion [46]. The majority of encapsulated/solid papillary carcinomas lack myoepithelial cells in their entirety (central and peripheral), which makes it difficult to differentiate between invasive and in situ components of these lesions. Therefore, although loss of myoepithelial cells can be used to distinguish malignant from benign papillary lesions, it should not be used by itself to differentiate in situ from invasive papillary carcinomas. Currently, there is no marker available that can differentiate between in situ and invasive papillary components, and until such a marker(s) is discovered, it is preferable to simply describe papillary carcinomas as either DCIS with a papillary variant or encapsulated or solid papillary carcinomas and to clearly state that invasion is present or absent (or indeterminate). When invasion is present, the type and size of the invasive component should be determined.

Risk of Recurrence

Papillary carcinomas of either DCIS papillary variant or encapsulated/solid papillary carcinomas are subject to the same risk of local recurrence and very low risk of obscure invasion that occur with other types of intraductal carcinomas. For instance, it has been reported that 8-year local recurrence rate of ductal carcinoma in situ varied from 2 % to 31 % [47–49] and distant metastasis rate from 1 % to 4 % [48, 49]. In a previous study which included 917 "encysted" papillary carcinomas, it was reported that the prognosis is excellent even if papillary carcinomas are associated with invasion [8]. However, complete local excision is important, and sentinel lymph node biopsy may be a prudent way to evaluate axillary involvement in such cases.

Invasive Papillary Carcinoma

The term invasive papillary carcinoma is reserved for invasive carcinomas exhibiting an exclusively papillary morphology in >90 % of the invasive tumor and should be distinguished from the other malignant papillary lesions described previously. Invasive non-papillary carcinoma associated with encapsulated or SPC should not be classified as invasive papillary carcinoma but categorized according to the individual invasive component. In such situations, invasive tumor size, histological grade, receptors, and other predictive parameters should be assessed in the invasive component rather than on the associated noninvasive papillary carcinoma component. Defined as such, invasive papillary carcinomas are extremely rare [9, 50–52] though it is possibly more frequent in the elderly [53]. Due to its rarity, no reliable epidemiologic data on invasive papillary carcinoma exist [9].

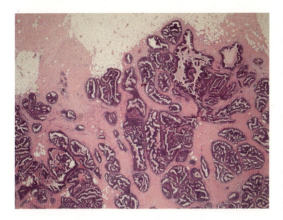

Fig. 11.4 A case of pure invasive papillary carcinoma

True invasive papillary carcinoma has no specific or known clinical characteristics or macroscopic features [9]. The microscopic features are similar to papillary DCIS but with frank invasive growth pattern, comprising mildly dilated ducts, glands, and microcysts containing papillary cores and lacking myoepithelial cells (Fig. 11.4). The size of the invasive structures may vary but typically small with no peripheral fibrous capsule/pseudocapsule unlike EPC or SPC. The stroma may show desmoplastic response. Solid invasive component or other special-type mammary carcinomas such as mucinous or lobular, if present, should comprise <10 % of the tumor.

True invasive papillary carcinoma should be differentiated from invasive micropapillary carcinoma, which is a clinically and pathologically separate entity; it lacks true fibrovascular cores, is characterized by neoplastic cells arranged in solid nests or tubules surrounded by clear spaces, and is considered an aggressive form of mammary carcinoma.

The prognosis of invasive papillary carcinoma appears to be related to tumor grade and stage. The good prognosis of invasive papillary carcinoma reported in literature was mainly derived from cases of encapsulated and SPC associated with invasion [8] and cannot be reliably used to reflect the behavior of true invasive papillary carcinoma as defined above.

The few cases that we have encountered in routine practice were hormone receptor positive and HER2 negative. Although some high-grade estrogen receptor-negative breast carcinomas may show papillary configuration, this is often focal and associated with tumor necrosis resulting in pseudopapillary morphology.

Papillary Carcinoma in Males

Several studies have reported a greater incidence of papillary carcinoma in males among the various histological tumor subtypes in the breast [8, 54, 55]. This is mainly related to encapsulated and SPC with or without associated stromal invasive disease. These studies suggested a twofold increase in the incidence of invasive papillary carcinoma in males and that invasive papillary carcinoma is the most frequent rare histological type encountered in males.

Immunohistochemistry of Papillary Lesions

The distinction of the different categories of papillary lesions including the distinction between benign and malignant entities based on hematoxylin and eosin (H&E) morphology can be challenging, and immunohistochemistry has to be used in many cases. The most important markers used in papillary lesions are those for myoepithelial cells, basement membrane, clonality, and neuroendocrine differentiation.

Markers related to epithelial cell clonality including estrogen receptor and basal CKs such as CK14 and CK5/CK6 can be used to differential clonal/neoplastic process seen in malignant papillary lesions (diffuse strong nuclear ER positivity together with lack of basal CK expression in low-grade neoplastic lesions) from hyperplastic processes seen in benign papillary lesions (heterogeneous mosaic expression of ER and basal CK in hyperplastic lesions). Although this immunophenotype can be also seen in some high-grade breast carcinoma, morphology in such cases is the clue to the correct diagnosis.

Myoepithelial markers including p63, myoid markers such as smooth muscle actin (SMA) and smooth muscle myosin heavy chain

(SMM-HC), CD10, calponin, and basal CKs can be used to differentiate between benign and malignant papillary lesions and between different types of malignant papillary lesions (Tables 11.1 and 11.3).

Neuroendocrine differentiation markers such as synaptophysin and chromogranin A are often used to demonstrate neuroendocrine differentiation in SPC but can also help in differentiating malignant from benign papillary lesions as expression of these markers in benign lesions is almost nonexistent.

Although basement membrane markers are reported in the diagnostic work-up of papillary lesions in some previous studies, we find them less useful due to the subjective interpretation of their expression.

Epithelial Displacement in Papillary Lesions

Epithelium displaced by a needle core or aspiration biopsy is more frequent in papillary lesions including benign and malignant entities because of their inherent friability. The epithelium can be dislodged and displaced into the surrounding stroma, often in the needle tract, and even into adjacent lymphatic channels mimicking lymphovascular invasion or be transported to axillary lymph nodes [56, 57]. It is important to be aware of the possibility of displacement after biopsy procedures to distinguish displaced epithelium from true stromal or lymphovascular invasion. The presence of prior biopsy site changes, degenerative changes in the "invasive" cell clusters, and the absence of reactive, altered stroma surrounding the fragments of epithelium are clues indicating epithelial displacement.

The nature of the displaced epithelium is best determined based on the nature of the underlying papillary lesion. In benign papillary lesions, lacking of peripheral myoepithelial cells around the displaced epithelial clusters should not be used as a criterion to define malignancy but rather mechanical effect during the process of displacement. Moreover, the presence of displaced epithelial clusters at the surgical margin in malignant papillary lesions should be disregarded during assessment of completeness of excision or tumor size measurement despite the fact that they are likely to be malignant.

References

1. O'Malley F, Visscher D, MacGrogan G, et al. Intraductal papilloma. In: Lakhani SR, Schnitt SJ, Tan PH, van de Vijver MJ, editors. WHO classification of tumors of the breast. 4th ed. Lyon: IARC press; 2012. p. 100–2.
2. Pal SK, Lau SK, Kruper L, et al. Papillary carcinoma of the breast: an overview. Breast Cancer Res Treat. 2010;122:637–45.
3. Ueng SH, Mezzetti T, Tavassoli FA. Papillary neoplasms of the breast: a review. Arch Pathol Lab Med. 2009;133:893–907.
4. Tan PH, Schnitt SJ, van de Vijver MJ, et al. Papillary and neuroendocrine breast lesions: the WHO stance. Histopathology. 2015;66:761–70.
5. Collins LC, Schnitt SJ. Papillary lesions of the breast: selected diagnostic and management issues. Histopathology. 2008;52:20–9.
6. Collins L, O'Malley FP, Visscher D, et al. Encapsulated papillary carcinoma. In: Lakhani SR, Schnitt SJ, Tan PH, van de Vijver MJ, editors. WHO classification of tumors of the breast. 4th ed. Lyon: IARC press; 2012. p. 106–7.
7. Rakha EA, Gandhi N, Climent F, et al. Encapsulated papillary carcinoma of the breast: an invasive tumor with excellent prognosis. Am J Surg Pathol. 2011;35:1093–103.
8. Grabowski J, Salzstein SL, Sadler GR, et al. Intracystic papillary carcinoma: a review of 917 cases. Cancer. 2008;113:916–20.
9. Tse G, Moriya T, Niu Y. Invasive papillary carcinoma. In: Lakhani SR, Schnitt SJ, Tan PH, van de Vijver MJ, editors. WHO classification of tumors of the breast. 4th ed. Lyon: IARC press; 2012. p. 64.
10. Pettinato G, Manivel CJ, Panico L, et al. Invasive micropapillary carcinoma of the breast: clinicopathologic study of 62 cases of a poorly recognized variant with highly aggressive behavior. Am J Clin Pathol. 2004;121:857–66.
11. Nusrat A, Parkos CA, Bacarra AE, et al. Hepatocyte growth factor/scatter factor effects on epithelia. Regulation of intercellular junctions in transformed and nontransformed cell lines, basolateral polarization of c-met receptor in transformed and natural intestinal epithelia, and induction of rapid wound repair in a transformed model epithelium. J Clin Invest. 1994;93:2056–65.
12. Rosen EM, Nigam SK, Goldberg ID. Scatter factor and the c-met receptor: a paradigm for mesenchymal/epithelial interaction. J Cell Biol. 1994;127:1783–7.

13. Hall JM, Bell ML, Finger TE. Disruption of sonic hedgehog signaling alters growth and patterning of lingual taste papillae. Dev Biol. 2003;255:263–77.

14. Twenty-second annual meeting of the association for chemoreception sciences. Chemical senses. 2000;25:593–688.

15. Ruco LP, Stoppacciaro A, Ballarini F, et al. Met protein and hepatocyte growth factor (HGF) in papillary carcinoma of the thyroid: evidence for a pathogenetic role in tumourigenesis. J Pathol. 2001;194:4–8.

16. Rakha EA. Morphogenesis of the papillary lesions of the breast: phenotypic observation. J Clin Pathol. 2016;69:64–9.

17. Koerner F. Papilloma and papillary carcinoma. Semin Diagn Pathol. 2010;27:13–30.

18. Li CI, Uribe DJ, Daling JR. Clinical characteristics of different histologic types of breast cancer. Br J Cancer. 2005;93:1046–52.

19. Louwman MW, Vriezen M, van Beek MW, et al. Uncommon breast tumors in perspective: incidence, treatment and survival in the Netherlands. Int J Cancer. 2007;121:127–35.

20. Solorzano CC, Middleton LP, Hunt KK, et al. Treatment and outcome of patients with intracystic papillary carcinoma of the breast. Am J Surg. 2002; 184:364–8.

21. Fayanju OM, Ritter J, Gillanders WE, et al. Therapeutic management of intracystic papillary carcinoma of the breast: the roles of radiation and endocrine therapy. Am J Surg. 2007;194:497–500.

22. Anderson WF, Chu KC, Chang S, et al. Comparison of age-specific incidence rate patterns for different histopathologic types of breast carcinoma. Cancer Epidemiol Biomarkers Prev. 2004;13:1128–35.

23. Rakha EA, Varga Z, Elsheik S, et al. High-grade encapsulated papillary carcinoma of the breast: an under-recognized entity. Histopathology. 2015;66:740–6.

24. Carter D, Orr SL, Merino MJ. Intracystic papillary carcinoma of the breast. After mastectomy, radiotherapy or excisional biopsy alone. Cancer. 1983;52:14–9.

25. Pathology and genetics of tumors of the breast and female genital organs. In: Tavassoli FA, Devilee P, editors. World Health Organization classification of tumors. Lyon: IACR Press; 2003.

26. Rosen PP. Rosen's breast pathology. 3rd ed. Philadelphia: Lippincott Williams & Wilkins; 2009.

27. Wei B, Bu H, Chen HJ, et al. Clinicopathologic study of solid papillary carcinoma of breast. Zhonghua Bing Li Xue Za Zhi. 2006;35:589–93.

28. Visscher D, Collins L, O'Malley FP, et al. Solid papillary carcinoma. In: Lakhani SR, Schnitt SJ, Tan PH, van de Vijver MJ, editors. WHO classification of tumors of the breast. 4th ed. Lyon: IARC press; 2012. p. 108–9.

29. MacGrogan G, Tse G, Collins L, et al. Intraductal papillary carcinoma. In: Lakhani SR, Schnitt SJ, Tan PH, van de Vijver MJ, editors. WHO classification of tumors of the breast. 4th ed. Lyon: IARC press; 2012. p. 103–5.

30. Tsang WY, Chan JK. Endocrine ductal carcinoma in situ (E-DCIS) of the breast: a form of low-grade DCIS with distinctive clinicopathologic and biologic characteristics. Am J Surg Pathol. 1996;20:921–43.

31. Tavassoli F, Devilee P. Papillary lesions. In: Tavassoli F, editor. Pathology of the breast. New York: McGraw-Hill; 1999. p. 325–72.

32. Rakha EA, Badve S, Eusebi V, et al. Breast lesions of uncertain malignant nature and limited metastatic potential: proposals to improve their recognition and clinical management. Histopathology. 2016;68:45–56.

33. Rakha EA, Tun M, Junainah E, et al. Encapsulated papillary carcinoma of the breast: a study of invasion associated markers. J Clin Pathol. 2012;65:710–4.

34. Hill CB, Yeh IT. Myoepithelial cell staining patterns of papillary breast lesions: from intraductal papillomas to invasive papillary carcinomas. Am J Clin Pathol. 2005;123:36–44.

35. Collins LC, Carlo VP, Hwang H, et al. Intracystic papillary carcinomas of the breast: a reevaluation using a panel of myoepithelial cell markers. Am J Surg Pathol. 2006;30:1002–7.

36. Nicolas MM, Wu Y, Middleton LP, et al. Loss of myoepithelium is variable in solid papillary carcinoma of the breast. Histopathology. 2007;51:657–65.

37. Maluf HM, Koerner FC. Solid papillary carcinoma of the breast. A form of intraductal carcinoma with endocrine differentiation frequently associated with mucinous carcinoma. Am J Surg Pathol. 1995;19:1237–44.

38. Leal C, Costa I, Fonseca D, et al. Intracystic (encysted) papillary carcinoma of the breast: a clinical, pathological, and immunohistochemical study. Hum Pathol. 1998;29:1097–104.

39. Wynveen CA, Nehhozina T, Akram M, et al. Intracystic papillary carcinoma of the breast: an in situ or invasive tumor? Results of immunohistochemical analysis and clinical follow-up. Am J Surg Pathol. 2011;35(1):1–14.

40. Mulligan AM, O'Malley FP. Metastatic potential of encapsulated (intracystic) papillary carcinoma of the breast: a report of 2 cases with axillary lymph node micrometastases. Int J Surg Pathol. 2007;15:143–7.

41. Lefkowitz M, Lefkowitz W, Wargotz ES. Intraductal (intracystic) papillary carcinoma of the breast and its variants: a clinicopathological study of 77 cases. Hum Pathol. 1994;25:802–9.

42. Harris KP, Faliakou EC, Exon DJ, et al. Treatment and outcome of intracystic papillary carcinoma of the breast. Br J Surg. 1999;86:1274.

43. Nassar H, Qureshi H, Volkanadsay N, et al. Clinicopathologic analysis of solid papillary carcinoma of the breast and associated invasive carcinomas. Am J Surg Pathol. 2006;30:501–7.

44. Duprez R, Wilkerson PM, Lacroix-Triki M, et al. Immunophenotypic and genomic characterization of papillary carcinomas of the breast. J Pathol. 2012;226:427–41.

45. Piscuoglio S, Ng CK, Martelotto LG, et al. Integrative genomic and transcriptomic characterization of papillary carcinomas of the breast. Mol Oncol. 2014;8: 1588–602.

46. Esposito NN, Dabbs DJ, Bhargava R. Are encapsulated papillary carcinomas of the breast in situ or invasive? A basement membrane study of 27 cases. Am J Clin Pathol. 2009;131:228–42.

47. Holmberg L, Garmo H, Granstrand B, et al. Absolute risk reductions for local recurrence after postoperative radiotherapy after sector resection for ductal carcinoma in situ of the breast. J Clin Oncol. 2008;26:1247–52.

48. Cutuli B, Fay R, Cohen-Solal-Le Nir C, et al. Ductal carcinoma in situ of the breast. Analysis of 882 cases. Presse Med. 2004;33:83–9.

49. Meijnen P, Oldenburg HS, Peterse JL, et al. Clinical outcome after selective treatment of patients diagnosed with ductal carcinoma in situ of the breast. Ann Surg Oncol. 2008;15:235–43.

50. Ellis IO, Galea M, Broughton N, et al. Pathological prognostic factors in breast cancer. II Histological type. Relationships with survival in a large study with long-term follow-up. Histopathology. 1992;20:479–89.

51. Rosen PP. The pathological classification of human mammary carcinoma: past, present and future. Ann Clin Lab Sci. 1979;9:144–56.

52. Dixon JM, Page DL, Anderson TJ, et al. Long term survivors after breast cancer. Br J Surg. 1985;72:445–8.

53. Fisher ER, Palekar AS, Redmond C, et al. Pathologic findings from the National Surgical Adjuvant Breast Project (protocol no.4). VI. Invasive papillary carcinoma. J Clin Pathol. 1980;73:313–22.

54. Anderson WF, Devesa SS. In situ male breast carcinoma in the surveillance, epidemiology, and end results database of the National Cancer Institute. Cancer. 2005;104:1733–41.

55. Burga AM, Fadare O, Lininger RA, et al. Invasive carcinomas of the male breast: a morphologic study of the distribution of histologic subtypes and metastatic patterns in 778 cases. Virchows Arch. 2006;449:507–12.

56. Youngson BJ, Cranor M, Rosen PP. Epithelial displacement in surgical breast specimens following needling procedures. Am J Surg Pathol. 1994;18:896–903.

57. Youngson BJ, Liberman L, Rosen PP. Displacement of carcinomatous epithelium in surgical breast specimens following stereotaxic core biopsy. Am J Clin Pathol. 1995;103:598–602.

Metaplastic Breast Carcinomas

12

Emad Rakha

Abstract

Metaplastic breast carcinomas comprise a wide spectrum of diseases with variable histological features and behavior and often present special challenges in diagnosis. As a "triple-negative" carcinoma, it falls within the "basal-like" phenotype of breast carcinomas. Immunohistochemistry is almost always essential in the diagnostic workup, and the differential diagnosis of metaplastic carcinoma on core biopsy is broad and includes both benign and malignant spindle cell lesions of the breast.

Keywords

Breast cancer • Metaplastic carcinoma • Histological types • Grade • Diagnosis • Outcome • Management

Introduction

Metaplastic breast carcinomas (MBCs) are a heterogeneous group of tumors characterized by the differentiation of the neoplastic epithelial cells into squamous and/or mesenchymal-looking elements including but not restricted to spindle, chondroid, osseous, and rhabdomyoid with or without conventional mammary adenocarcinoma component [1–11]. The carcinomatous component may be minimal, hard to find, or present only as carcinoma in situ. Given the variable histological appearances of MBC, a plethora of terms have been used to describe subgroups of MBC including spindle cell carcinoma, squamous cell carcinoma, adenosquamous carcinoma, matrix-producing carcinoma, carcinosarcoma, and carcinomas with pseudosarcomatous metaplasia, chondroid metaplasia, or osseous differentiation [1]. Other types with specific features have also been described including low-grade adenosquamous carcinoma, fibromatosis-like spindle cell metaplastic carcinoma or tumor, and variants of squamous cell carcinomas such as acantholytic variant and mucoepidermoid carcinoma. It is also important to note that metaplastic carcinomas with mixed morphology are common such

E. Rakha
Department of Cellular Pathology,
The University of Nottingham and Nottingham
University Hospitals NHS Trust, Nottingham City
Hospital, University of Nottingham, City Hospital
Campus, Hucknall Road, Nottingham NG5 1PB, UK
e-mail: Emad.Rakha@nottingham.ac.uk;
Emad.Rakha@nuh.nhs.uk

© Springer International Publishing Switzerland 2017
S. Shousha (ed.), *Breast Pathology*, DOI 10.1007/978-3-319-28655-6_12

as squamous cell carcinoma or matrix-producing carcinoma with spindle cell component [7, 8, 12–14].

The extent of metaplasia in breast carcinomas varies from a few microscopic foci in an otherwise typical mammary carcinoma to complete replacement of glandular growth by the metaplastic tumor pattern. When the metaplastic components form a significant proportion (usually >10%, although some authors have used different cutoffs including <10% [15], ≥20% [16], or ≥50% [4]), the term MBC is used. Breast carcinomas with metaplasia are usually derived from poorly differentiated ductal carcinomas [8, 17], but metaplasia can occur in well-differentiated tumors and, less commonly, in breast carcinomas of special type. For malignant mesenchymal-looking breast tumors completely lacking evidence of epithelial differentiation in the form of conventional mammary carcinoma component, including invasive or in situ elements, or molecular evidence of epithelial nature (e.g., cytokeratin expression), the term sarcoma is often applied. This includes primary breast sarcomas and metastatic sarcomas [14].

Although apocrine carcinomas, signet ring cell carcinomas, and carcinomas of salivary gland/skin adnexal differentiation are composed of metaplastic neoplastic cell population, they are not referred to as MBC and are not discussed in this chapter.

Epidemiology

MBC accounts for 0.2–1.5% of all invasive breast cancers [1–7]. However, the prevalence varies according to the different definitions adopted. Metaplastic carcinomas as defined here account for less than 1% of all invasive mammary carcinomas, but up to 5% of mammary carcinomas may undergo some (<10%) metaplastic change into a nonglandular growth pattern [18].

Similar to conventional mammary carcinomas, the vast majority occurs in postmenopausal female with mean age of 60 years (range 27–96) [7].

Clinical Features

The clinical presentation is like infiltrating ductal carcinoma of no special type (i.e., as a palpable breast mass usually in the 1- to 3-cm range, but occasionally as large tumors in the 20-cm range). The mean size of MBC is 3.9 cm (range 1 to >10 cm) [1]. Regarding tumor stage, 23% are TNM stage pT1, 53% are pT2, and 24% are pT3-4 [7]. Most metaplastic carcinomas appear as well-delineated mass densities. Microcalcifications are not a common feature but may be present, usually within a carcinoma in situ component. Ossification, suggesting osteosarcomatous differentiation, appears on mammography or as gritty areas on macroscopic examination.

Gross Pathology

Grossly most are firm and well delineated and have a solid cut surface. Squamous or chondroid differentiation is reflected as pearly white to firm glistening areas in the cut surface. Cystic change suggests squamous differentiation or areas of cavitated coagulation tumor necrosis. In our study of 405 MBCs, 70% of patients had axillary procedures with a median lymph node number of 9 (range 1–46). A third of these patients had positive nodes which were mainly few in number (median = 2) [7]. Forty-five percent of the positive nodes contained deposits of metaplastic elements as either pure (25%) or mixed with conventional carcinomas (20%); the remainder were involved by conventional adenocarcinoma of ductal/NST.

Microscopic Pathology

It had been customary to separate MBC into squamous, adenosquamous, matrix-producing, and spindle cell types. These morphologic distinctions are somewhat arbitrary because some metaplastic tumors exhibit multiple growth patterns, although one subtype may be predominant. Some authors considered that the presence of apparent microscopic overlapping and the lack of significant correlation between the microscopic pattern and prognosis support the concept that they are variants of a single entity [18]. However, some authors including our group demonstrated the presence of prognostic significance for the different subtypes of MBC, with matrix-producing carcinomas having the best outcome and high-grade spindle cell carcinomas having the worst outcome [7, 19, 20].

The World Health Organization (WHO; 2012 [1]) has classified MBC into two basic types, each with subcategories [1]. These include:

1. Carcinomas with squamous differentiation
2. Carcinomas with mesenchymal-looking differentiation
   • The squamous group includes:
     (a) Squamous carcinoma (large cell type with or without spindle cell metaplasia or acantholysis)
     (b) Adenosquamous (mixed squamous and adenocarcinomatous elements including high grade adenosquamous and mucoepidermoid) carcinoma
     (c) The good prognosis low-grade adenosquamous carcinoma
   • The mesenchymal-like carcinoma group includes:
     (a) Carcinoma with chondroid differentiation
     (b) Carcinoma with osseous differentiation
     (c) Carcinoma with rhabdomyosarcomatous differentiation

Squamous Cell Carcinoma and Variants

Small areas of squamous metaplasia may occur in an otherwise typical invasive ductal carcinoma, but only when squamous differentiation predominates that the case can be considered as representing a metaplastic squamous cell carcinoma.

Squamous cell carcinoma is the most frequent subtype of MBC. It usually presents as a cystic lesion where the cavity is lined by squamous cells with varying degrees of atypia. A spectrum of squamous differentiation may be present ranging from mature keratinizing epithelium (Fig. 12.1a, b) to poorly differentiated carcinoma with spindle cell, acantholytic, or sarcomatous areas, including various combinations of these features. Yet, the specific diagnosis of squamous cell carcinoma of the breast as a subtype of MBC is reserved for tumors composed entirely of keratinizing or nonkeratinizing malignant squamous cells [1, 19, 21]. In cases lacking in situ or conventional mammary carcinoma components, it is important to rule out adjacent cutaneous or metastatic squamous carcinoma to the breast from a distant site before making the diagnosis of primary disease. The most bland-appearing and well-differentiated cells often line cystic spaces; as the tumor cells emanate out to infiltrate the surrounding stroma, they become spindle shaped and lose their squamous features (Fig. 12.1c). Inflammatory infiltrate is usually prominent. A pronounced stromal reaction is often admixed with the spindled squamous carcinoma. Spindle cell transformation of squamous carcinoma is common but usually focal and inconspicuous. The squamous differentiation is retained in metastatic foci [8].

Acantholytic or pseudoangiomatous change has been reported and may lead to a mistaken diagnosis of angiosarcoma, and when present, acantholytic squamous carcinoma may follow a very aggressive clinical course [22]. The spindle cell and acantholytic/pseudoangiomatous variants require confirmation of their epithelial nature. They are positive for high molecular weight CKs (CK5, CK5/CK6, CK14, and 34βE12) and p63 but negative for vascular endothelial markers.

Like other MBCs, squamous cell carcinomas are negative for estrogen receptor (ER)/PgR/*HER2*. However, some metaplastic squamous cell carcinomas show weak mainly focal nuclear ER staining similar to that seen in some normal epidermal cell nuclei of uncertain significance (Fig. 12.1d). Squamous cell carcinoma can be graded based mainly on nuclear features.

Adenosquamous Carcinoma

Adenosquamous carcinoma of the breast is a rare invasive carcinoma that encompasses two subtypes with markedly different prognosis:

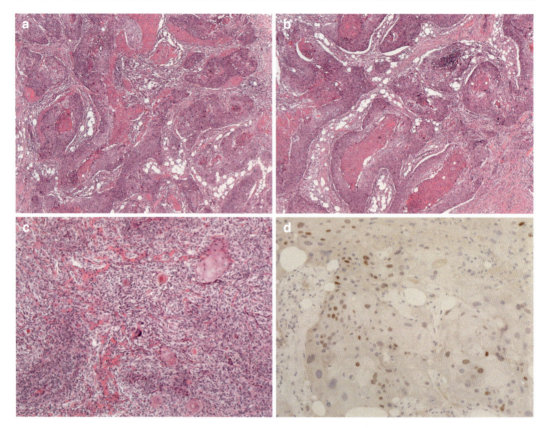

Fig. 12.1 (**a**) Metaplastic squamous carcinoma of the breast with keratin formation. (**b**) Demonstrates pure squamous differentiation while (**c**) showing mixed squamous and spindle cell mesenchymal-looking differentiation. (**d**) Shows focal estrogen receptor (ER) staining in the nuclei of metaplastic squamous cell carcinoma. Nuclear ER staining of variable intensity may be seen in some metaplastic squamous cell carcinoma, and its clinical significance is uncertain. Categorization of such cases into ER positive or ER negative is often challenging, and a repeat using a different ER antibody may validate the results

- **Low-grade adenosquamous carcinoma** or syringomatous squamous tumor that is morphologically similar to adenosquamous carcinoma of the skin and mucoepidermoid carcinoma. These have characteristic histological features and indolent behavior that are sufficient for them to be discussed separately in the fourth edition of the WHO book [1] and also in this chapter (see below) to avoid clinically misleading inclusion with the other aggressive subtypes of MBC.

- **High-grade adenosquamous carcinoma** is an aggressive tumor often presenting as a mixture of poorly differentiated squamous cell carcinoma and high-grade conventional mammary adenocarcinoma [5]. Because focal squamous differentiation can occur in up to 5 % of typical infiltrating ductal carcinomas of no special type, there should be a prominent admixture of invasive ductal and squamous carcinoma before the term *high-grade adenosquamous carcinoma* is used.

Spindle Cell Carcinoma

Spindle cell MBC is a rare invasive breast adenocarcinoma with abundant spindle cell transformation but with retention of their glandular nature. Electron microscopy reveals glandular lumina in the spindle cells. The spindle cells are arranged in a multitude of architectural patterns,

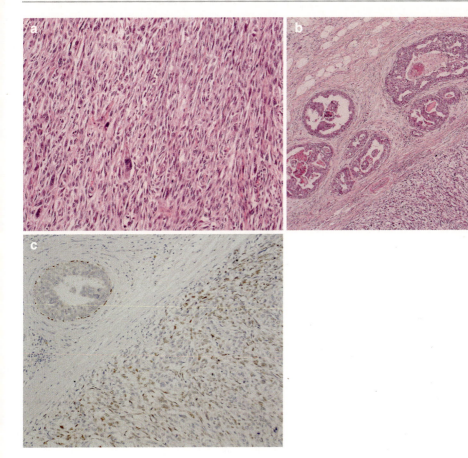

Fig. 12.2 (**a**) High-grade spindle cell metaplastic carcinoma. (**b**) Shows spindle cell carcinoma associated with DCIS confirming its primary mammary origin. (**c**) Shows positive expression of p63 in the malignant spindle cells and in the myoepithelial cells surrounding DCIS at the periphery of the tumor

show varying degrees of atypia and inflammatory infiltrate, and are typically immunoreactive with epithelial markers including luminal low molecular weight CKs such as CK7 and AE1/AE3 in addition to basal CKs and p63 (Fig. 12.2). Spindle cell MBC may include foci of epithelioid morphology or focal squamous or malignant myoepithelial differentiation, with some cases showing almost complete loss of epithelial/myoepithelial differentiation and greatly overlapping with sarcoma.

Similar to adenosquamous carcinoma, spindle cell carcinomas of the breast can be classified into low grade and high grade with different histological features and prognosis. Low-grade spindle cell "fibromatosis-like" MBC is typically composed of bland-looking spindle cell prolifer-

ation similar to fibromatosis and other benign spindle cell lesions of the breast but typically expressing high molecular weight basal-type CKs such as CK5/CK6 and CK14 and p63 (Fig. 12.3). Due to its indolent clinical behavior, this tumor is described separately (see below). On the other hand, high-grade spindle cell MBC is an aggressive type of MBC with variable degrees of positivity of CKs and other markers of squamous and myoepithelial differentiation.

Spindle cell MBC can be monophasic or biphasic. The monophasic pattern is composed of pure spindle cells or shows small cohesive foci of epithelioid cells. The biphasic pattern contains conventional carcinoma elements usually invasive carcinoma of no special type, ductal carcinoma in situ or squamous elements. Diagnostic

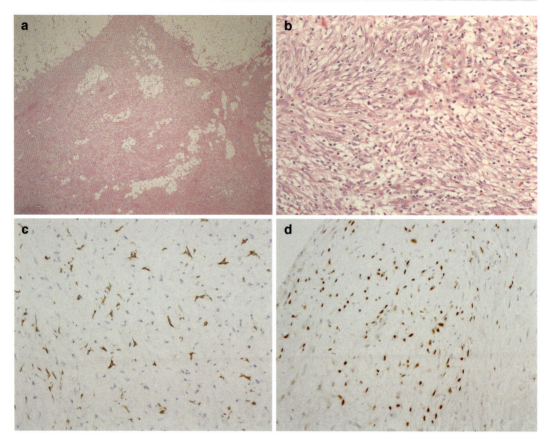

Fig. 12.3 Low-grade spindle cell metaplastic carcinoma (**a**, **b**) showing positive expression of CK14 (**c**) and p63 (**d**)

approach of mammary spindle cell lesions and the differential diagnosis of spindle cell MBC are discussed below.

Most spindle cell MBC occurs in postmenopausal women, presenting as discrete masses. The prognosis is determined by the tumor size and degree of differentiation as well as the pathologic stage. Many spindle cell MBCs are clearly high-grade tumors, easily recognizable as malignant; however, some varieties can appear deceptively benign [2, 6, 17]. These tumors are often misdiagnosed as nodular fasciitis, fibromatosis, granulation tissue reaction, or squamous metaplasia (see below). They can also be misclassified as low-grade sarcoma or fibrosarcoma. Yet most spindle cell carcinomas appear to have the same behavior as that of grade-matched infiltrating ductal carcinomas. The cumulative 5-year survival for spindle cell carcinoma of the breast has been reported at 64 % [7, 9]. Although large

tumors are more likely to recur, other histologic features such as grade, cellularity, mitotic activity, degree of differentiation, and inflammation do not seem to correlate with outcome [7]. Some authors have reported an aggressive behavior for spindle cell (sarcomatoid) carcinoma of the breast with a high rate of extranodal metastases, although they may have a significantly lower rate of nodal metastases than conventional ductal and lobular carcinomas [4, 23].

Matrix-Producing Metaplastic Carcinoma

This is a carcinoma with direct transition to a cartilaginous or osseous stromal matrix sometimes without an intervening spindle cell zone or osteoclastic cells [1], but more commonly with the heterologous areas developing from a spindle cell

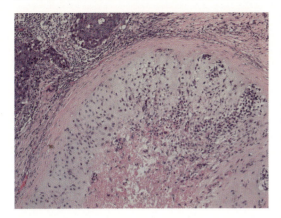

Fig. 12.4 Matrix-producing, metaplastic breast carcinoma. Note the presence of a chondrosarcomatous component

component (Fig. 12.4). Metaplastic cells in the osseous and cartilaginous matrix stain for S100 protein and vimentin, with variable and sometimes no reactivity for keratins and epithelial membrane antigen. Many of these tumors are negative for ER and PgR both in the mesenchymal and adenocarcinoma areas, although the latter may be occasionally hormone receptor positive. In some MBC, the mesenchymal element may show an admixture of different mesenchymal components or may show no clear line of differentiation. Angiosarcomatous, leiomyosarcomatous, osteosarcomatous, chondrosarcomatous, or rhabdomyosarcomatous patterns may be seen. Carcinomatous areas can be glandular, tubular, solid clusters or foci of squamous differentiation [1]. Extensive sampling may be needed to identify these diagnostic carcinomatous areas.

Matrix-producing MBC shows a variable degree of atypia which ranges from minimal atypia that overlaps with pleomorphic adenoma-like tumors of the breast [13] or mildly atypical cartilaginous tissue to overtly malignant high-grade lesions mimicking high-grade osteosarcomas or chondrosarcomas (Fig. 12.4). Metastases derived from a metaplastic carcinoma may be entirely adenocarcinoma, entirely metaplastic, or a mixture of both. A minority of axillary metastases actually contains heterologous components, but they are found more commonly in local recurrences on the chest wall and in visceral metastases [5].

Low-Grade Metaplastic Carcinomas

Despite the fact that low-grade adenosquamous carcinomas and fibromatosis-like MBC are discussed with other types of MBC, there is a view that these lesions should be considered as lesions of limited metastatic potential to reflect their indolent behavior [24]. Here we describe them in more details.

Low-Grade Adenosquamous Carcinoma

Low-grade adenosquamous carcinoma is a rare form of infiltrative breast tumors that commonly arise in association with benign proliferative complex sclerosing and papillary breast lesions [25]. It is characterized by well-developed tubule/gland formation often intimately admixed with solid nests of squamous differentiation in a spindle cell background. The carcinomatous glandular components often show rounded rather than angulated contour, and unlike tubular carcinomas they show expression of basal and luminal CKs and are ER negative. They are cytologically bland. The stromal component is of reactive nature and is typically "fibromatosis-like," being cellular and composed of bland spindle cells, but can be collagenous, hyalinized, or variably cellular. Clusters of lymphoid cells and lymphoid follicles are often present at the periphery of the lesion. The neoplastic glandular and squamous elements typically infiltrate the surrounding mammary structures and glands in long slender extension [1, 26]. Sometimes there appear to be immunoreactive myoepithelial cells at the edge of some tumor islands. The tumor cells lack hormone receptors.

Overlapping features between associated benign proliferative lesions and low-grade adenosquamous carcinoma exist [27]. Adenosquamous proliferation, stromal changes, and even clusters of lymphocytes can be seen within these benign proliferative lesions and are often described as reactive mimics or attributed to earlier biopsy. Differentiating benign proliferative lesions showing these features from low-grade adenosquamous carcinoma is often subjective. Previous studies have demonstrated that adenosquamous proliferation of reactive-looking lesions is morphologically and immunohistochemically indistinguishable from the neoplastic ducts of low-grade adenosquamous carcinoma [28].

Histologically low-grade adenosquamous carcinoma also needs to be differentiated from pure tubular carcinoma, adenomyoepithelioma, and syringomatous tumor of the nipple [29], while clinically it should be differentiated from the high-grade forms of metaplastic carcinoma and other triple-negative/basal-like carcinomas that are associated with an aggressive behavior [7]. A recent study reported molecular similarity between low-grade adenosquamous carcinoma and syringomatous tumor of the nipple [29].

Low-grade adenosquamous carcinoma has an excellent prognosis [24, 30]. To reflect its good prognosis, some authors preferred the term "infiltrating syringomatous adenoma" to avoid the term *carcinoma* as these lesions mainly recur after local excision with very low risk of metastasis. Although some examples have reached 8 cm in diameter, lymph node metastatic spread is extremely rare and was noted in only a single case.

Low-Grade Mucoepidermoid Carcinoma

Another very rare variant of squamous cell carcinoma has been reported as low-grade mucoepidermoid carcinoma of the breast, which is similar to those occurring in the salivary glands, lacking true keratinization or squamous pearls. It is characterized by central nests of epidermoid or mucus-secreting cells and cysts that are positive for low molecular weight CKs (CK7 and CK18) and lined by basaloid cells positive for high molecular weight CKs (CK14) and intermediate cells positive for CK5/CK6 and EGFR. Most mucoepidermoid carcinomas are low grade and behave as other indolent low-grade carcinomas. High-grade mucoepidermoid carcinoma behaves like other high-grade MBCs [31].

Low-Grade Fibromatosis-Like Metaplastic Carcinoma

Low-grade fibromatosis-like spindle cell carcinoma is a rare variant of spindle cell MBC that is associated with a favorable prognosis [32]. Local recurrence can occur after local excision and distant metastases occur occasionally [32, 33]. The tumor is characterized by the proliferation of low-grade, cytologically bland spindle cells, which compose at least 95 % of the total tumor area and histologically resemble fibromatosis [32, 34]. Differentiation between these two entities in routine practice is often based on expression of epithelial markers.

In a recent copy number analyses study, Takano et al. [35] demonstrated that low-grade fibromatosis-like spindle cell carcinomas are characterized by low genomic instability and share no copy number aberrations with other MBCs. They suggested that this entity is a unique group of tumors, and their genotype belies their apparent homogeneous morphology and phenotype [35]. Despite its indolent behavior that is similar to some locally aggressive lesions with very low metastatic potential [32, 34], such as fibromatosis, a malignant diagnosis using the term carcinoma or metaplastic carcinoma with triple-negative status may trigger inappropriate use of aggressive adjuvant systemic chemotherapy [32, 36]. However, caution is advised as larger tumors, even if they show low-grade spindle cell areas, are likely to be heterogeneous, and higher-grade component if present can be associated with aggressive behavior [23, 33].

Diagnosing Metaplastic Carcinoma with Extensive "Mesenchymal-Like" Differentiation

It is important to note that some mesenchymal-like MBCs show extensive metaplastic differentiation up to the degree that mammary epithelial origin is difficult to confirm. The presence of one or more of the following three features is often used as evidence of the epithelial origin of mesenchymal-like (matrix-producing and spindle cell) malignant tumors of the breast:

1. Coexistence of invasive carcinomatous components (i.e., ductal NST, lobular).
2. Associated ductal carcinoma in situ (DCIS). In a previous study of 405 MBCs, we found that conventional-type carcinomatous element was present in 57 % of cases, while DCIS was identified in 42 % of cases [7].
3. Molecular demonstration of epithelial differentiation using ultrastructural features or immunohistochemistry with epithelial-specific markers (i.e., cytokeratins and epithelial membrane antigen). In a previous study of 103 matrix-producing MBCs, immunohistochemistry was available for 45 cases. Of those 43 cases showed positivity for one or more epithelial-associated biomarkers including all cases (18 cases) without morphologically (H&E) identifiable epithelial features, whereas two cases lacked such evidence, and they were diagnosed as primary mammary osteosarcoma and atypical osteoid tumor, respectively [14]. However inappropriate expression of epithelial antigens by pure mesenchymal tumors and the presence of occasional tight junctions and desmosomes in unquestionable benign and malignant mesenchymal cells have been documented, despite the fact that these findings are typically limited to isolated cells and are sporadic in nature. Therefore care should be exercised when diagnosing a case as MBC based purely on focal expression of epithelial biomarkers [14]. Davis and coworkers [37] have suggested that metaplastic sarcomatoid carcinomas that lack or have only a minimal overt invasive carcinomatous component have a biologic behavior similar to that of sarcomas. In addition to systemic treatment, early aggressive local therapy is recommended because these patients have a high rate of local relapse.

Differential Diagnoses

Diagnostic difficulties of MBC stem not only from the existence of multiple histological subtypes but also from the overlapping histological features with multiple entities ranging from reactive/benign to aggressive malignant tumors. These entities can simply be classified into groups equivalent to the different histological subtypes of MBC.

Low-grade metaplastic squamous cell carcinoma should be differentiated from reactive/benign squamous lesions in the breast. Squamous cells may be seen as metaplastic changes in cysts, papillary lesions, phyllodes tumor, and gynecomastia particularly following trauma, biopsy procedure, inflammation, or infarction. Breast abscesses and chronic breast inflammation may lead to squamous metaplasia [38, 39].

High-grade metaplastic squamous cell carcinoma should be differentiated from metastatic squamous cell carcinoma particularly those of the lung, skin, esophagus, and cervix and from primary cutaneous squamous cell carcinoma infiltrating the breast. Clinical history, imaging findings, tumor location in the breast, and histological findings together with any coexisting lesions can help in making the correct diagnosis. The presence of ductal carcinoma in situ (DCIS) or conventional invasive mammary carcinoma components and location within the interstitial tissue of the breast favor primary breast origin, while superficial location with adjacent epidermal dysplasia may point out toward primary skin lesion. History of metastatic or previous squamous cell carcinoma elsewhere favors non-breast primary origin. Immunohistochemistry may not be very helpful in making a definite diagnosis as most of squamous cell carcinomas of the breast share a similar immunoprofile regardless of its site of origin with positivity of p63 and high molecular weight cytokeratins (CK5/6 and CK14), and 20–30 % express luminal cytokeratins (CK7). They are negative for TTF1 and CDX2 [40].

Acantholytic and pseudoangiomatous variants of squamous cell carcinomas should be differentiated from angiosarcoma. The expression of vascular markers (e.g., CD31, CD34, factor VIII) and negative expression of p63, CK5/CK6, and CK14 help in making a diagnosis [41].

A significant spindle cell component can be found in many breast lesions, both benign and malignant. Even though these lesions may not be entirely spindle celled (e.g., phyllodes tumor), sampling error caused by a core biopsy may sample predominantly spindled areas without the other identifying components being present.

Bland-looking spindle cell MBC should be differentiated from reactive/benign lesions that can have a significant spindle cell component including fibromatosis, some examples of sclerosing adenosis, benign phyllodes tumors, adenomyoepithelioma (spindle cell variant), inflammatory myofibroblastic tumor (also called inflammatory pseudotumor), myofibroblastoma, leiomyoma, spindle cell lipoma, cellular angiolipoma, pseudoangiomatous stromal hyperplasia, and repair reaction to a prior biopsy site or traumatic fat necrosis [12, 42–45].

Malignant-looking spindle cell MBC should be differentiated from other malignant lesions that can have a significant spindle cell component including malignant phyllodes tumor, periductal stromal sarcoma, CD10+ stromal sarcoma, primary breast sarcomas (also called stromal sarcoma), and angiosarcoma [12].

Generally the diagnostic approach in assessing breast spindle cell lesions should include the following points:

(a) Component cells: pure spindle cells or mixed with other cells, including adipose tissue, muscle cells, inflammatory cells, or parenchymal elements, including epithelial cells and myoepithelial cells, ducts, and/or lobules.
(b) Growth pattern: fascicular, storiform, diffuse, or whirling.
(c) Margins: infiltrating or well defined.
(d) Cellularity: low, moderate, or high.
(e) Cytonuclear atypia: high-grade cytonuclear atypia indicates a malignant process with a differential diagnosis of MBCs, sarcomas, melanomas, and metastatic spindle cell tumors. In contrast, absent or low-grade atypia may represent a reactive, benign, or low-grade malignant process. Frequent mitotic figures, including atypical forms, are a feature of high-grade MBC and other malignant spindle cell tumors. Although some reactive spindle cell breast lesions, such as nodular fasciitis, may show frequent mitotic figures, these are typically of normal forms and not associated with cytonuclear atypia.

(f) Immunohistochemistry: this is very helpful in challenging cases. Biomarkers indicating epithelial differentiation are particularly important. Immunohistochemistry can be used for the diagnosis of specific lesions or to rule out other entities.
(g) Other features: the presence of thick bundles of hyalinized collagen between the spindle cells is an important feature of myofibroblastoma. Necrosis is usually seen in high-grade malignant lesions. The presence of in situ carcinoma or conventional mammary-type invasive carcinoma in the surrounding breast tissue favors the diagnosis of MBC. Some MBCs are associated with papillomas or radial scars [46]. Patient age, lesion size, location in relation to skin and deep structures, and rate of growth are additional helpful features.

Diagnosis of MBC on Core Biopsy

Diagnosis of squamous cell carcinoma on needle core biopsy (NCB) is often based on the identification of squamous cells and atypia sufficient for a malignant diagnosis. It is more difficult to make a diagnosis of a bland-looking squamous cell lesion on NCB, and caution should be taken as the differential diagnosis includes benign and malignant entities. Similarly caution should be taken on diagnosing matrix-producing breast lesions, overdiagnosis of pleomorphic adenoma-like tumors of the breast as MBC has been reported [13], and underdiagnosis as benign cartilaginous lesions has also been documented. Diagnosis of high-grade lesion is often more straightforward despite the frequent difficulty of typing such lesions as MBC and primary or metastatic sarcomas.

Diagnosis of breast spindle cell lesions on NCBs is more difficult and is often based on awareness of the clinical setting, careful examination of the hematoxylin- and eosin-stained sections, and immunohistochemistry [12]. The commonest spindle cell lesion of the breast, in our experience, is a scar. The presence of hemosiderin-laden macrophages or fat necrosis is an important clue to this diagnosis. Sometimes, making a definite diagnosis is difficult, because the fibroblasts show atypia or there is no fat necrosis or there are no hemosiderin macrophages to support the diagnosis. In such cases, it is prudent to categorize the lesion as B3 (lesions of uncertain malignant potential) and recommend further core biopsy or diagnostic excision.

At the malignant end of the spectrum, MBC is the commonest diagnosis. A malignant diagnosis (B5b) can be made if there is definite epithelial differentiation on morphology or immunohisto-chemistry. The immunohistochemical panel in such cases should include epithelial differentia-tion markers, including multiple low and high molecular weight CKs, and other markers to help exclude other entities in the differential diagnosis based on morphology and clinical history. Occasionally, the features are clearly malignant, but a definite diagnosis is not possible. Recommendation for node biopsy or consider-ation of neoadjuvant therapy is not possible in such cases, and a definite diagnosis should await examination of the excised specimen.

Treatment and Prognosis

Some early reports indicated that MBC has a poor survival rate, possibly in the range of 35 % at 5 years follow-up, and this poor survival occurred even though MBCs metastasize to lymph nodes less frequently than would be expected with invasive ductal carcinomas of no special type and of similar size and grade [9]. However, more recent survival studies have found that, in comparison with matched typical breast cancer cases, there is no major difference in treatment patterns, recurrence, or survival [7, 23]. In a large multicenter study of 405 MBC cases [7], we found that the outcome of MBC is not different from matched ductal/NST carci-noma, but the performance of the established prognostic variables in MBC is different. Lymph

node stage, lymphovascular invasion, and histo-logic subtype are associated with outcome, but tumor size and grade are not. Chemotherapy was associated with longer survival although this effect was limited to early-stage disease. In that study no association between radiotherapy and outcome was identified, and the outcome of MBC diagnosed in Asian countries was more favorable than those in Western countries. Multivariate analysis of MBC shows that histologic subtype is an independent prognostic feature [7]. Another study suggested that the overall survival rate of MBC was 83 % at 5 years, and it was not different to a control group of patients with infiltrating ductal carcinoma [20].

MBC often shows more advanced stage at pre-sentation compared to conventional-type mam-mary adenocarcinoma but less frequent lymph node metastasis than those of similar size and grade. Treatment is primarily surgical removal with or without polyagent chemotherapy. Some reports suggest that MBCs have lower response rate to conventional chemotherapy than other types of triple-negative conventional carcinomas [1].

Genetics of Metaplastic Breast Carcinoma

Benign and malignant mammary glandular cells show a high degree of phenotypic plasticity [8, 18, 47]. Squamous, spindle, and heterologous matrix-producing transdifferentiation of mammary epi-thelial/myoepithelial cells is seen in both benign and malignant lesions [48–50]. MBC showing mesenchymal differentiation with or without het-erologous elements originates from carcinomas that undergo sarcomatous neometaplasia as a result of further genetic instability or mutations. Zhuang and colleagues [51] have demonstrated identical clonality of the carcinomatous and spin-dle cell components as well as a focus of ductal carcinoma in situ (DCIS) that was present in one case. The authors concluded that the two invasive components and its precursor were clonal and that the sarcomatous component arose from mutation of the carcinoma. Likewise, after an investigation

40. Pereira TC, Share SM, Magalhaes AV, et al. Can we tell the site of origin of metastatic squamous cell carcinoma? An immunohistochemical tissue microarray study of 194 cases. Appl Immunohistochem Mol Morphol. 2011;19:10–4.

41. Parramore B, Hanly M, Yeh KA, et al. Acantholytic variant of squamous cell carcinoma of the breast: a case report. Am Surg. 1999;65:467–9.

42. Loose JH, Patchefsky AS, Hollander IJ, et al. Adenomyoepithelioma of the breast. A spectrum of biologic behavior. Am J Surg Pathol. 1992;16:868–76.

43. Ebrahim L, Parry J, Taylor DB. Fibromatosis of the breast: a pictorial review of the imaging and histopathology findings. Clin Radiol. 2014;69:1077–83.

44. Ali M, Fayemi AO, Braun EV, et al. Fibromatosis of the breast. Am J Surg Pathol. 1979;3:501–5.

45. Rito M, Schmitt F, Pinto AE, et al. Fibromatosis-like metaplastic carcinoma of the breast has a claudin-low immunohistochemical phenotype. Virchows Arch. 2014;465:185–91.

46. Gobbi H, Simpson JF, Jensen RA, et al. Metaplastic spindle cell breast tumors arising within papillomas, complex sclerosing lesions, and nipple adenomas. Mod Pathol. 2003;16:893–901.

47. Wang X, Mori I, Tang W, et al. Metaplastic carcinoma of the breast: p53 analysis identified the same point mutation in the three histologic components. Mod Pathol. 2001;14:1183–6.

48. Smith BH, Taylor HB. The occurrence of bone and cartilage in mammary tumors. Am J Clin Pathol. 1969;51:610–8.

49. Rosen PP. Rosen's breast pathology. 3rd ed. Philadelphia: Lippincott Williams & Wilkins; 2009.

50. Spagnolo DV, Shilkin KB. Breast neoplasms containing bone and cartilage. Virchows Arch A Pathol Anat Histopathol. 1983;400:287–95.

51. Zhuang ZI, Lininger RA, Man YG, Albuquerque A, Merino MJ, Tavassoli FA. Identical clonality of both components of mammary carcinosarcoma with differential loss of heterozygosity. Mod Pathol. 1997;10:354–62.

52. Lien HC, Lin CW, Mao TL, et al. p53 overexpression and mutation in metaplastic carcinoma of the breast: genetic evidence for a monoclonal origin of both the carcinomatous and the heterogeneous sarcomatous components. J Pathol. 2004;204:131–9.

53. Geyer FC, Weigelt B, Natrajan R, et al. Molecular analysis reveals a genetic basis for the phenotypic diversity of metaplastic breast carcinomas. J Pathol. 2010;220:562–73.

54. McCarthy A, Savage K, Gabriel A, et al. A mouse model of basal-like breast carcinoma with metaplastic elements. J Pathol. 2007;211:389–98.

55. Sarrio D, Rodriguez-Pinilla SM, Hardisson D, et al. Epithelial-mesenchymal transition in breast cancer relates to the basal-like phenotype. Cancer Res. 2008;68:989–97.

56. Leibl S, Gogg-Kammerer M, Sommersacher A, et al. Metaplastic breast carcinomas: are they of myoepithelial differentiation?: immunohistochemical profile of the sarcomatoid subtype using novel myoepithelial markers. Am J Surg Pathol. 2005;29:347–53.

57. Weigelt B, Ng CK, Shen R, et al. Corrigendum: metastatic breast carcinomas display genomic and transcriptomic heterogeneity. Mod Pathol. 2015;28:607.

Sami Shousha

Abstract

The breast is occasionally the site of metastatic tumors from elsewhere in the body. This chapter reviews the literature about the subject, outlines the features that would help differentiating such metastatic lesions from primary breast cancer, and provides illustrated examples. Differentiating metastatic ovarian carcinoma from primary breast carcinoma is discussed in more detail, as well as differentiating metastatic neuroendocrine tumors from primary breast carcinomas with neuroendocrine differentiation.

Keywords

Breast • Metastatic carcinoma • Immunohistochemistry • Melanoma • Ovarian carcinoma • Neuroendocrine tumors • Renal cell carcinoma • Leiomyosarcoma

Introduction

Although metastatic carcinoma to the breast is quite rare, it is important to keep it always in mind, particularly when dealing with core biopsies, as its management is usually completely different from the management of primary breast carcinoma. It is not surprising therefore that review articles about the subject appear regularly in *Pathology Journals*, as well as numerous case reports and collection of cases. According to

Silverman and Oberman [1], the first ever review was written by Charache in 1942 [2]. The majority of patients in these older reports had metastatic malignant melanoma. In an autopsy study of 12 cases published in 1991, four were malignant melanoma and two ovarian, two renal, two gastric, one pulmonary, and one pancreatic carcinoma [3]. In a survey of 60 secondary neoplasms of the breast published in the twentieth century, around half (31 cases) were hematologic malignancies, including lymphomas and leukemias, which were reported mostly in the later part of that period [4]. The remaining cases in that report included 6 melanomas and 11 lung, 4 stomach, 3 kidney, and 1 each for pancreatic, uterus, esophagus, thyroid, and skin squamous cell carcinoma. A series of 18 non-hematological cases reported

S. Shousha
Department of Histopathology,
Charing Cross Hospital & Imperial College,
Fulham Palace Road, London W6 8RF, UK
e-mail: s.shousha@imperial.ac.uk

from Nottingham, UK, covering a 10-year period and published in 2007 included five lung carcinomas, four melanomas, four ovarian carcinomas, and one each for kidney, esophagus, thyroid, small intestine, and prostate carcinoma [5]. The author estimated the incidence of metastatic carcinomas to the breast during the reported period to be 0.3 % of all malignant mammary tumors.

Perhaps the largest reported series is the one published in 2007 from M.D. Anderson Cancer Center in Houston, Texas, and included 169 patients with metastases from solid neoplasms [6]. The lesions were clinically palpable in 77 % of patients and were diagnosed by radiology in 14 %, either as a single (52.7 %) or multiple (24 %) nodules. Fifteen percent of patients had bilateral breast involvement. A prior history of cancer was known in only 88 % of patients at the time of diagnosing the breast metastases. Around one third of patients (65) had melanomas and around 25 % had metastases from respiratory tract tumors. The patients in that series had an age range of 13–85 years with a median of 51 years. The median survival from the time the breast metastases were diagnosed was 10 months with a range of 0.4–192.7 months. Survival was better in patients who had no evidence of other diseases at the time of diagnosis, patients with neuroendocrine tumors, and patients who underwent surgical resection of the breast metastases.

A more recent report of 85 cases of metastases to the breast and axillary lymph nodes diagnosed between 1990 and 2010 at the Memorial Sloan Kettering Cancer Center, New York, included 72 women and 13 men [7]. The metastases were diagnosed before the primary tumor was detected in 11 % of patients. Seventy-seven percent had other metastases at the time of diagnosis. The median age was 54 years (range 15–83). Fifteen percent had multiple nodules and the metastases were bilateral in 12 %. The size of the metastases varied between 5 and 180 mm with a median size of 16.8 mm. Twenty-two percent of patients had melanomas, 17 % ovarian carcinoma, 13 % pulmonary tumors, 8 % gastrointestinal tumors, and 6 % each from genitourinary tract, gynecologic tract, and uterine leiomyosarcoma. Melanoma was the commonest metastases in male as well as female patients. Follow-up was available for 55 patients (65 %), of whom 52 (96 %) died of the disease, with a median survival of 15 months and a range of 1–83 months.

To summarize, metastatic tumors in the breast are rare, but it is important to be aware of their presence. Only one or two cases per year will be seen in a hospital that sees 500 patients with breast cancer every year. Melanomas are the most common cause of metastases to the breast followed by ovarian and lung cancers, although metastases from tumors almost anywhere in the body can occur. The metastases present mostly as a single unilateral nodule, but around 15 % of patients will have multiple or bilateral lesions. Prognosis is poor, but is generally better in patients who have no evidence of disease elsewhere at the time of diagnosing the breast metastases and particularly those who can tolerate surgical excisions.

How to Diagnose Metastases in the Breast

Perhaps the most important step is for the referring clinician to mention in the request form sent with the biopsy the fact that the patient has a history of a previous or current cancer elsewhere in the body. However, in many cases, the referring clinician, mostly a radiologist, might not be aware of the full clinical history, and in around 10 % of patients there is no history of a previous cancer [6, 7]. In these cases the pathologist has to rely on intrinsic features present in the, usually core, biopsy sections.

Starting with the hematoxylin and eosin (H&E)-stained sections, an unusual morphological pattern would be the first noticeable feature. Most primary breast cancers have familiar patterns whether they are ductal, lobular, tubular, mucinous, or any other less common forms. A pattern which does not fit with that of known breast cancer patterns should alert the pathologist to the possibility of metastases, for example, the diffuse sheets of cells with pale-stained cytoplasm and pleomorphic vesicular nuclei with prominent nucleoli that can be seen in melanoma (Fig. 13.1a, b); the unusual glandular structures

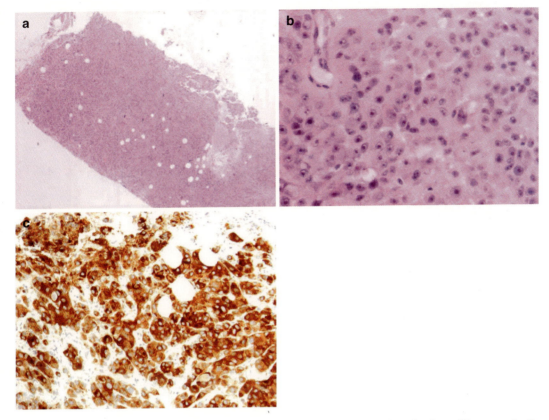

Fig. 13.1 Metastatic malignant melanoma. A 35-year-old female presented with a suspicious lesion of the left breast. She had a past history of malignant melanoma. (**a**) Core biopsy diffusely infiltrated with sheets of neoplastic cells. (**b**) High-power view showing solid groups of cells with abundant eosinophilic cytoplasm with pleomorphic nuclei having prominent nucleoli. (**c**) The cells are positive for Melan A

that can be seen in ovarian (Fig. 13.2a), colonic (Fig. 13.3a), salivary gland (Fig. 13.4a), or renal cell (Fig. 13.5a, b) carcinomas; or the bundles of spindle cells with pleomorphic "cigar"-shaped nuclei of leiomyosarcoma (Fig. 13.6a, b). The absence of DCIS elements and elastosis would enhance the possibility of metastases [5].

The next alarm bell usually rings when the routine immunostained sections for breast cancer, ER, PgR, and HER2, arrive. This is particularly the case for a negative ER staining of a glandular tumor that can be easily mistaken for a primary breast carcinoma, e.g., colonic (Fig. 13.3b) or salivary gland (Fig. 13.4b) metastases. At this stage it might be helpful to contact the referring physician asking if there is information about the patient having a history of extra-mammary carcinoma. Such information would help in limit-ing the number of immunostains that have to be requested to establish the diagnosis.

The final step is to subject the biopsy to a panel of immunostains, trying to identify the primary site of origin of the tumor. The panel will be tailored according to individual circumstances, but usually includes, in addition to ER and GATA3 (for breast carcinoma), CK7, CK20, and CDX2 (for gastrointestinal tumors); TTF1 (for lung tumors); WT1, CA125, and PAX8 (for ovarian tumors, see below); CA19.9 (for pancreatic and hepatobiliary tumors); RCC and CD10 for renal cell carcinoma (Fig. 13.5d, e); chromogranin and synaptophysin (for neuroendocrine tumors); and at least one melanoma marker like S100, Melan A (Fig. 13.1c), or HMB 45. Additional immunostains may be needed like CD45, to exclude lymphomas.

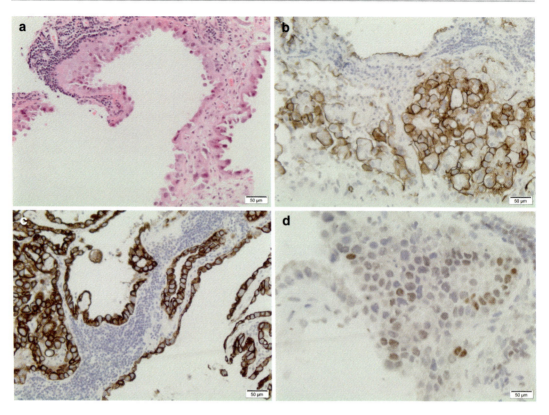

Fig. 13.2 Metastatic clear cell ovarian carcinoma. A 61-year-old female presented with a complex cystic breast lesion. She had a recent history of ovarian carcinoma, clear cell type. (**a**) Core biopsy showing cystic lesion lined by neoplastic clear cells with pleomorphic nuclei. (**b**) The cells are positive for CA125 and (**c**) CK7. (**d**) There was also focal positive staining for GATA3

Six examples are illustrated representing some of the metastases encountered at our hospital during the last few years. These include a metastatic melanoma (Fig. 13.1); clear cell ovarian carcinoma (Fig. 13.2); colonic adenocarcinoma (Fig. 13.3); parotid adenocarcinoma, not otherwise specified (Fig. 13.4); renal cell carcinoma (Fig. 13.5); and uterine leiomyosarcoma (Fig. 13.6). Examples of non-mammary metastases in axillary lymph nodes are illustrated in Chap. 14.

Distinguishing Ovarian Metastases from Primary Breast Carcinoma

This can be difficult because of the overlap of the morphological and immunohistochemical features of breast and ovarian carcinoma that com-monly lead to initial misdiagnosis [7]. Most metastatic ovarian carcinomas are of the serous type and can show a papillary architecture. The presence of prominent psammoma bodies is in favor of ovarian origin. Both tumors are mostly ER and CK7 positive, so these will not be of great help, although a strong ER staining is more commonly seen in breast carcinoma.

The majority of ovarian serous carcinomas are positive for WT1 and CA125, but these can be occasionally positive in breast carcinoma. However, WT1 is strongly and diffusely expressed in 95 % of serous ovarian carcinomas [8], but its expression in the breast seems to be restricted to mucinous carcinomas [8, 9], which are unlikely to be confused with metastatic ovarian carcinoma because of their characteristic morphology. Also, CA125 is strongly expressed in up to 95 % of serous ovarian carcinomas, but it

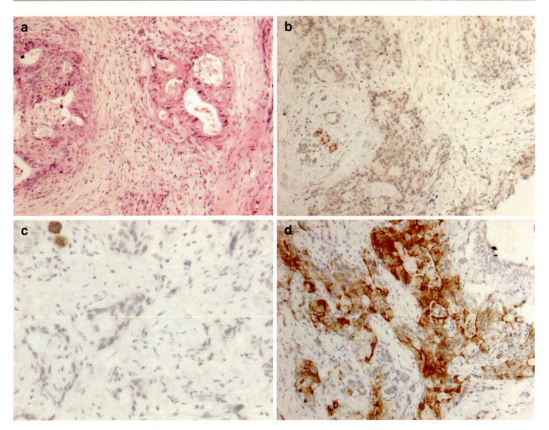

Fig. 13.3 Metastatic colonic adenocarcinoma. A 45-year-old female presented with 2-cm palpable breast lump. Later told she had colonic adenocarcinoma removed 2 years earlier. (**a**) Core biopsy showing a moderately dif- ferentiated adenocarcinoma. The glandular pattern is not typical of what is usually seen in primary breast carci- noma. (**b**) The tumor is ER negative, (**c**) CK7 negative, and (**d**) CK20 positive

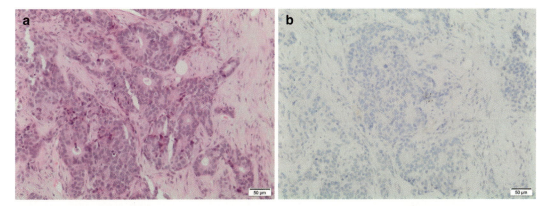

Fig. 13.4 Metastatic parotid adenocarcinoma. A 56-year- old female presented with two small densities in the lower inner aspect of the left breast, 2 cm apart. She had a his- tory of parotid adenocarcinoma, not otherwise specified with lymph node metastasis, removed 2 years earlier. (**a**) Core biopsy showing a moderately differentiated adeno- carcinoma with focal cribriform pattern unlike that com- monly seen in primary cribriform breast carcinoma. (**b**) The tumor is ER negative

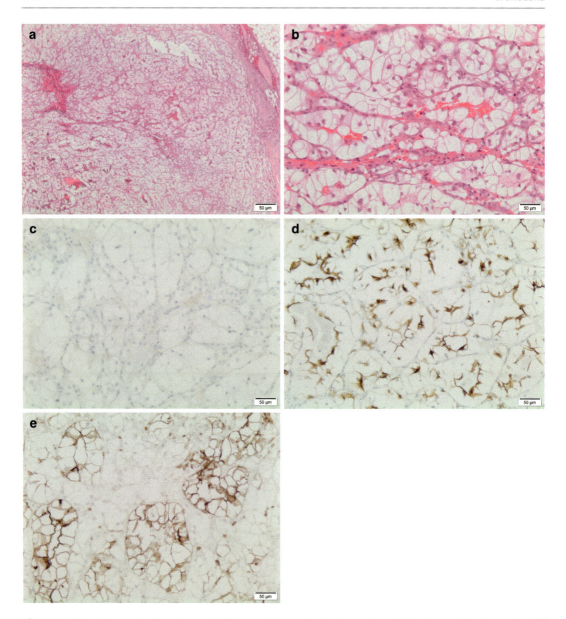

Fig. 13.5 Metastatic renal cell carcinoma. A 82-year-old female who had a history of left breast and renal carcinomas. She presented with a small local recurrence in the left mastectomy scar. (**a**) The lesion was well circumscribed and consists of closely packed clear cells. (**b**) High-power view showing the clear cytoplasm and relatively small nuclei. (**c**) The cells are ER negative, (**d**) RCC Ag positive, and (**e**) CD10 positive

is only expressed focally and weakly in up to 16 % of breast carcinomas [8, 10]. Thus the presence of WT1 and CA125 positivity very strongly favors an ovarian origin [8].

GATA3 and PAX8 are two useful additional markers that have been more recently introduced for that purpose. GATA3 is positive in up to 95 % of breast carcinomas [11, 12] and in only 6–7 % of ovarian serous carcinomas [11, 12] and 13 % of clear cell ovarian carcinoma (Fig. 13.2) [11]. PAX8 is expressed in 99 % of high-grade ovarian serous carcinoma and 71 % of non-serous ovarian carcinoma [13] and was not detected in any of a total of 362 breast carcinomas of various types in two large series of cases [13, 14].

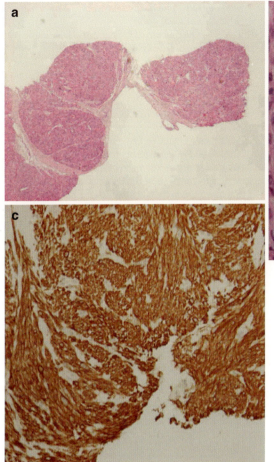

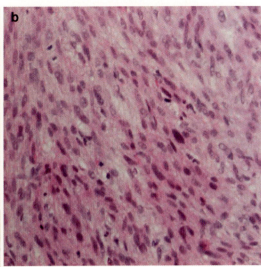

Fig. 13.6 Metastatic leiomyosarcoma. A 59-year-old woman presented with a suspicious breast lesion. She had a previous history of uterine leiomyosarcoma. (**a**) Core biopsy showing sheets of a spindle cell lesion. (**b**) High-power view showing closely packed spindle-shaped cells with pleomorphic cigar-shaped nuclei and scattered mitotic figures. The cells were cytokeratin negative and (**c**) desmin strongly positive

Distinguishing Neuroendocrine Metastases from Primary Breast Carcinoma with Neuroendocrine Differentiation

Primary neuroendocrine tumors of the breast are rare (discussed in Chap. 18). They are classified into three subtypes, well-differentiated (carcinoid-like) and poorly differentiated (small-cell) neuroendocrine tumors and invasive breast carcinoma with neuroendocrine differentiation [15]. They have morphological patterns similar to those seen in neuroendocrine tumors arising in other organs (nests, trabeculae, and minimal glands) and contain similar chromogranin-/synaptophysin-positive granules. Differentiation on morphological grounds can be impossible and relies mainly on immunohistochemistry. In a study of 22 cases of metastatic neuroendocrine tumors to the breast (15 well and 7 poorly differentiated), mainly from the lung and gastrointestinal tract, ER was positive (weak) in only 2 out of 16 cases examined, and GATA3 was negative in all 9 cases studied [16]. In addition, most well-differentiated tumors expressed site-specific markers including TTF1 positivity in seven out of ten lung metastases and CDX2 positivity in all five small intestinal metastases.

References

1. Silverman EM, Oberman HA. Metastatic neoplasms in the breast. Surg Gynecol Obstet. 1974;138:6–28.
2. Charache H. Metastatic tumors in the breast. Ann Surg. 1942;115:47–50.
3. Di Bonito L, Luchi M, Giarelli L, Falconieri G, Viehl P. Metastatic tumors to the female breast. An autopsy study of 12 cases. Pathol Res Pract. 1991;187:432–6.
4. Georgiannos SN, Aleong JC, Goode AW, Sheaff M. Secondary neoplasms of the breast. A survey of the 20th century. Cancer. 2001;92:2259–66.
5. Lee AHS. The histological diagnosis of metastases to the breast from extramammary malignancies. J Clin Pathol. 2007;60:1333–41.
6. Wiliams SA, Ehlers II RA, Hunt KK, Yi M, Kuerer HM, Singletary SE, et al. Metastases to the breast from nonbreast solid neoplasms. Presentation and determinants of survival. Cancer. 2007;110:731–7.
7. DeLair DF, Corben AD, Catalano JP, Vallejo CE, Brogi E, Tan LK. Non-mammary metastases to the breast and axilla: a study of 85 cases. Mod Pathol. 2013;26:343–9.
8. Tornos C, Soslow R, Chen S, Akram M, Hummer AJ, Abu-Rustum N, et al. Expression of WT1, CA125 and GCDFP-15 as useful markers in the differential diagnosis of primary ovarian carcinomas versus metastatic breast cancer to the ovary. Am J Surg Pathol. 2005;29:1482–9.
9. Domfeh AB, Carley AL, Striebel JM, Karabakhtsian RG, Florea AV, McManus K, et al. WT1 immunoreactivity in breast carcinoma: selective expression in pure and mixed mucinous subtypes. Mod Pathol. 2008;21:1217–23.
10. Loy TS, Quesenberry JT, Sharp SC. Distribution of CA125 in adenocarcinomas. Am J Clin Pathol. 1992;98:175–9.
11. Clark BZ, Beriwal S, Dabbs DJ, Bhargava R. Semiquantitative GATA-3 immunoreactivity in breast, bladder, gynecologic tract and other cytokeratin 7-positive carcinomas. Am J Clin Pathol. 2014;142:64–71.
12. Miettinen M, McCue PA, Sarlomo-Rikala M, Rys J, Czpiewski P, Wazny K, et al. GATA3: a multispecific but potentially useful marker in surgical pathology. A systematic analysis of 2500 epithelial and nonepithelial tumors. Am J Clin Pathol. 2014;38:13–22.
13. Laury AR, Perets R, Pio H, Krane JF, Barletta JA, French C, et al. A comprehensive analysis of PAX8 expression in human epithelial tumors. Am J Surg Pathol. 2011;35:816–26.
14. Nonaka D, Chiriboga L, Soslow RA. Expression of Pax8 as a useful marker in distinguishing ovarian carcinomas from mammary carcinomas. Am J Clin Pathol. 2008;32:1566–71.
15. Tan PH, Schnitt SJ, van de Vijver MJ, Ellis IO, Lakhani SR. Papillary and neuroendocrine breast lesions: the WHO stance. Histopathology. 2015;66:761–70.
16. Mohanty SK, Kim SA, DeLair DF, Bose S, Laury AR, Chopra S et al. Comparison of metastatic neuroendocrine neoplasms to the breast and primary invasive mammary carcinomas with neuroendocrine differentiation. Modern Pathol 2016;29:788–798.

Sami Shousha

Abstract

This chapter deals with the current practices of assessing the axillary lymph node status of patients with breast carcinoma. Many patients undergo an axillary node core biopsy or fine needle aspiration prior to surgery. This may be followed, later on, by sentinel node biopsy and/or axillary node clearance depending on the result of the provisional node assessment. Methods for dealing with these different biopsy types are discussed. The chapter ends with a discussion of carcinoma of unknown primary (CUP) origin occasionally seen in axillary lymph nodes.

Keywords

Breast carcinoma • Metastatic carcinoma • Axillary lymph nodes • Sentinel lymph nodes • OSNA • Microbubbles • Carcinoma of unknown primary (CUP) origin • Immunohistochemistry • Benign inclusions in lymph nodes

Current Scheme for Dealing with Axillary Lymph Nodes in Patients with Breast Carcinoma

- Preoperatively, fine needle aspirate (FNA) or core biopsy is carried out if there are lymph nodes that are clinically or radiologically suspicious of malignancy.
- If the FNA or core biopsy is positive for malignancy, axillary dissection can be carried out at the time of breast surgery.

S. Shousha (✉)
Department of Histopathology, Charing Cross Hospital & Imperial College,
Fulham Palace Road, London 6 8RF, UK
e-mail: s.shousha@imperial.ac.uk

- If the FNA or core biopsy is negative for malignancy, sentinel lymph node biopsy is carried out at the time of surgery or, in some occasions, prior to starting neoadjuvant chemotherapy.
- Intraoperative assessment of sentinel nodes is carried out, by varying methods, in some centers, but is not generally recommended as discussed below. However, occasionally intra-operative frozen section may be performed if the node was clinically highly suspicious and the FNA or core biopsy was inconclusive, and the patient has agreed before the operation to proceed with axillary dissection if the frozen section was positive.
- Otherwise, the sentinel lymph node is processed for routine examination.
- If the sentinel node is negative, no further axillary procedures are done.
- If the sentinel node is positive, axillary node clearance may be carried out later on in some patients, depending on the extent of nodal involvement as described below.

Preoperative Ultrasound-Guided Axillary Node Core Biopsy

This is carried now more frequently by radiologists at the time of taking a breast core biopsy if there is a radiologically abnormal lymph node. The yield from a core biopsy is usually better than that of FNA [1, 2]. Although the specificity of both methods is reported to be 100 %, the sensitivity of core biopsy is higher than FNA (88.2 % versus 72.5 %, respectively) [2].

As in breast core biopsies, we initially cut three levels of the axillary lymph node core biopsy and stain them with hematoxylin and eosin (H&E). This is usually enough to detect the tumor if it were there. Occasionally, we may resort to cutting deeper sections or stain a section for pan-cytokeratin (e.g., AE1/AE3), if there are only a few suspicious cells in the original sections. We also cut and examine deeper sections if no tumor was detected in the original set of slides. A problem arises sometimes when the axillary core biopsy consists entirely of carcinoma with no normal lymph node

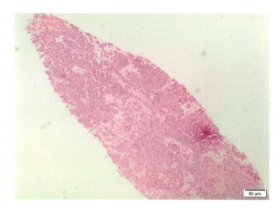

Fig. 14.1 Ultrasound-guided core biopsy of an axillary lymph node. The biopsy consists entirely of tumor with no identifiable lymph node tissue

tissue included (Fig. 14.1). We report the presence of malignancy and discuss the case in our weekly multidisciplinary meeting to ascertain that this is a lymph node metastasis rather than a second primary focus in the breast or its tail.

Preoperative Microbubble Contrast-Enhanced Axillary Sentinel Node Core Biopsy

Microbubbles are ultrasound contrast agents, each smaller than a red blood cell, that act as reflectors of the ultrasound beam. They were initially used for cardiac imaging and their use was later expanded to include hepatic and other organ imaging [3–5]. They have been used for the localization of sentinel nodes, after intradermal injection, in patients with breast cancer and no radiologically abnormal lymph nodes [4]. Once the sentinel node is identified, an ultrasound-guided FNA or core biopsy can be undertaken [5]. In a study of 136 patients, the sentinel node was successfully identified in 93 % of patients [5]. Seventeen patients (13 %) had positive nodes, and these were treated by axillary node clearance. The remaining patients underwent sentinel lymph node biopsies in the usual way. Nine of these (8 %) had positive nodes, four of which were micrometastases. In another study carried out by the same authors, the sensitivity of the test was 61 % and the specificity 100 % [6].

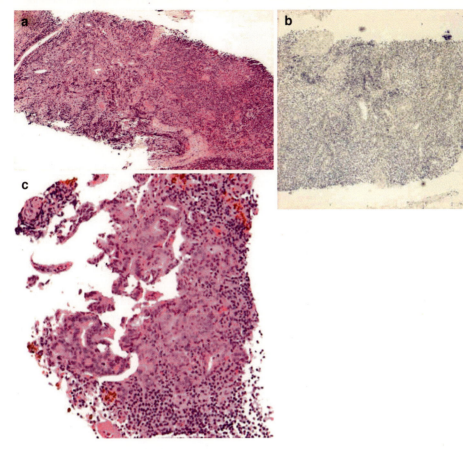

Fig. 14.2 Microbubble-enhanced ultrasound-guided core biopsy of sentinel lymph node. (**a**) A negative core (H&E). (**b**) Same case stained for pan-cytokeratin (AE1/ AE3) confirming the absence of metastasis. (**c**) A positive core biopsy containing metastatic carcinoma (H&E)

We have used the technique at Charing Cross Hospital in a few patients and obtained reasonably sized core biopsies from the enhanced nodes (Fig. 14.2). Because of the inherent limited size of the specimen, a negative biopsy necessitates a conventional sentinel node biopsy, and in some positive cases, it was difficult to assess whether the node had a micro- or macrometastasis. The technique would be most useful if wider biopsy needles are used.

Sentinel Lymph Nodes

The sentinel lymph node is the first node to which lymph drainage and metastasis from breast cancer occur [7, 8]. It is usually situated in level I, but it could be in level II or III, intramammary, interpectoral, and internal mammary node or even a supraclavicular node. The node is identified by injecting a radiolabeled isotope (usually technetium Tc 99m-labeled colloid) or a blue dye or both in the breast skin and then locating the node surgically in the axilla either by a handheld probe that detects gamma ray emission and/or the blue dye color.

Eighty-five percent of patients have a single sentinel node with 15 % having two or more. It has been shown that in the hands of experienced surgeons, the sentinel node, because of its location at the forefront of all other draining nodes, reflects the true axillary lymph node status in 95 % of appropriately selected patients (usually those with tumors less than 3 cm in diameter and clinically negative axilla) [7]. Thus, if the senti-nel node is free of tumor, the patient can be spared from further axillary dissection with its associated high morbidity. The procedure can be applied to patients who had neoadjuvant chemo-therapy prior to their surgery [9].

Radiation Risk

A Consensus Conference statement expressed no objections to the immediate processing of sentinel nodes as "they contain radioactivity (that) results in a level of personal exposure that is a small fraction of the maximum allowable yearly dose." The American Association of Directors of Anatomic and Surgical Pathology have also concluded that delaying the dealing with sentinel lymph nodes does not appear to be justified [10].

However, monitoring the level of radiation in the laboratory and in the examined specimens is recommended as increased radioactivity in the submitted specimens has been noted in some institution over time [11]. In general, it is advis-able that sentinel lymph nodes be dealt with in a special area of the cut-up room. Any contami-nated material used (plastic bag containers and blades) should be disposed of in a special con-tainer according to specific guidelines drawn in accordance with the hospital's radiation safety policy. These safety issues do not arise if only blue dye is used for localization.

Sampling

The current trend in the UK, emphasized by the UK National Guidelines, is toward the routine processing of sentinel nodes, as there are doubts about the accuracy of intraoperative assessment [12]. The nodes are fixed in 10 % neutral formalin and cut, either before or after fixation, into 2-mm-thick slices. This would ensure the detection of all macrometastasis, those larger than 2 mm, as well as most large micrometastases. The slices from each node are placed in one or more cas-settes, according to the node's size, embedded in

paraffin wax, and sections are cut and stained with hematoxylin and eosin (H&E). The UK guidelines recommend cutting and staining just one section from each paraffin block. Some cen-ters, however, cut and stain step sections, usually three, from each block. If the node is very small, less than 5 mm, it is embedded intact and step sections examined.

Immunohistochemistry

The UK guidelines do not recommend the use of cytokeratin immunohistochemistry as a routine to detect occult metastasis, as the yield is very low. Some centers, however, find it advisable to stain at least one section for pan-cytokeratin (AE1/AE3) if the H&E-stained sections are neg-ative [13, 14]. As would be expected, if the lymph node is cut into 2-mm-thick slices, cytokeratin immunohistochemistry of H&E-negative nodes will only identify smaller micrometastases and isolated tumor cells, the significance of which is not known (Fig. 14.3a) [15]. In general, immuno-histochemistry is indicated when worrying cells are seen in H&E-stained sections (Fig. 14.3b, c) particularly in cases of invasive lobular carci-noma where metastatic tumor cells can be diffi-cult to identify.

Microscopic Classification

Microscopically, the metastases are classified into macrometastasis (more than 2 mm across), micrometastasis (0.2–2.0 mm), and isolated tumor cells (less than 0.2 mm or less than 200 tumor cells). If the metastases are present as sep-arate clusters, only the largest cluster is measured and the node classified according to its largest dimension [16]. If the metastases are present as a continuous string of tumor cells, as occurs some-times in metastatic lobular carcinoma, the metas-tasis is classified according to the length of the string. The location of the metastasis, whether nodal, subcapsular, capsular (Fig. 14.3d), or extracapsular (Fig. 14.3e), is not a factor in clas-sification [16].

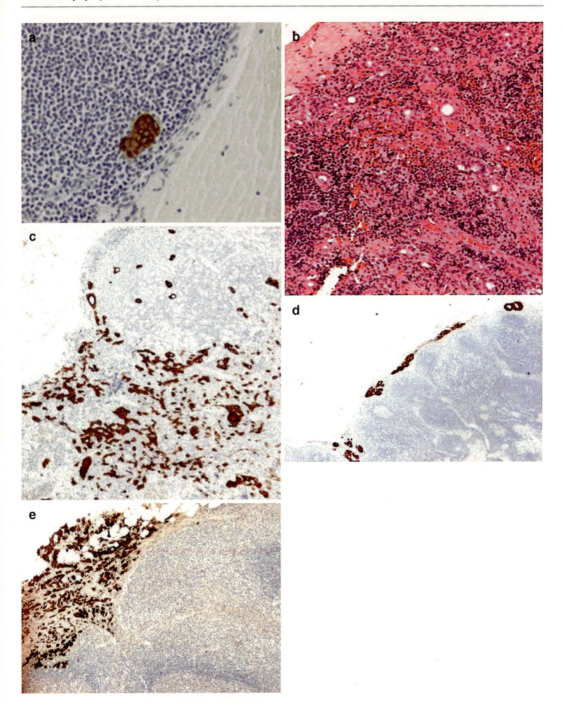

Fig. 14.3 (**a**) A small group of isolated tumor cells identified by pan-cytokeratin (AE1/AE3) immunostaining. (**b**) H&E-stained section of a lymph node containing difficult to see suspicious cells. (**c**) Same case stained with AE1/ AE3 showing a scatter of positively stained malignant cells. (**d**) Capsular metastasis stained with AE1/AE3. The metastasis is classified according to the size of the largest cluster. (**e**) Extracapsular metastasis stained with AE1/AE3

Intraoperative Assessment of Sentinel Nodes

Frozen Section and Imprint Cytology

Some surgeons prefer to have an immediate "intraoperative" result, so that if the node is positive, axillary clearance can be carried out while the patient is still in theater. In this case, a frozen section, cytology imprint, or both can be carried out and the result given to the surgeon within 20 min or so. These morphological intraoperative methods of assessment have a high incidence of false-negative results. The false-negative rate for frozen sections is reported to be as high as 25–40 %, mostly for cases of lobular carcinoma, micrometastasis, and isolated tumor cells. Lymph nodes largely replaced by fat are difficult to cut and assess in frozen sections. Imprint cytology and smears may have higher false-negative rates. However, in our institution, frozen sections are sometimes carried out on clinically highly suspicious lymph nodes in patients whom preoperative diagnosis of axillary lymph nodes was unsuccessful, and the patient has consented for an axillary clearance if the frozen section proved to be positive.

Intraoperative Molecular Assessment

There are more recently introduced "molecular" techniques for the intraoperative assessment of sentinel nodes. The one that is widely available in Europe is called the OSNA system (One-Step Nucleic Acid Amplification; Sysmex Corporation GmbH) [17]. This system relies on detecting and amplifying cytokeratin 19 messenger RNA that is expressed by benign and malignant breast epithelial cells, but not by lymphoid or hemopoietic cells (Fig. 14.4a, b) [18, 19]. The lymph node is received fresh in the laboratory, dissected from the surrounding fat, and homogenized in a test tube, which is then inserted in the device for the assessment. The whole process takes between 30 and 40 min, and up to three lymph nodes can be examined at the same time. We have found 96 % concordance between OSNA and routine histology [20]. The method has the big advantage of meticulously testing the entire lymph node for metastases. A quantitative result is obtained which correlates with the tumor burden in the lymph node. This helps to define the metastasis, when present, as a micro- or a macrometastasis and might also help in predicting the presence or absence of metastases in non-sentinel nodes [21, 22]. If this is validated in a large study, it would help in deciding which patient with positive sentinel node can avoid having axillary clearance. However, there are a few drawbacks for using molecular techniques that have to be kept in mind:

- To give full assessment, the whole node has to be processed, with no tissue left to produce a histology section for permanent record. If part

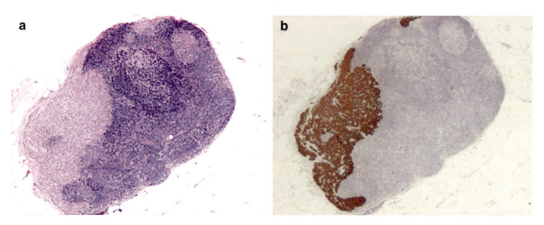

Fig. 14.4 (**a**) An H&E-stained section showing a lymph node with a macrometastasis. (**b**) Same node showing the macrometastasis staining strongly positive for cytokeratin 19. The lymphoid tissue is negative

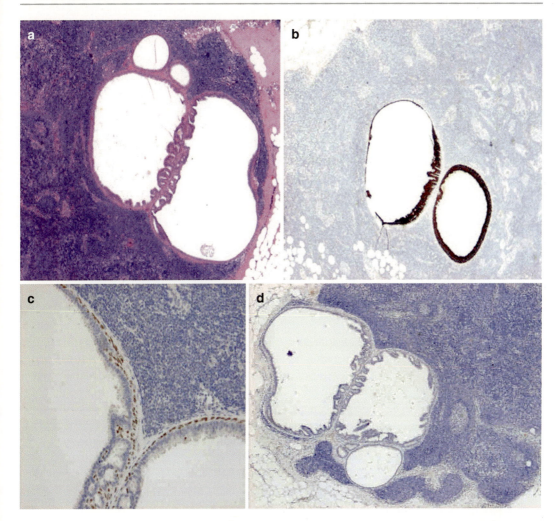

Fig. 14.5 Benign epithelial inclusions in a sentinel lymph node. (**a**) H&E-stained section of the lymph node showing cystically dilated glands within the lymph node. (**b**) Section from the same node showing strong positive staining for pan-cytokeratin (AE1/ AE3), confirming the epithelial nature of the inclusions. (**c**) Positive staining of myoepithelial cells around the cysts with p63 establishes their benign nature. (**d**) Negative staining of the cysts with WT1 indicates that the inclusions are of mammary-like rather than Mullerian-like (endosalpingiosis) tissue which would be WT1 positive and lack myoepithelial cells

of the node is used for histology, "allocation bias" might arise.

- Rarely, benign breast inclusions may be present in lymph nodes (Fig. 14.5), and these may be scored as positive, as the technique cannot differentiate between benign and malignant epithelial elements.
- There are rare breast carcinomas, some medullary, high-grade invasive ductal, papillary, and metaplastic, that are cytokeratin 19 negative [23–25]. For this reason, it has been suggested to stain core biopsies of breast carcinomas beforehand for CK 19 if the OSNA system is going to be used for assessing the sentinel lymph node status [25].
- The presence of other diseases in the lymph node, for example, lymphoma or a granulomatous inflammation, would be missed.

Non-sentinel Nodes, Axillary Sampling, and Clearance

These specimens can be handled while fresh or after overnight fixation, with no need for using clearing techniques. The number of lymph nodes in axillary clearances varies from one patient to another, as well as on the extent of the surgical clearance and thoroughness of the pathological dissection. Small lymph nodes can be missed by less experienced pathologists or less meticulous examination of the specimen, but these are usually the ones not involved by tumor, as the presence of malignancy hardens the node and makes it easily palpable. The average number of lymph nodes in the axilla is around 24, with an average of 11 in level I, 8 in level II (behind the pectoralis minor muscle), and 5 in level III (infraclavicular).

All the nodes in the specimen are identified by palpation, dissected, and dealt with according to their size.

- If they are big enough to be bisected (>5 mm), this is done along the presumed site of their hilum, and both halves are processed in one cassette.
- If the nodes are too small for bisection, they are processed intact, and in this case more than one lymph node may be processed in the same cassette.
- If a lymph node is too big to be included in a cassette and there is obvious tumor involvement, only one slice of that node is processed.
- If the enlarged node does not show obvious macroscopic deposits, the whole node is sectioned horizontally into 2-mm-thick slices and processed in two or more cassettes.

The whole idea is to keep track of the number of lymph nodes dissected from the specimen, so it is vital to record in the block description the number of nodes in each cassette. We usually examine one H&E-stained section from each paraffin block. However, we do immunohistochemistry for pan-cytokeratin, particularly in lobular carcinoma, if suspicious cells are seen in an otherwise negative-looking H&E-stained section (Fig. 14.3b, c).

Can Axillary Lymph Node Dissection Be Avoided?

Axillary lymph node dissection is a staging procedure with little or no impact on survival or mortality. The need for axillary clearance in sentinel node-positive patients is being questioned. Growing evidence indicates that omission of axillary clearance in patients with positive sentinel node is safe [26]. The (UK) Association of Breast Surgery and American Society of Clinical Oncology recommended omitting axillary clearance in patients with micrometastases and in selected patients with one or two positive nodes who are going to undergo conservative surgery followed by radiotherapy [27].

Carcinoma of Unknown Primary (CUP)

Occasionally abnormal axillary lymph nodes are detected by radiologists in patients with no evidence of breast cancer. Core biopsies are usually taken. Many of these will prove on histological examination to be reactive in nature. A few would have a lymphoproliferative hematological disorder that needs referring to a hematologist. Only a rare case would show a carcinoma, and as there is no known carcinoma in the breast, the pathologist's advice would be sought regarding the possible primary site of origin.

Morphology

The commonest primary site for a metastatic carcinoma in an axillary lymph node is the

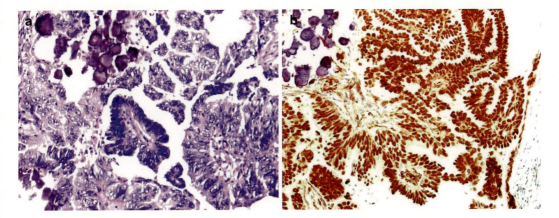

Fig. 14.6 Metastatic ovarian adenocarcinoma in a core of an axillary lymph node. (**a**) H&E sections showing a prominent papillary pattern associated with a group of psammoma bodies. (**b**) The tumor cells are strongly positive for WT1

breast. The morphology of the tumor in H&E-stained sections would give a preliminary idea whether the tumor could be of an occult mammary or extra-mammary origin. As in metastases to the breast, the commonest extra-mammary metastases to the axillary lymph nodes include melanomas followed by ovarian and lung carcinomas, but metastases from many other organs have also been reported [28]. As discussed in Chap. 13, certain morphologies sometimes point to specific organs and that would help in selecting the immunohistologic tests that would be most useful in reaching a conclusion. For example, a papillary pattern associated with psammoma bodies would be highly suggestive of an ovarian origin (Fig. 14.6)

Immunohistochemistry

It has been estimated that immunohistochemistry is successful in detecting the primary origin of the tumor in 66 % of cases [29]. The immunohistochemical panel used should always include ER and GATA3 to investigate the possibility of a metastasis from an occult primary breast carcinoma or, in very rare instances, a breast carcinoma arising in ectopic breast tissue

in the axilla or lymph nodes. CK7 and CK20 are also routinely included to cover a variety of organs including the breast, lung, hepatobiliary tract, stomach, and colorectum. Also included is one or more of the melanoma markers Melan A, S100, and HMB45 (Fig. 14.7); TTF1 for lung cancer (Fig. 14.8); one or more of the ovarian markers WT1, C125, and PAX8; one or both of the neuroendocrine markers chromogranin and synaptophysin; CD10 for urological tumors; and CD45 to exclude lymphoma. The tumor is sometimes so poorly differentiated that morphology is of no help and identification will depend solely on immunohistochemistry (Fig. 14.9). In around a third of cases, morphology and immunohistochemistry fail to identify the primary site of origin, and other means have to be tried including radiology and molecular pathology.

Further Radiological Investigations

If the histology is strongly in favor of a primary breast origin, breast MRI is carried out looking for an occult tumor. Otherwise, CT scans are performed to confirm the histologically suggested primary site of origin or to identify a hidden site that histology failed to pinpoint.

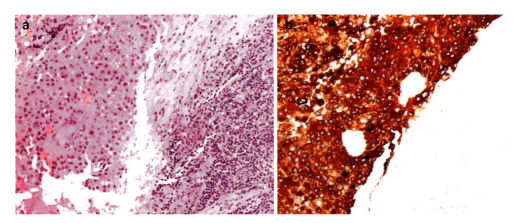

Fig. 14.7 Metastatic melanoma (**a**) H&E sections showing the lymph node with a sheet of melanoma cells on the left. (**b**) The melanoma cells show strong positive staining with HMB45

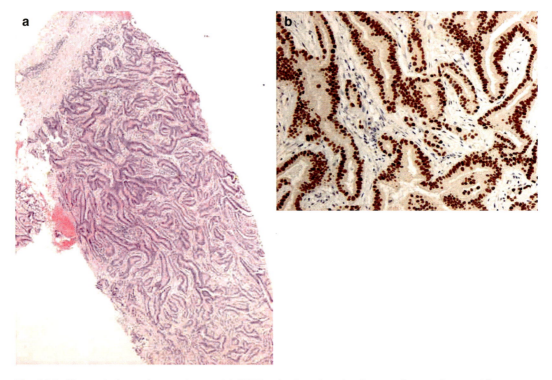

Fig. 14.8 Metastatic lung adenocarcinoma. (**a**) H&E-stained section showing an adenocarcinoma with a pattern different from that expected in the breast. (**b**) The primary lung origin is confirmed by this strong TTF1 expression

Molecular Studies

A variety of molecular techniques are available to identify the primary site of origin using gene expression profiling [30]. More recently, it has been suggested that next-generation sequencing may ultimately be used to determine the specific molecular signature of the tumor (*rather than its primary site of origin*) upon which the treatment can be based [31, 32].

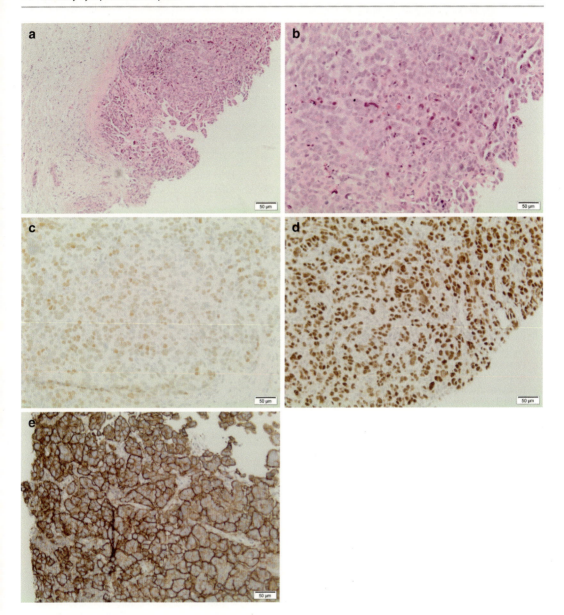

Fig. 14.9 Axillary lymph node with metastatic carcinoma. (**a**) Low-power view of an H&E-stained sections. The tumor is poorly differentiated and could be of primary breast origin. (**b**) High-power view of the same section. (**c**) The tumor was weakly ER positive (**d**) but showed strong expression of WT1 and (**e**) CA125 confirming a primary ovarian origin

References

1. Houssami N, Ciatto S, Turner RM, Cody III HS, Macaskill P. Preoperative ultra-sound guided needle biopsy of axillary nodes in invasive breast cancer. Meta-analysis of its accuracy and utility in staging the axilla. Ann Surg. 2011;254:243–51.

2. Rautiainen S, Masarwah A, Sudah M, Sutela A, Pelkonen O, Joukainen S, et al. Axillary lymph node biopsy in newly diagnosed invasive breast cancer: comparative accuracy of fine-needle aspiration biopsy versus core-needle biopsy. Radiology. 2013;269: 54–60.

3. Wilson SR, Burns PN. Microbubble-enhanced US in body imaging: what rule? Radiology. 2010;257:24–39.

4. Sever AR, Mills P, Jones SE, Cox K, Weeks J, Fish D, Jones PA. Preoperative sentinel node identification with ultrasound using microbubbles in patients with breast cancer. AJR. 2011;196:251–6.
5. Sever AR, Mills P, Weeks J, Jones SE, Fish D, Jones PA, Mali W. Preoperative needle biopsy of sentinel lymph nodes using intradermal microbubbles and contrast-enhanced ultrasound in patients with breast cancer. AJR. 2012;198:465–70.
6. Cox K, Sever A, Jones S, Weeks J, Mills P, Devalia H, Fish D, Jones P. Validation of a technique using microbubbles and contrast enhanced ultrasound (CEUS) to biopsy sentinel lymph node (SLN) in preoperative breast cancer patients with a normal greyscale axillary ultrasound. Eur J Surg Oncol. 2013;39:760–5.
7. Veronesi U, Viale G, Paganelli G, Zurrida S, Luini A, Galimberti V, et al. Sentinel lymph node biopsy in breast cancer. Ten-year results of a randomized controlled study. Ann Surg. 2010;251:595–600.
8. Jaffer S, Bleiweiss IJ. Evolution of sentinel lymph node biopsy in breast cancer, in and out of vogue? Adv Anat Pathol. 2014;21:433–42.
9. Kuehn T, Bauerfeind I, Fehm T, Fleige B, Housschild M, Helms G, et al. Sentinel-lymph-node biopsy in patients with breast cancer before and after neoadjuvant chemotherapy (SENTINA): a prospective, multicenter cohort study. Lancet Oncol. 2013;14:609–18.
10. Fitzgibbons PL, Livolsi VA, on behalf of the Surgical Pathology Committee of the College of Anatomic Pathologists and the Association of directors of Anatomic and Surgical Pathology. Recommendations for handling radioactive specimens obtained by sentinel lymphadenectomy. Am J Surg Pathol. 2000;24:1549–51.
11. Ranshaw AA, Kish R, Gould EW. Increasing radiation from sentinel node specimens in pathology over time. Am J Clin Pathol. 2010;134:299–302.
12. Dixon JM, Rutgers E, Hunt KK. Intraoperative assessment of axillary lymph nodes in patients with breast cancer. Time to abandon? BMJ. 2014;349:g6803.
13. Yared MA, Middleton LP, Smith TL, Kim HW, Ross MI, Hunt KK, Sahin AA. Recommendations for sentinel lymph node processing in breast cancer. Am J Surg Pathol. 2002;26:377–82.
14. Verma R, Rajan SS, Verghese ET, Horgan K, Hanby AM, Lane S. Pathological evaluation of the staging axillary lymph nodes for breast cancer: a national survey in the United Kingdom. Histopathology. 2014;65:707–11.
15. Klevesath MB, Bobrow LG, Pinder SE, Purushotham AD. The value of immunohistochemistry in sentinel lymph node histopathology in breast cancer. Br J Cancer. 2005;92:2201–5.
16. Turner RR, Weaver DL, Cserni G, Lester SC, Hirsch K, Elashoff DA, et al. Nodal stage classification for breast carcinoma: improving interobserver reproduc-

ibility through standardized histologic criteria and image-based training. J Clin Oncol. 2008;26:258–63.
17. Tsujimoto M, Nakabayashi K, Yoshidome K, Kaneko T, Iwase T, Akiyama F, et al. One step nucleic acid amplification for intraoperative detection of lymph node metastasis in breast cancer patients. Clin Cancer Res. 2007;13:4807–16.
18. Schoenfeld A, Luqmani Y, Smith D, O'Reilly S, Shousha S, Sinnett HD, Coombes RC. Detection of breast cancer micrometastases in axillary lymph nodes by using polymerase chain reaction. Cancer Res. 1994;54:2986–90.
19. Schoenfeld A, Luqmani Y, Sinnett HD, Shousa S, Coombes RC. Keratin 19 mRNA measurement to detect micrometastasis in lymph nodes in breast cancer patients. Br J Cancer. 1996;74:1639–42.
20. Snook K, Layer G, Jackson P, deVries C, Shousha S, Nigar E, et al. Multicentre evaluation of intraoperative molecular analysis of sentinel lymph nodes in breast carcinoma. Br J Surg. 2011;98:527–35.
21. Osako T, Iwase T, Kimura K, Horii R, Akiyama F. Sentinel node tumour burden quantified based on cytokeratin19 mRNA copy number predicts non-sentinel node metastases in breast cancer: molecular whole-node analysis of all removed nodes. Eur J Cancer. 2013;49:1187–95.
22. Peg V, Espinosa-Bravo M, Vieittes B, Vilardell F, Antunez JR, de Salas MS, et al. Intraoperative molecular analysis of total tumor load in sentinel lymph node: a new predictor of axillary status in early breast cancer patients. Breast Cancer Res Treat. 2013;139:87–93.
23. Dalal P, Shousha S. Keratin 19 in paraffin sections of medullary carcinoma and other benign and malignant breast lesions. Mod Pathol. 1995;8:413–6.
24. Alvarenga CA, Paravidino PI, Alvarenga M, Dufloth R, Gomes M, Zeferino LC, Schmitt F. Expression of CK19 in invasive breast carcinomas of special histological types: implications for the use of one-step nucleic acid amplification. J Clin Pathol. 2011;64:493–7.
25. Vilardell F, Novell A, Martin J, Santacana M, Velasco A, Diez-Castro MJ, et al. Importance of assessing Ck19 immunostaining in core biopsies in patients subjected to sentinel node study by OSNA. Virchows Arch. 2012;460:569–75.
26. Barry M, Kell MR. Breast cancer: can axillary lymph node dissection be avoided? Eur J Surg Oncol. 2012;38:6–7.
27. Lyman GH, Tamin S, Edge SB, Newman LA, Turner RR, Weaver DI, et al. Sentinel lymph node biopsy for patients with early stage breast cancer. American Society of Clinical Oncology clinical practice guideline update. J Clin Oncol. 2014;32:1365–83.
28. DeLair DF, Corben AD, Catalano JP, Vallejo CE, Brogi E, Tan LK. Non-mammary metastases to the breast and axilla: a study of 85 cases. Mod Pathol. 2013;26:343–9.

29. Anderson GG, Weiss LM. Determining tissue of origin for metastatic cancers. Meta-analysis and literature review of immunohistochemistry performance. Appl Immunohistochem Mol Morphol. 2010;18:3–8.
30. Monzon FA, Lyons-Weiler M, Buturovic LJ, Ted Rigl C, Henner WD, Sciulli C, et al. Multicenter validation of a 1,550-gene expression profile for identification of tumor tissue of origin. J Clin Oncol. 2009;27:2503–8.
31. Silverman JF, Elsheikh TM. The value of molecular analysis for the workup of metastasis of unknown primary origin. Pathol Case Rev. 2014;19:8–12.
32. Dolled-Filhart MP, Rimm DL. Gene expression array analysis to determine tissue of origin of carcinoma of unknown primary: cutting edge or already obsolete. Cancer Cytopathology. 2013;3:129–35.

A Practical Approach to the Use of Immunohistochemistry in the Diagnosis and Management of Breast Disease

15

Colin A. Purdie

Abstract

This chapter provides comprehensive information concerning the use of immunohistochemistry in breast pathology. It starts with outlining the general principles and quality assurance issues that should be followed concerning tissue fixation and processing and result interpretation. Various antibodies used for the diagnosis of breast diseases including those used for providing prognostic and predictive information are then dealt with individually supported by ample illustrations.

Keywords

Breast cancer • Breast pathology • Immunohistochemistry • Differential diagnosis • Biomarker • Protein expression

Abbreviations

AVL	Atypical vascular lesion
DCIS	Ductal carcinoma in situ
EGFR	Epidermal growth factor receptor
EMA	Epithelial membrane antigen
EQA	External quality assurance
ER	Estrogen receptor
FISH	Fluorescent in situ hybridization
GCDFP	Gross cystic disease fluid protein
HER2	Human epidermal growth factor receptor 2
IDC	Invasive ductal carcinoma
IHC	Immunohistochemistry
ILC	Infiltrating lobular carcinoma
LCIS	Lobular carcinoma in situ
Mwt	Molecular weight
NBF	Neutral buffered formalin
PR	Progesterone receptor
SMMHC	Smooth muscle myosin heavy chain

C.A. Purdie
Department of Pathology, Ninewells Hospital &
Medical School, University of Dundee,
Dundee DD1 9SY, UK
e-mail: colin.purdie@nhs.net

© Springer International Publishing Switzerland 2017
S. Shousha (ed.), *Breast Pathology*, DOI 10.1007/978-3-319-28655-6_15

Introduction

Background

The use of antibodies to label and visualize antigens *in situ* within cells and tissues was first described in 1941 using antibodies fused to a fluorescent molecule [1]. Since that first description, the techniques have become more refined and exact with the use of monoclonal antibodies and ever more sensitive detection systems.

Immunohistochemistry (IHC) has become central to the diagnosis and management of breast disease. The identification of the proteins expressed by individual cells as well as their cellular localization allied to the tissue morphology permits a much more precise diagnosis to be reached permitting better management decisions and therapy.

In particular, IHC is essential to the management of breast cancer both in qualitative (diagnostic) and quantitative (predictive) terms. Breast IHC gives information central to the diagnosis of breast cancer, provides prognostic information, and also predicts response to specific targeted therapies. As distinct biological subtypes of breast cancer are identified using gene expression profiling, IHC shows promise as a cheaper and faster way to subclassify breast cancers into groups with specific behaviors and response to different therapies that should lead to improved patient survival and quality of life

General Issues

The basic principles of good IHC in breast disease are the same as those for IHC in any other cellular pathology setting. The potential problems break down into three areas: tissue preparation and processing (pre-analytical), immunostaining (analytical), and interpretation (post-analytical). All of these can be important in different settings and to a variable degree (Table 15.1). It is, therefore, important to minimize the impact of each of them by optimizing all steps in the process and aiming for maximum consistency to maintain diagnostic integrity:

1. *Pre-analytical:*
   - *Time to fixation*: The time between obtaining the specimen and entering fixative should be as short as possible (this is usually straightforward for core biopsies, and, for this reason, core biopsies usually give the most consistent immunostaining). Delays in fixation adversely affect breast IHC [2]. Resection specimens should be incised as soon as possible after they are removed from the patient to permit rapid fixation (this is vital for good histology as well as IHC). Adequate volumes of fixative should be used, but the most important issue is that the lesion of interest is exposed to fixative quickly and adequately. Thus, tumors should be incised or sliced usually within 30–60 min or may be refrigerated for a short period (without any appreciable loss in morphology or antigenicity) prior to preparation for fixation.
   - *Type of fixative*: For almost all IHC purposes, neutral buffered formalin (NBF) is the fixative of choice. NBF does have the disadvantage (as far as breast pathology is concerned) of being aqueous. This means that it penetrates fatty tissue relatively slowly, again emphasizing the importance of timely specimen preparation prior to immersion in fixative.
   - *Duration of fixation*: This should be sufficient to allow the specimen to completely fix. NBF penetrates tissues at roughly 1 mm per hour. Thus, a 2 mm diameter core biopsy will usually be adequately fixed in 1 h. However, the tumor in an unincised wide local excision or mastectomy would be autolyzed before the fixative had penetrated the tissue sufficiently to permit tumor fixation. The greater the surface-to-volume ratio, the more rapid and complete will be fixation – tumors sliced into 5 mm thick slice will be adequately fixed in 10 h or less. For this reason, sequential 5 mm slicing is the method of choice in this author's practice. Overfixation can also be an issue in that it can lead to loss of antigenicity although this is antigen and antibody

Table 15.1 Summary of factors involved in producing a consistent, high-quality IHC service

Timing	Factor	Recommendation	Significance	Comments
Pre-analytical	Time to fixation	As soon as possible; 30–60 min	Delays in fixation cause tissue autolysis resulting in poor tissue morphology and loss of antigenicity	Periods of refrigeration prior to preparation and fixation do not seem to cause problems with IHC
	Fixative	Neutral buffered formalin (NBF)	Cheap and plentiful. Preserves tissue leaving proteins, DNA, and RNA intact and available for in situ analysis permitting morphological correlation	Also allows the use of other techniques such as in situ hybridization and gene expression studies
	Tissue preparation	Most specimens larger than a core or vacuum biopsy should be sliced or incised through the tumor. This increases the surface-to-volume ratio facilitating fixation	As an aqueous fixative, NBF penetrates fatty tissue poorly meaning that the tumor would autolyze before the fixative reached and fixed the tumor if it were not incised	All breast specimens should be prepared for fixation on the day of surgery
	Duration of fixation	6–72 h	Underfixation results in poor processing; Overfixation can cause reduced antigenicity	This recommendation is for ER and HER2 IHC but is sensible to apply to all breast specimens
	Tissue processing	Standard overnight protocols	Little published data; Good processing is important for consistent IHC	Shortened, rapid processing protocols require formal validation of IHC prior to diagnostic use
Analytical	Antibody	Use validated antibodies with known sensitivity and specificity; Test for batch-to-batch consistency with new batches of antibody	Even commercial antibodies can show batch-to-batch variation in sensitivity	
	Immunostainers	Consider the use of automated immunostainer	Computer-controlled immunostainers remove (from certain aspects of IHC) the risk of human error	Automated immunostainers provide high levels of consistency
	Controls	Use appropriate positive (on-slide) and negative controls	This provides evidence that the IHC has worked and is of adequate specificity to permit interpretation	For ER and HER2, positive controls with a range of expression levels should be used
	Quality assurance	IHC performance should be subject to external QA	Without external validation, IHC performance may gradually deteriorate unnoticed	Participation in EQA ensures constant vigilance regarding IHC and helps to maintain good performance
Post-analytical	Interpretation	All pathologists require appropriate training in the interpretation of IHC	The interpretation is at least partly subjective and requires experience and training	
	Audit	All IHC should be subject to regular audit; The frequency of ER and HER2 IHC should be subject to continuous ongoing audit	Audit helps to reassure that all aspects of IHC are functioning adequately	

specific [3]. The effects of overfixation may be overcome by prolonged antigen retrieval, but this is at the expense of analytical consistency. For ER and HER2 testing, at least, the recommendations are for fixing excisional specimens for between 6 and 72 h [4], and it seems sensible to adopt these guidelines for all breast specimens.

- *Tissue processing*: There are few data on this variable. Consistent tissue processing of adequately fixed tissue is required for reliable, good-quality IHC. Most modern, automated tissue processors provide this. A change to the use of short, rapid process cycles would require a period of revalidation to ensure that the results of IHC on tissue derived from the new process are directly comparable to those from the previously validated cycle.

2. *Analytical:*
- *Validated antibodies*: All antibodies require validation prior to diagnostic use. They should be applied to a test tissue with known levels of expression to ensure that the appropriate tissues are staining adequately and that non-expressing tissues are truly negative. Each new batch of antibody should be tested in parallel with the previous batch to ensure batch-to-batch consistency. Most antibodies in current diagnostic use can be supplied by commercial organizations with good levels of quality control. However, validation of new antibodies and between batches is still necessary.
- *Automated immunostainers*: These provide high levels of consistency and reliability and are particularly useful in laboratories with large volumes of diagnostic IHC. Running costs for these may be high due to the requirement for the use of prefilled reagents only available from the manufacturer. The use of computer control of all of the stages along with bar-coded slide and reagent recognition does remove many of the potential "human error" problems.
- *Controls*: All IHC assays require both a positive and negative control:
  - The negative control goes through the entire IHC process but without the addition of the primary antibody, just the

antibody buffer. This controls for non-specific (i.e., non-primary antibody-related) staining which could be caused by many factors including endogenous peroxidase activity or nonspecific binding of any of the other components in the detection system.
  - The positive control should, ideally, be on the same slide as the test section to ensure that it undergoes exactly the same process as the test section (Fig. 15.1). The positive control tissue should include expressing and non-expressing tissues to provide information on the specificity of the staining. In assays (such as ER and HER2) where the level of expression is critical, and not simply the presence or absence of expression, then several tissues with varying levels of expression should be used. These should include, at least, tissue with no expression, high expression, and intermediate levels of expression. It is worth bearing in mind that, even with on-slide controls, the test and control sections may not be treated in exactly the same way despite being very close to each other and on the same slide. Close attention should always be paid to the pattern of expression in the test tissue even if the positive control looks adequate. Incomplete coverage of the slide by reagents at any stage in the process can cause inconsistencies between test and control. For instance, close scrutiny for ER expression in benign epithelial elements should be sought before calling a tumor ER negative even if the on-slide control is satisfactory.
- *Laboratory procedures*: It is clearly vital that the histotechnology staff are well trained and understand the importance of all stages of the IHC process. This is particularly important in troubleshooting when things go wrong. The ability to analyze the various components in the IHC process is vital to testing each one when there are problems in order to identify where the problem is located. Clear, written standard operating procedures (SOPs) are

important to maintain a consistent level of IHC output that is so heavily relied upon by pathologists.

3. *Post-analytical:*
- *Audit*: All IHC processes should be subject to audit. However, this is particularly important for those biomarkers which are used to guide adjuvant therapy in breast cancer management (ER and HER2). A rolling audit of levels of positivity for ER and HER2 should be carried out and the frequencies of positivity compared to published national values to ensure that problems are identified and corrected. Where there is a confirmatory test (such as HER2 FISH), then this should also be audited and compared to the IHC and national published values.
- *Quality assurance*: External quality assurance (EQA) is central to a robust and responsive IHC service. This involves the independent, external review of IHC carried out on tissue from the host institution and that supplied by the EQA organization. Such a system allows benchmarking against large numbers of similar institutions and helps to maintain quality and consistency as well as providing early warning of problems either with the submitting organization or, in some cases, with a commercial product supplied to a number of laboratories.
- *Pathologist performance*: All pathologists require training in the assessment of IHC. This occurs during their specialist postgraduate training. However, in order to avoid interpretational drift, trained pathologists require interobserver rates of reporting IHC to be monitored to ensure consistency.
- *Reporting*: In areas of qualitative assessment, this is dependent on ongoing training, professional discussion, case review, attendance at training meetings, and continuing professional development. However, when the assessment is quantitative (ER and HER2), then there is requirement for clear, published guidelines (discussed in the relevant sections) and audit (discussed above).

Fig. 15.1 Low-power view of a core biopsy stained for HER2. The test section (core biopsy of breast) is on the *right*-hand side, and a control section is on the *left*-hand side which shows positive tumor cells and negative non-neoplastic cells. This provides confirmation that the IHC has worked (on this particular slide) and that the appropriate cells are stained positively or negatively. This is of importance when the test section shows no staining with a particular antibody and contains no internal control tissue

General Principles

Since its first discovery, IHC has become central to the diagnosis and management of breast disease. In general terms, IHC should usually be carried out in panels with more than one antibody to a particular antigen or class of antigens. A diagnosis that depends on the staining of one antibody alone should be viewed with caution and corroboration sought by other means.

Although the utility of IHC in breast cancer pathology has been developed empirically over more than 30 years, the advent of gene expression profiling in 2000 [5, 6] has revealed a novel way of molecular subtyping breast cancer that produces useful data for prognostication and therapy response prediction. Indeed, some have claimed that these molecular subtypes are associated with distinct clinical presentations, sites of relapse, histological features, responses to chemotherapy, and outcomes [7, 8]. Gene expression profiling is currently too expensive and too demanding in terms of technical expertise and logistics to be put into clinical practice. However, IHC can be used to provide surrogates for this molecular taxonomy [9] providing further information to guide diagnosis and therapy in breast cancer.

In the following sections, the antibodies that are useful in the management of breast disease will be discussed. The diagnostic categories used are those in the most recent edition of the *WHO Classification of Tumours of the Breast* [10].

Cytokeratins

Background

Cytokeratins (CKs) are the intermediate filament proteins that form the intracytoplasmic cytoskeleton of epithelial cells. Cytokeratins have important roles in mechanical stability within the cell but are also involved in processes such as mitosis, cell migration, and differentiation. They are located in the cytoplasm and, although usually referred to as "cytokeratins," are, more accurately, termed simply "keratins" since the development of a new consensus nomenclature [11]. However, in view of its common usage in pathological publications, "cytokeratin" will be used in this chapter.

A total of 54 cytokeratin genes exist, and they are expressed in highly specific patterns related to the epithelial type and stage of cellular differentiation [12]. Cytokeratins are subdivided into two groups: type I (acidic) and type II (basic or neutral). They are typically found in pairs comprising one of each subtype. The first classification divided them into type I (CK 9–19) and type II (CK1-8) [13], but since then many more have been discovered culminating in a new nomenclature [11]. Cytokeratins may also be classified on the basis of their molecular weight (mwt). This section will confine its discussion to those

cytokeratins with utility in the diagnosis of breast disease (Table 15.2).

When epithelial cells undergo neoplastic transformation, they tend to maintain their original pattern of CK expression making CK IHC a useful tool for diagnosing and classifying tumors. Antibodies directed against different CKs have a variety of uses depending upon their specificities.

General (Broad-Spectrum) Cytokeratins

The general or broad-spectrum CKs are those which identify a large number of cytokeratins of both low and high molecular weight thus giving the best chance of picking up the expression of any cytokeratin while using the fewest number of assays. They have a number of uses in breast disease (Table 15.3).

Identification of Occult Carcinoma

- This can be of particular importance in the identification of infiltrating lobular carcinoma within stroma or adipose tissue. In cases where there is a clinical or imaging abnormality but no obvious tumor in a biopsy or within foci of fat necrosis, CK IHC can reveal invasive carcinoma (Fig. 15.2).
- Biopsies showing crush artifact where the nature of cells cannot be ascertained on morphology.

Table 15.2 Cytokeratin antibodies of diagnostic utility in the management of breast disease

	Antibody	CK Moll No.	Comments
General	AE1/3	1–8, 10, 15, 16, and 19	A useful and dependable wide-spectrum CK antibody
	Cam 5.2	8, 18, and ?7	Mainly stain luminal epithelium
	CK 7	7	
	MNF116	5, 6, 8, 17, and 19	A useful and dependable wide-spectrum CK antibody
Luminal	CK 8	8	Ductal (luminal) epithelium (benign and malignant)[a]
	CK 18	18	
Basal	CK 5	5	Basal (myoepithelial) cells and benign luminal epithelial cells
	CK 14	14	
	34βE12	1, 5, 10, and 14	

[a]May be negative in basal-like cancers

- Necrotic tumor showing only cell "ghosts" may still retain sufficient cytoplasmic CK to be "resurrected" and reveal their epithelial nature.

Identification of Microinvasion

This would be carried out in conjunction with basal (myoepithelial) or basement membrane markers. Microinvasion is usually diagnosed in the context of high-grade ductal carcinoma in situ (DCIS). Surrounding the colonized ducts in such cases, there is often a dense lymphoid infiltrate making identification of low-volume microinvasive disease impossible using only morphology. In these cases, individual epithelial cells and small clusters can be highlighted by CK IHC (Fig. 15.3). It is also necessary, in such cases, to confirm that the cells in question have lost their attendant myoepithelial cells or basement membrane (see later section).

Identification of Low-Volume Residual Malignant Disease Post-chemotherapy

Neoadjuvant chemotherapy is being used increasingly frequently both within the context of T4 disease and to downstage T2 and T3 tumors to allow conservation surgery. With response rates of up to 87 % [14] and pathological complete responses (pCR, no residual in situ, invasive or lymph node metastatic disease) in up to 39 % (especially in HER2-positive and triple-negative disease) [15], the tumor bed can be difficult to assess. Individual, residual carcinoma cells may resemble macrophages (and vice versa), but this can be resolved easily using CK IHC. This permits an accurate assessment of the residual disease which has proven prognostic significance [14].

Table 15.3 Summary of usefulness of general (broad-spectrum) cytokeratins

Utility	Caveats
Identification of occult carcinoma	Will not differentiate benign from malignant
Identification of microinvasion	Requires to be used in conjunction with myoepithelial marker
Identification of residual disease post-chemotherapy	Endogenous peroxidase activity in macrophages
Identification and confirmation of metastatic carcinoma in lymph nodes	Requires morphological and IHC differentiation from benign nodal inclusions

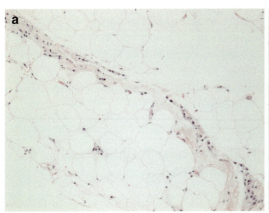
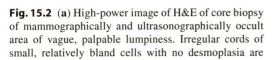
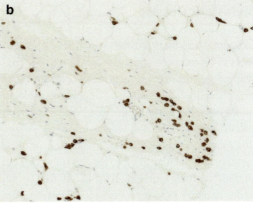

Fig. 15.2 (**a**) High-power image of H&E of core biopsy of mammographically and ultrasonographically occult area of vague, palpable lumpiness. Irregular cords of small, relatively bland cells with no desmoplasia are visible. (**b**) IHC with AE1/3 shows that these cells are epithelial in origin and were ultimately shown to be an infiltrating lobular carcinoma

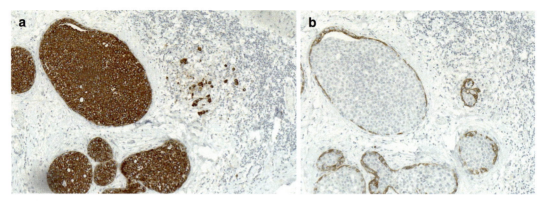

Fig. 15.3 (a) AE1/3 staining of an area of carcinoma in situ (*left*) with cells in adjacent stroma largely obscured by a dense inflammatory cell infiltrate. (b) These are confirmed to represent microinvasion by the absence of any surrounding myoepithelium on CK5 staining

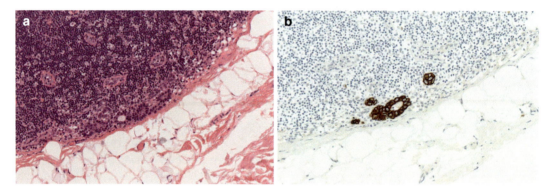

Fig. 15.4 (a) H&E showing low-volume metastatic disease in an axillary lymph node. (b) This is confirmed on AE1/3 and no further occult metastatic disease found resulting in staging as pN0(i+), isolated tumor cells only

Identification and Accurate Classification of Lymph Node Metastatic Disease

In nodes where there are cells which are difficult to identify on morphological grounds alone, CK IHC will provide the necessary certainty (Fig. 15.4). As even small-volume disease (including isolated tumor cells) has a measurable detrimental effect on outcome, this analysis is worthwhile [16]. Again, this may be of particular help when the primary carcinoma is lobular in type; indeed some authors suggest carrying out CK IHC in all the lymph nodes draining lobular cancers [17]. However, not all CK-positive cells found within a lymph node represent metastatic carcinoma, and vigilance is required not to overdiagnose benign nodal epithelial inclusions (Fig. 15.5).

An antibody cocktail (such as AE1/3 which contains a mixture of AE1 and AE3) is highly useful in these situations as it gives the greatest coverage of CK mwt types. MNF116 also detects a broad spectrum of CKs and is a useful backup. Either of these antibodies would be recommended for most of the situations described in this section (Table 15.3).

High Molecular Weight (Basal) Cytokeratins

These largely comprise CKs 5 and 14 in breast disease with 34βE12 as a less specific alternative (Table 15.2). These antibodies have four principal uses in the diagnosis and classification of breast disease (Table 15.4):

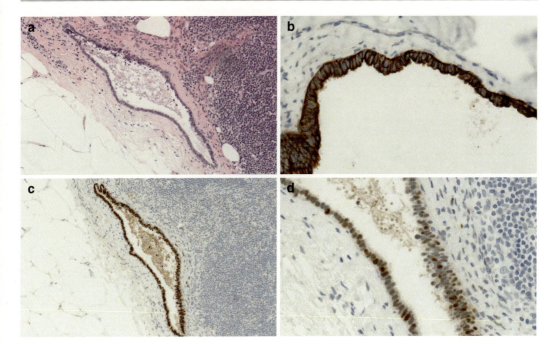

Fig. 15.5 (**a**) H&E of a morphologically epithelial tubular structure in the capsule of an axillary sentinel node. (**b**) The cells are confirmed to be epithelial on cytokeratin staining (AE 1/3). (**c**) They are also ER positive. (**d**) However, they also stain with WT1 and have the morphological features of fallopian tubal epithelium. This is a case of nodal endosalpingiosis (benign tubal epithelial nodal inclusion). Parenthetically, the cells also expressed CK19 and would have given a positive result with intraoperative real-time PCR sentinel node analysis

Table 15.4 Summary of the usefulness of high mwt cytokeratins

Utility	Caveats
Identification of benign (IHC positive) versus atypical or malignant (IHC negative) epithelium	Some benign epithelial processes are negative – columnar cell change, apocrine metaplasia
Identification of myoepithelial cells to differentiate in situ from invasive carcinoma	May be attenuated in DCIS
	In some tumors myoepithelial cells may be genuinely absent yet the tumor be regarded as in situ (encapsulated papillary carcinoma)
	In basal-like carcinomas, the malignant cells are positive
Identification of basal-like carcinoma	There are no agreed IHC criteria for defining basal-like carcinomas
Identification of the myoepithelial component of adenomyoepithelial tumors	

- They stain benign luminal epithelial cells positively with a rather variegated pattern (Fig. 15.6), which is particularly useful in differentiating usual-type hyperplasia from atypical intraductal proliferations or in situ carcinoma (of ductal or lobular types).
- They stain myoepithelial cells which surround intact ducts lying between the luminal epithelial cells and the basement membrane. They are useful, therefore, as a surrogate for assessing whether the basement membrane has been breached or tumor is invading the stroma (Fig. 15.3).
- The identification of basal-like carcinomas of the breast including metaplastic carcinoma (Fig. 15.7) and salivary gland-type tumors (Fig. 15.8).

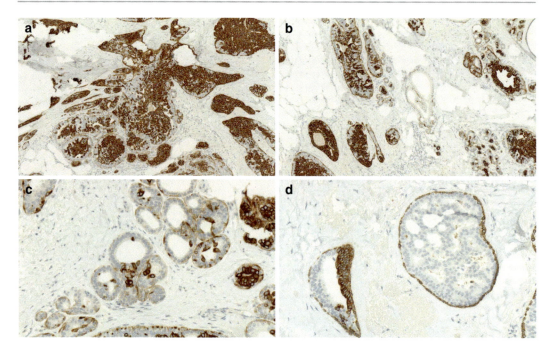

Fig. 15.6 (a) Immunohistochemistry for CK5 showing the typical pattern of positive, but somewhat variegated, staining in foci of epithelial hyperplasia of usual type. (**b**) A similar pattern of positive staining in usual-type hyperplasia along with a focus of apocrine metaplasia centrally; this is benign but is CK5 negative. (**c**) Benign columnar cell change showing largely negative staining. (**d**) The *left*-hand duct shows positive staining in an area of usual-type hyperplasia along with partial involvement by CK5-negative columnar cells showing flat epithelial atypia. The *right*-hand duct shows low-grade DCIS which is CK5 negative

- The identification of the myoepithelial component in adenomyoepithelial tumors (with low mwt CK staining the epithelial cells in a mirror image) (Fig. 15.9).

  There are a number of *caveats*, however, in the use and interpretation of high mwt CK expression (Table 15.4):

- Some normal, entirely benign epithelial cells stain negatively. These include columnar cells and apocrine cells (Fig. 15.6), and, as in all IHC interpretations, the patterns of immunostaining must be considered in the context of the tissue and cellular morphology.
- Some DCIS may express high mwt CKs. This is usually high grade and of basal cell phenotype and relatively easily identified morphologically; again morphology takes precedence over IHC.

- Some basal-like carcinomas only express a limited range of CKs, and a large panel should be employed when this diagnosis is suspected (see later section).
- Some of the rarer, invasive special-type carcinomas (such as adenoid cystic and low-grade adenosquamous carcinomas) may appear low grade but express high mwt CKs causing diagnostic confusion (especially in needle core biopsies). These tumors tend to be triple negative, for hormone receptors and HER2 expression, and the use of another myoepithelial marker, such as smooth muscle myosin heavy chain (SMMHC), will demonstrate the invasive nature of the tumor.
- The myoepithelial cell layer around a duct containing DCIS may become severely attenuated making its identification by high mwt CK staining difficult. In these circumstances, the use of another (non-CK) marker of myoepithelial differentiation (such as p63 or

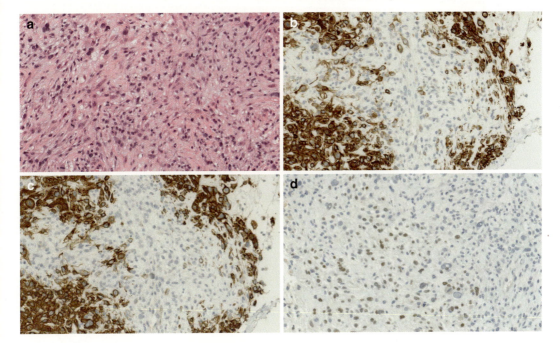

Fig. 15.7 (**a**) H&E of metaplastic (spindle cell) carcinoma. The tumor is morphologically malignant and composed of spindle cells; thus the differential diagnosis would include sarcoma and malignant phyllodes tumor. (**b**) CK5 shows positive (but variable) staining, as does CK14 (**c**) in a similar pattern. (**d**) Staining for p63 is also positive. The stromal component of phyllodes tumors is occasionally positive for CK and p63, so a careful search for an epithelial component is required; this may be particularly challenging in core biopsies

SMMHC) may be helpful (Fig. 15.10; see later section).

- In some tumors, the absence of myoepithelium may not be considered synonymous with stromal invasion. Some carcinomas showing a papillary morphology fall into this category. The WHO has identified the encapsulated papillary carcinoma as a papillary carcinoma defined by "the presence of a thick fibrous capsule that surrounds the tumour" with "myoepithelial cells that are absent within the papillae as well as around the periphery of the tumour" [18]. Thus, WHO has decided that, despite the absence of myoepithelial cells around this tumor and the fact that it can invade locally into pectoralis muscle and (rarely) metastasize to the regional lymph nodes, bone, or lung [19], it should be regarded as in situ carcinoma and be treated as such (a luxury not afforded to tubular carcinoma, an invasive carcinoma which has an equally excellent prognosis).

Low Molecular Weight (Luminal) Cytokeratins

Antibodies to these CKs can be used as alternatives to the broad-spectrum CKs discussed above although they do risk missing basal-like carcinomas. They can be helpful in identifying the cells of Paget's disease in the epidermis of the nipple. Keratinocytes express high mwt cytokeratins and will be picked up by broad-spectrum CKs meaning that both the epidermal cells and the Paget's cells will be positive. However, by using a luminal CK, only the Paget's cells will be positive. The only *caveat* is that benign (Toker) cells have the same CK expression pattern as Paget's cells (Table 15.5). In order to avoid misdiagnosis, it should be clear that Paget's cells are usually cytologically high grade (being associated with HG DCIS) and, in >95 % of cases, HER2 positive (see later section) [27].

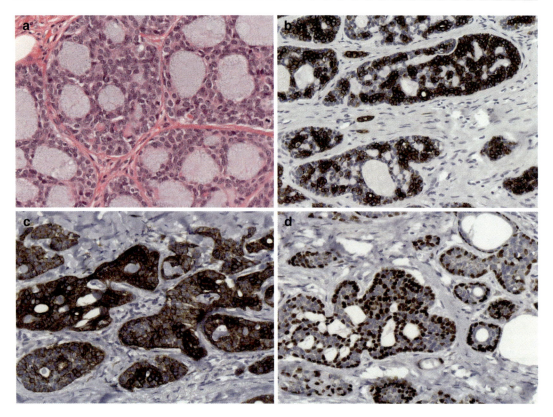

Fig. 15.8 (a) H&E of adenoid cystic carcinoma showing the typical morphology of cribriform structures composed of luminal and basaloid cells. (b) CK7 highlights the luminal cells, whereas CK5 (c) and p63 (d) highlight the basaloid cells

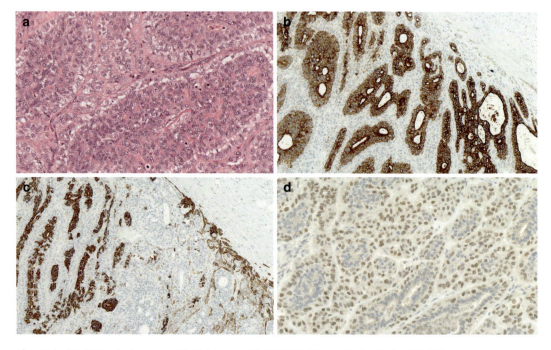

Fig. 15.9 (a) H&E of adenomyoepithelial tumor. (b) CK18 highlights the luminal, epithelial component whereas CK14 (c) and p63 (d) the myoepithelial component

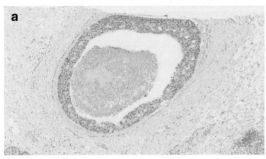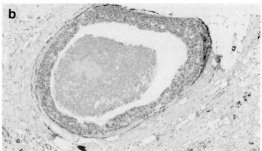

Fig. 15.10 (a) Duct containing high-grade DCIS stained for CK5. The malignant epithelium is negative, but there are no myoepithelial cells staining raising the possibility of stromal invasion although morphologically the disease appears to be in situ. (b) Staining of the same duct for SMMHC shows clear staining of an attenuated myoepithelial cell layer. This is particularly clear around the upper part of the duct. Some of the staining around the lower part represents staining of lymphovascular channels which needs to be differentiated from true myoepithelial staining

Table 15.5 Antibodies of diagnostic utility in identifying myoepithelial cells

Marker	Utility	Comments	Caveats
CK 5 and 14 [20]	Stains myoepithelial cells	Malignant epithelial cells are usually negative	Also stains basal-like carcinoma cells (in situ or invasive)
		Does not stain myofibroblasts	See Table 15.3
		See Table 15.3	
34βE12 [20]	Stains myoepithelial cells	Malignant epithelial cells are usually negative	Also stains basal-like carcinoma cells (in situ or invasive)
		Does not stain myofibroblasts	Less specific than CK5 and CK14
p63 [21, 22]	Stains myoepithelial cells	p53 homologue	Not as sensitive as some other markers
	Clean nuclear staining that is easy to interpret	Does not stain myofibroblasts	May be positive in adenoid cystic, metaplastic, and basal-like carcinomas
Smooth muscle myosin heavy chain (SMMHC) [22]	Stains myoepithelial cells	Highly sensitive	Also stains other muscle tissues including blood vessels
		Stromal myofibroblasts are usually negative	
		Negative in basal-like carcinomas and therefore useful in identifying in situ carcinoma in such tumors	
Smooth muscle actin (SMA) [23]	Stains myoepithelial cells		Also stains myofibroblasts limiting its usefulness
CD10 [24]	Stains myoepithelial cells	Common acute lymphoblastic leukemia antigen (CALLA)	Less sensitive and specific than SMMHC
		Highly sensitive	
Calponin [23]	Stains myoepithelial cells	Good sensitivity	Stains some myofibroblasts
S100 [25]	Stains myoepithelial cells	Low specificity	Stains many other tissues including some epithelial cells
H-caldesmon [23]	Stains myoepithelial cells	SMA-binding protein	
P-cadherin [26]	Stains myoepithelial cells	Cell adhesion molecule	
		Highly sensitive	
		Stromal myofibroblasts are negative	

Myoepithelial Markers

In addition to high mwt CKs, there are a number of other markers that can be used to identify myoepithelial cells. Their identification is important in the differentiation of in situ from invasive carcinoma. These markers are also useful in detecting myoepithelial expression in (adeno-) myoepithelial tumors. Each has its own advantages and disadvantages (Table 15.6).

A number of these markers will cross-react with other antigens, or the antigens are expressed by cells other than myoepithelial cells. As such, care must be applied to their interpretation to take into account these differing characteristics. Again morphology must take precedence. An approach employing two (or more) markers at the same time is often helpful. Using two markers from different groups will give different and complementary information. Thus a useful approach is to use a basal cytokeratin (which will also give information about the nature of the epithelium including basal-like expression) along with SMMHC (which does not usually stain basal-like tumors or any epithelial components).

Basal-Like Markers

Gene expression profiling identified a number of different breast cancer subtypes which include the basal-like group. These are characterized by the expression of high mwt cytokeratins (as well as EGFR in a proportion) but no expression of ER, PR, and HER2 (triple negative). However,

Table 15.6 Summary of the usefulness of low mwt cytokeratins

Utility	Caveats
Identification of Paget's cells in the epidermis of the nipple	Benign (Toker) cells present within the epidermis of the nipple (however, these are HER2 negative)
Identification of the epithelial component in adenomyoepithelial tumors and salivary-type tumors	

this immunophenotype marks a rather heterogeneous group of tumors, including medullary-like, metaplastic (including spindle cell, squamous and adenosquamous cancers), and adenoid cystic carcinomas as well as benign and malignant myoepithelial/adenomyoepithelial tumors. Of particular note are the spindle cell carcinomas which are difficult to differentiate morphologically from benign or malignant mesenchymal tumors. The fibromatosis-like subtype of spindle cell carcinoma is particularly challenging, and the diagnostic workup of any spindle cell breast lesion (no matter how bland) should include a broad panel of cytokeratins including especially those in the broad-spectrum and high molecular weight groups. In addition, p63 is particularly useful as it is highly sensitive in identifying spindle cell carcinoma (Fig. 15.7) [28].

Markers of Lobular Neoplasia

Tumors of lobular type are characterized by a population of intermediate-sized cells showing poor cell-to-cell cohesion. The in situ component fills the acinar units of lobules (hence the name), and the invasive component shows a diffuse, infiltrative growth pattern as individual or narrow cords of cells. The characteristic pattern of discohesive growth appears to be the result of aberrations in cell-cell adhesion caused by dysregulation of the pathway involving the transmembrane glycoprotein E-cadherin and its interactions with several catenin proteins including β-catenin, α-catenin, γ-catenin, and p120 catenin. Infiltrating lobular carcinomas (ILC) are characterized by loss of E-cadherin expression caused by aberrations in the *CDH1* gene that encodes E-cadherin. In the majority of cases, there is mutation of one copy of the *CDH1* gene along with deletion of the wild-type copy, although homozygous deletion and promoter hypermethylation may also be involved in some cases [29]. These CDH1 alterations are also seen in lobular carcinoma in situ (LCIS) indicating that this change occurs early in lobular carcinogenesis [30].

E-cadherin is strongly expressed by normal ductal epithelium of the breast in a clean membranous pattern which acts as an excellent internal control. IHC for E-cadherin shows absent expression in 94 % of LCIS and 84–98 % of ILC [31, 32]. In some cases, there is diminished, but not completely absent, staining or it may appear granular. These patterns are, however, relatively uncommon. By contrast, strong membrane staining is detected in 96 % of invasive ductal carcinoma (IDC) and 98 % of DCIS with focal loss of staining in the remainder [32]. Absent expression has been described in 7 % of IDC associated with grade 3, ER-negative tumors, and reduced expression is relatively common in basal-like, triple-negative ductal cancers (unpublished observation).

In tumors that appear lobular in type but still express E-cadherin, p120-catenin IHC may demonstrate an aberration in another part of the cell adhesion pathway. In ILC p120 catenin shows a switch in expression pattern from a membrane location (similar to E-cadherin) to cytoplasmic (Table 15.7). Thus it provides its own internal control, as some staining is always present. Normal ductal epithelium shows a membranous pattern analogous to E-cadherin (Fig. 15.11) [33].

The diagnosis of lobular carcinoma remains one based ultimately on morphology, as this is the technique used to define the tumor type in all clinical studies to date. However, the use of E-cadherin and/or p120-catenin IHC may be helpful in some situations. It can help in the differentiation of low-grade DCIS from LCIS which is particularly important in small diagnostic core biopsies where the management is very different for these two entities. Where the distinction is between cytologically high-grade in situ lesions (DCIS versus pleomorphic LCIS), it is, perhaps, less important as both entities are currently managed as high-grade DCIS; nonetheless, accurate categorization is always to be encouraged in order to study the natural history of these disease processes.

Although ILC and IDC are treated similarly, the management pathways are not identical. Where a preoperative diagnosis of ILC is made, many centers will undertake breast MRI to exclude clinically and mammographically occult multifocality or bilaterality. Furthermore, the natural history of lobular carcinoma is somewhat different with a greater tendency to metastasize to the bones, GI tract, uterus (including the cervix), meninges, ovary, peritoneum/retroperitoneum, and pleura [34, 35]. There is also limited evidence that lobular carcinomas are less sensitive to neoadjuvant chemotherapy although some of this effect may be due to the fact that they are usually strongly ER positive [36]. Thus, accurate subtyping is important and E-cadherin and/or p120-catenin IHC may aid this process.

Nonetheless, it should be stressed that the diagnosis of ductal and lobular carcinomas is primarily morphological, and, where there is a discrepancy between the pathological typing and the IHC expression pattern for E-cadherin or p120 catenin, then the morphology takes precedence.

Table 15.7 Summary of the usefulness of markers of lobular neoplasia

Antigen	Utility	Caveats
E-cadherin	Positive membranous staining in non-lobular tumors	The diagnosis of lobular-type tumors is still based on morphology
		Some lobular carcinomas are E-cadherin positive
		Some non-lobular carcinomas are negative
		Positive controls (internal or external) are important in interpreting negative staining
p120 catenin	Membranous staining in non-lobular tumors, cytoplasmic staining in lobular tumors	Acts as its own internal control as staining is either membranous or cytoplasmic
	Identifies some lobular tumors that show membranous E-cadherin staining	Staining not as clean as E-cadherin

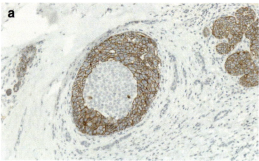

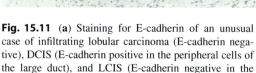

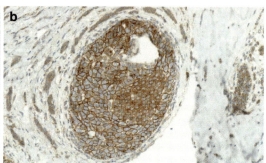

Fig. 15.11 (a) Staining for E-cadherin of an unusual case of infiltrating lobular carcinoma (E-cadherin negative), DCIS (E-cadherin positive in the peripheral cells of the large duct), and LCIS (E-cadherin negative in the central cells of the large duct). (b) Staining for p120 catenin shows a change in the pattern of staining from membranous to cytoplasmic in the infiltrating lobular carcinoma and LCIS

Proliferation Markers

There is good evidence that proliferation correlates strongly with prognosis. The significance of mitotic counting was first appreciated in 1925 [37] and has been a standard part of tumor grading for decades [38]. More recently, attempts have been made to use IHC for markers of cell proliferation to assess the role of proliferation in a new way. IHC using Ki67 antibodies has been extensively studied and shows that higher Ki67 counts correlate with poorer breast cancer survival [39]. This staining is clean and nuclear in type making assessment relatively straightforward. Furthermore, there has been considerable interest in the utility of this technique for differentiating the luminal A and B groups identified by gene expression profiling (both are ER+, HER2−, but luminal B cancers have a higher proliferation fraction). Using IHC as a surrogate for the expensive and technically demanding gene expression profiling would have many advantages, and it has been suggested that a cutoff of 14 % Ki67-positive cancer cells could be used to separate ER+, HER2− cancers into luminal A and B [40].

However, there is no standardization of technique between laboratories for the analysis of Ki67 staining. In particular, it is not clear what constitutes a positive cell, how many cells should be counted, or which part of the tumor should be assessed (center or advancing edge, staining hot spots, or average of whole tumor). The recommendations from the International Ki67 Breast Cancer Working Group state [41] that "… no established quality assurance schemes are in place to ensure that the procedures for Ki67 analysis in one laboratory lead to scores comparable to those in others. Thus, the direct application of specific cutoffs for decision making must be considered unreliable unless analyses are conducted in a highly experienced laboratory with its own reference data. The same issues prohibit comparisons of Ki67 data between clinical trials."

The assessment of proliferation by Ki67 IHC may well become normal practice in the future once standardized protocols for the staining and counting have been devised, and there is an external quality assurance program in place to ensure that interlaboratory variation is minimized. Until such time, this technique must be considered as a research tool unless the individual laboratory has considerable experience and their own robust reference data with clinical outcomes as evidence of its value.

Neuroendocrine Markers

The expression of neuroendocrine markers (chromogranin A, synaptophysin, CD56, and NSE) is seen in up to 30 % of primary breast carcinomas [18]. In order to be described as a neuroendocrine tumor, there should be expression in >50 % of cells; otherwise the tumor is simply classified morphologically with a rider mentioning the NE

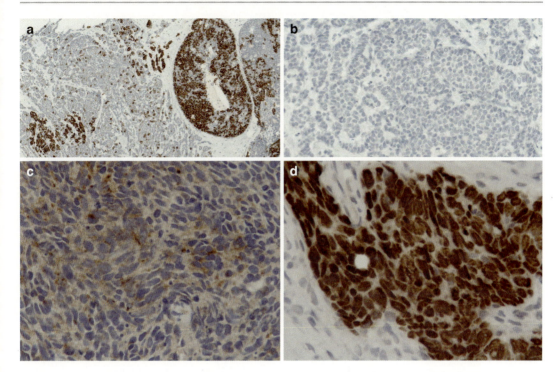

Fig. 15.12 (**a**) Staining for synaptophysin in an invasive carcinoma showing neuroendocrine differentiation. (**b**) This tumor is negative for chromogranin emphasizing the importance of using more than one antibody. DCIS is present confirming that this tumor is primary to the breast.

(**c**) A different tumor showing weak positive staining for chromogranin. (**d**) The same tumor also stains positively for TTF1 and is a primary, poorly differentiated neuroendocrine carcinoma/small-cell carcinoma

marker expression. Only chromogranin A and synaptophysin should be used to confirm NE differentiation with CD56 and NSE being used as a screening tool due to their higher sensitivity but lower specificity (Fig. 15.12).

Low-grade NE tumors in the breast must be differentiated from metastatic tumors (particularly from the GI tract). Primary breast NE tumors may have an in situ component and are almost always strongly and evenly ER positive as well as expressing GCDFP. GI tract NE tumors usually express CDX-2 and are CK 7 negative. The poorly differentiated/small-cell carcinomas of the breast are morphologically similar to those in the lung. Again, the presence of an in situ component is helpful in confirming a primary site in the breast. TTF1 may be positive in such primary breast tumors and so is unhelpful (Fig. 15.12). Clinical assessment and CT scanning the thorax may be advisable to rule out a lung primary as radical surgery to the breast and axilla in patients

with metastatic, small-cell carcinoma of the lung would be inappropriate.

Other invasive carcinomas of the breast may also express NE markers. Some of these will be ductal carcinomas of no special type, whereas others tend to be of mucinous or solid papillary types. These tumors are almost all strongly ER positive and HER2 negative. The NE marker expression is of doubtful significance with regard to prognosis but should be described in order that any recurrence or metastasis can be characterized [18].

Hormone Receptors

Estrogen receptor (ER) and progesterone receptor (PR) are steroid hormone receptors that act as transcriptional activators when they bind estrogen or progesterone, respectively. The binding of estrogen to ER is required for PR to function properly. The expression of ER in breast cancers is prognostic (ER+ cancers have a better prognosis) and predictive of response to selective ER modulators (SERMs). PR expression also provides prognostic information; again expression is associated with better prognosis. Almost all PR+ cancers are also ER+, but cancers that are ER+PR− have a worse prognosis than those that are ER+PR+ even when both groups receive SERM therapy [42].

IHC for ER and PR is nuclear in localization. Its level of expression and the proportion of cells are predictive of SERM response, and a number of scoring systems exist which combine these two parameters in different ways [43–45]. However, current guidance would suggest that any tumor with more than 1 % of the invasive cells expressing ER should be considered positive and be eligible for SERM therapy [46].

In addition to its use as a prognostic and predictive marker in the management of invasive breast cancer, ER IHC can be used as a diagnostic tool. It is strongly and evenly positive in clonal epithelial proliferations as seen in low-grade DCIS and LCIS. It is useful in the distinction of cribriform carcinoma (usually strongly positive) from adenoid cystic carcinoma which is uniformly negative. ER may be helpful in identifying metastases as being of breast origin (Fig. 15.13), but it should be noted that many other tissues and tumors may also express ER: ovarian and endometrial cancers, vulval and vaginal tumors, some melanomas, thyroid tumors, desmoid tumors, and meningioma. This list is not comprehensive, and all factors should be taken into account when considering ER expression in a tumor. Some benign breast tumors such as myofibroblastoma and leiomyoma also express ER (Fig. 15.13).

As the data on ER (and to a certain extent PR) are used for treatment planning as well as prognostication, then it is vital that the entire ER testing pathway (from tissue acquisition through fixation, processing, immunostaining, and interpretation) is quality assured. Particular care must be taken with internal controls: positive staining should be seen in benign ductal epithelium, and on-slide positive and negative control tissues are also very useful. In addition, a rolling internal audit of ER expression levels is recommended with comparison to published positivity levels for

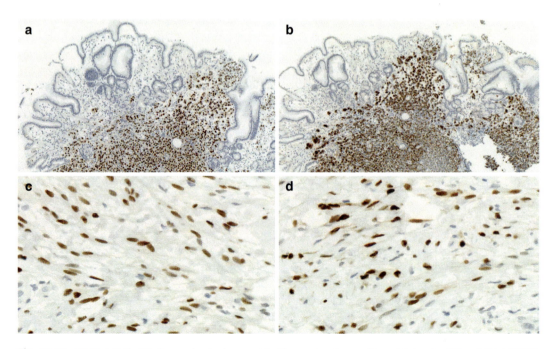

Fig. 15.13 (a) Metastatic lobular carcinoma in a gastric biopsy showing positive staining for ER and (b) GCDFP. (c) Myofibroblastoma staining positively for ER and (d) PR

both screening and symptomatic breast cancer populations. Rigorous audit allied to both internal and external quality control is vital to maintaining a safe and accredited ER and PR IHC testing service.

HER2

HER2 (also known as ERBB2 or *neu*) is part of the *h*uman *e*pidermal growth factor *r*eceptor family. It is a transmembrane receptor tyrosine kinase which usually heterodimerizes with other members of the HER family. HER2 does not bind a ligand, but ligands bind to another HER family member, and following heterodimerization with HER2, there is activation of phosphorylation pathways controlled by the intracellular domain of HER2. HER2 activation results in cell proliferation. HER2 overexpression and gene amplification are seen in approximately 15 % of breast cancers, and these changes are associated with higher grade and stage as well as poorer prognosis [47]. HER2 is the target for a number of specific therapeutic agents including trastuzumab and lapatinib. These agents are only licensed for the treatment of patients with tumors showing HER2 protein overexpression and/or HER2 gene amplification (Figs. 15.1 and 15.14).

In a manner analogous to ER and PR, HER2 IHC is both prognostic and predictive (of response to targeted therapies) and, as such, is subject to very similar guidelines, audit, and both internal and external quality assurance constraints. There are clear and precise guidelines for the assessment of HER2 IHC and when cases should be referred for HER2 gene amplification analysis: usually by dual-color *f*luorescent *in situ h*ybridization (FISH) [48] (Fig. 15.14).

HER2 IHC may also be useful diagnostically in the assessment of nipple biopsies as it is strongly positive in 95 % of Paget's disease of the nipple. It may also be helpful in delineating low-volume in situ and invasive carcinoma in specimens resected following neoadjuvant chemotherapy. In this setting (if the tumor is known to be HER2 positive), HER2 IHC will pick up low-volume residual disease and also demonstrate that it is malignant where there may be difficulty in differentiating residual tumor cells from nonneoplastic cells showing chemotherapy changes.

Vascular Markers

Vascular markers are useful in identifying lymphovascular invasion (LVI) and vascular differentiation in tumors.

LVI is an independent prognostic factor for both disease-free and breast cancer-specific survival. This is true for node-negative and

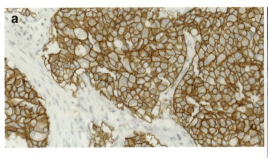
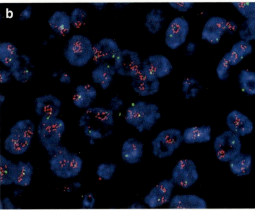

Fig. 15.14 (**a**) Positive staining for HER2 at the 3+ level. (**b**) Dual-color HER2 FISH. The green signals are from a control probe on the same chromosome as HER2 (Alphasatellite CEP17), and the red signals are from HER2. Counting signals gives a HER2 copy number and HER2/CEP17 ratio which are used to define HER2 gene amplification

node-positive disease [49, 50] making it particularly important to accurately identify and confirm its presence. This is especially valuable in node-negative disease where the presence of LVI may alter adjuvant therapy planning. There are a number of methods of identifying LVI which all have advantages and disadvantages (Table 15.8). Most studies indicate that the use of IHC increases the frequency of LVI detection but that both the H&E-detected and IHC-detected LVI have prognostic significance. Where differential markers for lymphatic and blood vessels have been employed, the majority of vascular invasion is lymphatic [51].

The main differential diagnosis for LVI is retraction artifact surrounding an area of stromal invasion or DCIS. In such cases, a combined approach using antibodies to endothelial cells (such as CD31), as well as myoepithelial cells (CK5, p63), will accurately categorize these different processes. SMMHC is a very sensitive marker for myoepithelial cells but does also stain smooth muscle in the walls of blood vessels (even those of small caliber with thin walls) meaning that it should be avoided in this particular situation.

Vascular tumors may occur in the breast in a manner analogous to those elsewhere and should be assessed in the same way. The increase in breast cancer incidence along with the identification of cancers at an earlier stage by screening has resulted in escalating numbers of patients who have received adjuvant whole breast radiotherapy following breast-conserving surgery. One of the most contentious issues in breast pathology is the assessment of post-radiotherapy vascular changes. These changes occur predominantly in the breast skin and range from radiation dermatitis through atypical vascular lesions (AVLs) to angiosarcoma [52, 53]. The differentiation of these entities can be very difficult. Their vascular nature can be demonstrated by positive IHC using factor VIII, CD34, and CD31 (Fig. 15.15). Ki67 IHC can be useful in showing proliferative activity. It is now clear that almost all post-radiotherapy angiosarcomas show MYC gene amplification by FISH, but this is not seen in AVLs (Fig. 15.15). FISH is probably the best method, but IHC shows a strong correlation with MYC protein expression which appears to be 100 % in cases showing *MYC* amplification [54, 55]. Approximately 54–100 % of post-radiotherapy angiosarcomas show *MYC* amplification and MYC protein expression, but no cases of AVL show either feature. Thus, if present, MYC protein expression in a vascular tumor is highly suggestive of secondary angiosarcoma; however, its absence does not completely exclude this diagnosis.

Markers of Breast Differentiation

There are no absolute markers of breast differentiation. The most frequently used are gross cystic disease fluid protein (GCDFP), mammaglobin, and, more recently, GATA3.

GCDFP is also expressed by salivary glands, some skin adnexal tumors, and prostatic adenocarcinomas but highly suggestive of the breast (if these other possibilities can be excluded) with a specificity of 98 % but a relatively low sensitivity of 62–77 % [56, 57]. As few as 23 % of breast carcinomas may be positive [57], although this figure will be higher in tumors with apocrine features. Thus, positive staining is helpful in suggesting a possible breast origin, but a negative result does not exclude the breast (Fig. 15.13).

Mammaglobin is a protein which is expressed by human mammary epithelium and showed early promise as a human mammary-specific

Table 15.8 Stains used for identifying lymphovascular invasion

Marker	Comments
H&E	Not specific, false negative and positive
EVG	Not good for small vessels
Factor VIII	BV and LV, weak in small vessels
CD34	BV and LV, weaker in LV, stromal cells in breast
CD31	BV and LV, variable expression in LV
Podoplanin/D2-40	LV but not BV, also stains myoepithelial cells

EVG Elastica van Gieson, *BV* blood vessel, *LV* lymphatic vessel

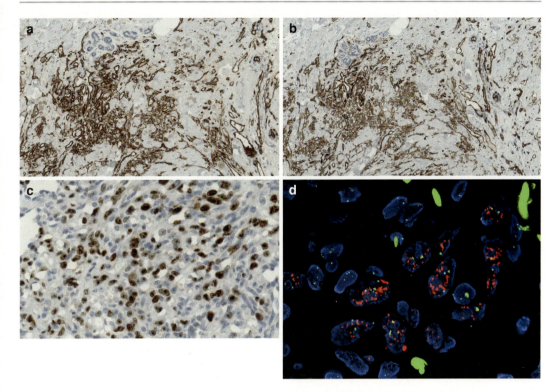

Fig. 15.15 (**a**) Post-radiotherapy angiosarcoma showing positive staining for CD31 and (**b**) CD34. (**c**) The tumor is highly proliferative as shown by staining for

Ki67. (**d**) FISH for myc (*red*), IgH (*green*), and CEP8 (*blue*) shows myc amplification

marker [58]. Mammaglobin expression by IHC is cytoplasmic in localization and is detected in 55–83 % of breast carcinomas [57, 59]. However, it is also detectable in normal endometrium and 17 % of endometrial carcinomas [59]. Furthermore, another study identified mammaglobin staining in 8 % of non-breast tumors including melanoma, ovarian serous carcinoma, endometrial carcinoma, sweat gland, and salivary gland tumors [57]. Thus, mammaglobin is more sensitive than GCDFP but less specific.

GATA3 is one of the six members of a family of transcription factors that contain zinc finger DNA-binding domains. They play an important role in the cellular differentiation of many tissues, and GATA3 plays a specific role in the differentiation of breast luminal epithelial cells. It is expressed strongly in approximately 95 % of primary breast carcinomas in one study [60], but in a recent review, the positivity ranged from 91 to 100 % in ER+ disease and 3–83 % in ER− dis-

ease with an average of about 47 % in roughly comparable studies [61]. The differing methodologies, cutoffs, and volumes of tissue used in these studies make comparison difficult and probably underlie the wide range of positivity frequency. In metastatic breast cancer, GATA3 is expressed in 73–95 % of cases, and, when the primary is positive, the metastasis is almost always positive [61]. Furthermore, GATA3 appears to be more sensitive than either GCDFP or mammaglobin. GATA3 is expressed by other carcinomas including urothelial carcinomas, cutaneous squamous cell, and adnexal carcinomas in addition to squamous cell carcinomas of the cervix, larynx, and bronchus. However, these tumors can usually be differentiated from breast carcinoma on morphological or clinical grounds. GATA3 staining is, therefore, highly sensitive for carcinomas of the breast and urothelium but not specific. It should be used in combination with a panel of other antibodies in cases of metastatic disease to suggest a likely primary. In the breast itself, it may be very useful in biopsies of high-grade, ER– carcinoma with no in situ disease to confirm that it is a breast primary and not a mammary metastasis from another site.

No single antibody will give a definitive answer to the origin of a tumor, and, once again, this highlights the importance of using a panel of antibodies to give guidance to the clinical team. If the pattern of IHC is not helpful, then a non-definitive report is issued.

Miscellaneous Markers

Epidermal Growth Factor Receptor (EGFR)

Epidermal growth factor receptor (EGFR/HER1/ErbB1) is a glycoprotein which forms part of a family of transmembrane, tyrosine kinase receptors. It comprises an extracellular domain that binds a number of ligands (including EGF and TGF-α), a transmembrane domain, and an intracellular domain that is a tyrosine kinase. Ligand binding results in EGFR dimerization and a change in the tyrosine kinase to an active conformation. This, in turn, results in multiple responses including alterations in cell growth, differentiation, and migration. Dysregulation in EGFR is observed in many human tumor types including carcinomas of the head and neck, bladder, ovary kidney, colon, lung, as well as breast [62].

Overexpression of EGFR is observed in approximately 20 % of breast cancers and is associated with higher grade, increasing tumor size, and poorer prognosis [63]. It is particularly prevalent in triple-negative and basal-like cancers as well as inflammatory cancers where it is observed in up to 50 % [64]. These tumors are aggressive and carry a poor prognosis in the absence of systemic therapy. However, overexpression is also prevalent in adenoid cystic carcinoma (which has a good prognosis) with a frequency of 65 % [65]. Although the EGFR pathway appeared to be a good target for therapeutic intervention, the data so far have not shown definite benefit for such

agents even when there is overexpression [64]. Thus, EGFR expression may be of some help diagnostically, but it is not (currently) a useful prognostic or predictive marker.

KIT (CD117)

KIT overexpression in breast cancer is very rare (3 %) and is not related to gene mutation [66]. As such, it does not appear to be a suitable target for imatinib. However, adenoid cystic carcinoma, epithelial-myoepithelial carcinomas, and malignant phyllodes tumors do express KIT meaning that it may be of some utility in the diagnostic setting but not as a marker of response to specific therapy [67–69].

Epithelial Membrane Antigen

Epithelial membrane antigen (EMA), also known as MUC1, is a mucinous glycoprotein which is widely expressed by most glandular and ductal epithelial cells as well as some hemopoietic cells and many tumors showing epithelial or epithelioid differentiation. In the breast, it is usually expressed along the luminal (secretory) aspect of ductal and acinar epithelial cells (the cell border facing the lumen). However, this pattern is reversed in invasive micropapillary carcinoma where the expression of EMA is localized to the stromal (outer) aspect of the cell clusters resulting in the so-called "inside-out" morphology with a space around the cell groups rather than within them (Fig. 15.16). EMA also inhibits the formation of the E-cadherin/beta-catenin complex [70]. This can be visualized by IHC for E-cadherin in micropapillary carcinoma (Fig. 15.16), and the combination of EMA and E-cadherin IHC may be helpful in confirming this diagnosis [71].

The intraepidermal adenocarcinoma cells of Paget's disease of the nipple usually express EMA [72]. However, EMA is also expressed by benign Toker's cells within the epidermis of the nipple. As such, EMA expression is not helpful in this situation, and the diagnosis should be

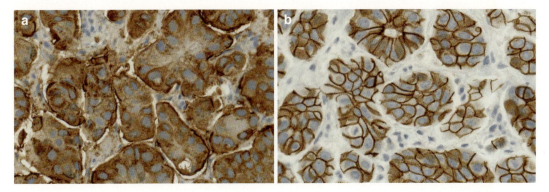

Fig. 15.16 (**a**) Invasive micropapillary carcinoma stained for EMA. (**b**) The same tumor stained for E-cadherin

confirmed by the presence of cytological atypia and the expression of luminal cytokeratins and (usually) HER2.

Conclusion

In recent years, immunohistochemistry has become essential to the diagnosis and management of breast disease. It is used both qualitatively as an aid to reaching a robust diagnosis and quantitatively to guide the management of breast cancer.

As detailed above, this can usually be achieved using a relatively small repertoire of antibodies. Their use must be governed by the appreciation of the importance of adequate internal and external controls (both positive and negative) as well as audit and compliance with high standards of quality assurance and control.

In general terms, IHC is an aid to diagnosis, but morphological considerations should still be regarded as the diagnostic gold standard. Any diagnosis that depends on the staining of a single antibody (especially if it is not corroborated by the morphology or other antibodies) should be regarded with extreme caution. Thus, the use of panels of antibodies that give different but overlapping information is particularly helpful. For instance, instead of using CK5 and CK14 to look for myoepithelial cells, using CK5 and SMMHC or CK5 and p63 will give complementary information by examining the myoepithelial cells in two different ways. Furthermore, for some diagnostic issues such as looking for epithelial expression in spindle cell tumors, a large number of different antibodies to cytokeratin should be employed as the cells may only express one or two of them.

IHC has become a vital part of the pathological workup of many breast specimens (particularly small diagnostic biopsies), but it must be used rationally and with special regard to its potential weaknesses and failings. However, armed with a sound knowledge of the pitfalls backed up by audit and external quality assurance, IHC is a key tool in the diagnosis and management of breast disease.

References

1. Coons AH, Creech HJ, Jones RN. Immunological properties of an antibody containing a fluorescent group. Proc Soc Exp Biol Med. 1941;47:200–2.
2. Khoury T, Sait S, Hwang H, et al. Delay to formalin fixation effect on breast biomarkers. Mod Pathol. 2009;22:1457–67. doi:10.1038/modpathol.2009.117
3. Arber DA. Effect of prolonged formalin fixation on the immunohistochemical reactivity of breast markers. Appl Immunohistochem Mol Morphol. 2002;10:183–6.
4. Wolff AC, Hammond MEH, Hicks DG, et al. Recommendations for human epidermal growth factor receptor 2 testing in breast cancer: American Society of Clinical Oncology/College of American Pathologists clinical practice guideline update. J Clin Oncol. 2013;31:3997–4013. doi:10.1200/JCO.2013.50.9984
5. Sørlie T, Perou CM, Tibshirani R, et al. Gene expression patterns of breast carcinomas distinguish tumor subclasses with clinical implications. Proc Natl Acad Sci USA. 2001;98:10869–74. doi:10.1073/pnas.191367098

6. Perou CM, Jeffrey SS, van de Rijn M, et al. Distinctive gene expression patterns in human mammary epithelial cells and breast cancers. Proc Natl Acad Sci USA. 1999;96:9212–7.

7. Chang JC, Wooten EC, Tsimelzon A, et al. Gene expression profiling for the prediction of therapeutic response to docetaxel in patients with breast cancer. Lancet. 2003;362:362–9. doi:10.1016/S0140-6736(03)14023-8

8. van de Vijver MJ, He YD, van't Veer LJ, et al. A gene-expression signature as a predictor of survival in breast cancer. N Engl J Med. 2002;347:1999–2009. doi:10.1056/NEJMoa021967

9. Tang P, Skinner KA, Hicks DG. Molecular classification of breast carcinomas by immunohistochemical analysis: are we ready? Diagn Mol Pathol. 2009;18:125–32. doi:10.1097/PDM.0b013e31818d107b

10. Lakhani S, Ellis I, Schnitt SJ, et al. WHO classification of tumours of the breast. 4th ed. Lyon: IARC; 2012.

11. Schweizer J, Bowden PE, Coulombe PA, et al. New consensus nomenclature for mammalian keratins. J Cell Biol. 2006;174:169–74. doi:10.1083/jcb.200603161

12. Moll R, Divo M, Langbein L. The human keratins: biology and pathology. Histochem Cell Biol. 2008;129:705–33. doi:10.1007/s00418-008-0435-6

13. Moll R, Franke WW, Schiller DL, et al. The catalog of human cytokeratins: patterns of expression in normal epithelia, tumors and cultured cells. Cell. 1982;31:11–24.

14. Symmans WF, Peintinger F, Hatzis C, et al. Measurement of residual breast cancer burden to predict survival after neoadjuvant chemotherapy. J Clin Oncol. 2007;25:4414–22. doi:10.1200/JCO.2007.10.6823

15. Houssami N, Macaskill P, von Minckwitz G, et al. Meta-analysis of the association of breast cancer subtype and pathologic complete response to neoadjuvant chemotherapy. Eur J Cancer. 2012;48:3342–54. doi:10.1016/j.ejca.2012.05.023

16. de Boer M, van Deurzen CHM, van Dijck JAAM, et al. Micrometastases or isolated tumor cells and the outcome of breast cancer. N Engl J Med. 2009;361:653–63. doi:10.1056/NEJMoa0904832

17. Cserni G, Bianchi S, Vezzosi V, et al. The value of cytokeratin immunohistochemistry in the evaluation of axillary sentinel lymph nodes in patients with lobular breast carcinoma. J Clin Pathol. 2006;59:518–22 doi:10.1136/jcp.2005.029991

18. Tan P-H, Schnitt SJ, van de Vijver MJ, et al. Papillary and neuroendocrine breast lesions: the WHO stance. Histopathology. 2015;66:761–70. doi:10.1111/his.12463

19. Rakha EA, Gandhi N, Climent F, et al. Encapsulated papillary carcinoma of the breast: an invasive tumor with excellent prognosis. Am J Surg Pathol. 2011;35:1093–103. doi:10.1097/PAS.0b013e31821b3f65

20. Dewar R, Fadare O, Gilmore H, Gown AM. Best practices in diagnostic immunohistochemistry: myoepithelial markers in breast pathology. Arch Pathol Lab Med. 2011;135:422–9. doi:10.1043/2010-0336-CP.1

21. Barbareschi M, Pecciarini L, Cangi MG, et al. p63, a p53 homologue, is a selective nuclear marker of myoepithelial cells of the human breast. Am J Surg Pathol. 2001;25:1054–60.

22. Werling RW, Hwang H, Yaziji H, Gown AM. Immunohistochemical distinction of invasive from noninvasive breast lesions: a comparative study of p63 versus calponin and smooth muscle myosin heavy chain. Am J Surg Pathol. 2003;27:82–90.

23. Lazard D, Sastre X, Frid MG, et al. Expression of smooth muscle-specific proteins in myoepithelium and stromal myofibroblasts of normal and malignant human breast tissue. Proc Natl Acad Sci U S A. 1993;90:999–1003.

24. Moritani S, Kushima R, Sugihara H, et al. Availability of CD10 immunohistochemistry as a marker of breast myoepithelial cells on paraffin sections. Mod Pathol. 2002;15:397–405. doi:10.1038/modpathol.3880536

25. Egan MJ, Newman J, Crocker J, Collard M. Immunohistochemical localization of S100 protein in benign and malignant conditions of the breast. Arch Pathol Lab Med. 1987;111:28–31.

26. Kovács A, Walker RA. P-cadherin as a marker in the differential diagnosis of breast lesions. J Clin Pathol. 2003;56:139–41.

27. Sek P, Zawrocki A, Biernat W, Piekarski JH. HER2 molecular subtype is a dominant subtype of mammary Paget's cells. An immunohistochemical study. Histopathology. 2010;57:564–71. doi:10.1111/j.1365-2559.2010.03665.x

28. Reis-Filho JS, Milanezi F, Steele D, et al. Metaplastic breast carcinomas are basal-like tumours. Histopathology. 2006;49:10–21. doi:10.1111/j.1365-2559.2006.02467.x

29. Berx G, Cleton-Jansen AM, Nollet F, et al. E-cadherin is a tumour/invasion suppressor gene mutated in human lobular breast cancers. EMBO J. 1995;14:6107–15.

30. Vos CB, Cleton-Jansen AM, Berx G, et al. E-cadherin inactivation in lobular carcinoma in situ of the breast: an early event in tumorigenesis. Br J Cancer. 1997;76:1131–3.

31. Rakha EA, Patel A, Powe DG, et al. Clinical and biological significance of E-cadherin protein expression in invasive lobular carcinoma of the breast. Am J Surg Pathol. 2010;34:1472–9. doi:10.1097/PAS.0b013e3181f01916

32. Acs G, Lawton TJ, Rebbeck TR, et al. Differential expression of E-cadherin in lobular and ductal neoplasms of the breast and its biologic and diagnostic implications. Am J Clin Pathol. 2001;115:85–98. doi:10.1309/FDHX-L92R-BATQ-2GE0

33. Sarrió D, Pérez-Mies B, Hardisson D, et al. Cytoplasmic localization of p120ctn and E-cadherin loss characterize lobular breast carcinoma from preinvasive to metastatic lesions. Oncogene. 2004;23:3272–83. doi:10.1038/sj.onc.1207439

34. Borst MJ, Ingold JA. Metastatic patterns of invasive lobular versus invasive ductal carcinoma of the breast. Surgery. 1993;114:637–41. discussion 641–2.

35. Harris M, Howell A, Chrissohou M, et al. A comparison of the metastatic pattern of infiltrating lobular carcinoma and infiltrating duct carcinoma of the breast. Br J Cancer. 1984;50:23–30.
36. Cortazar P, Zhang L, Untch M, et al. Pathological complete response and long-term clinical benefit in breast cancer: the CTNeoBC pooled analysis. Lancet. 2014;384:164–72. doi:10.1016/S0140-6736(13)62422-8
37. Greenhough RB. Varying degree of malignancy in cancer of the breast. J Cancer Res. 1925;9:453–63.
38. Bloom H. Histological grading and prognosis in breast cancer. Br J Cancer. 1959;11:359–77
39. de Azambuja E, Cardoso F, de Castro G, et al. Ki-67 as prognostic marker in early breast cancer: a meta-analysis of published studies involving 12,155 patients. Br J Cancer. 2007;96:1504–13. doi:10.1038/sj.bjc.6603756
40. Cheang MCU, Chia SK, Voduc D, et al. Ki67 index, HER2 status, and prognosis of patients with luminal B breast cancer. J Natl Cancer Inst. 2009;101:736–50. doi:10.1093/jnci/djp082j
41. Dowsett M, Nielsen TO, A'hern R, et al. Assessment of ki67 in breast cancer: recommendations from the international ki67 in breast cancer working group. J Natl Cancer Inst. 2011;103:1656–64. doi:10.1093/jnci/djr393
42. Purdie CA, Quinlan P, Jordan LB, et al. Progesterone receptor expression is an independent prognostic variable in early breast cancer – a population based study. Br J Cancer. 2014;110:565–72. doi:10.1038/bjc.2013.756
43. Detre S, Saclani Jotti G, Dowsett M. A "quickscore" method for immunohistochemical semiquantitation: validation for oestrogen receptor in breast carcinomas. J Clin Pathol. 1995;48:876–8.
44. Harvey JM, Clark GM, Osborne CK, Allred DC. Estrogen receptor status by immunohistochemistry is superior to the ligand-binding assay for predicting response to adjuvant endocrine therapy in breast cancer. J Clin Oncol. 1999;17:1474–81.
45. Goulding H, Pinder S, Cannon P, et al. A new immunohistochemical antibody for the assessment of estrogen receptor status on routine formalin-fixed tissue samples. Hum Pathol. 1995;26:291–4.
46. Hammond MEH, Hayes DF, Dowsett M, et al. American Society of Clinical Oncology/College Of American Pathologists guideline recommendations for immunohistochemical testing of estrogen and progesterone receptors in breast cancer. J Clin Oncol. 2010;28:2784–95. doi:10.1200/JCO.2009.25.6529
47. Purdie CA, Baker L, Ashfield A, et al. Increased mortality in HER2 positive, oestrogen receptor positive invasive breast cancer: a population-based study. Br J Cancer. 2010;103:475–81. doi:10.1038/sj.bjc.6605799
48. Rakha EA, Pinder SE, Bartlett JMS, et al. Updated UK recommendations for HER2 assessment in breast cancer. J Clin Pathol. 2015;68:93–9. doi:10.1136/jclinpath-2014-202571
49. Mohammed RAA, Martin SG, Mahmmod AM, et al. Objective assessment of lymphatic and blood vascular invasion in lymph node-negative breast carcinoma: findings from a large case series with long-term follow-up. J Pathol. 2011;223:358–65. doi:10.1002/path.2810
50. Gujam FJA, Going JJ, Edwards J, et al. The role of lymphatic and blood vessel invasion in predicting survival and methods of detection in patients with primary operable breast cancer. Crit Rev Oncol Hematol. 2014;89:231–41. doi:10.1016/j.critrevonc.2013.08.014
51. Mohammed RAA, Martin SG, Gill MS, et al. Improved methods of detection of lymphovascular invasion demonstrate that it is the predominant method of vascular invasion in breast cancer and has important clinical consequences. Am J Surg Pathol. 2007;31:1825–33. doi:10.1097/PAS.0b013e31806841f6
52. Weaver J, Billings SD. Postradiation cutaneous vascular tumors of the breast: a review. Semin Diagn Pathol. 2009;26:141–9. doi:10.1053/j.semdp.2009.10.001
53. Brenn T, Fletcher CDM. Radiation-associated cutaneous atypical vascular lesions and angiosarcoma: clinicopathologic analysis of 42 cases. Am J Surg Pathol. 2005;29:983–96.
54. Fraga-Guedes C, André S, Mastropasqua MG, et al. Angiosarcoma and atypical vascular lesions of the breast: diagnostic and prognostic role of MYC gene amplification and protein expression. Breast Cancer Res Treat. 2015;151:131–40. doi:10.1007/s10549-015-3379-2
55. Ginter PS, Mosquera JM, MacDonald TY, et al. Diagnostic utility of MYC amplification and anti-MYC immunohistochemistry in atypical vascular lesions, primary or radiation-induced mammary angiosarcomas, and primary angiosarcomas of other sites. Hum Pathol. 2014;45:709–16. doi:10.1016/j.humpath.2013.11.002
56. Lerwill MF. Current practical applications of diagnostic immunohistochemistry in breast pathology. Am J Surg Pathol. 2004;28:1076–91.
57. Bhargava R, Beriwal S, Dabbs DJ. Mammaglobin vs GCDFP-15: an immunohistologic validation survey for sensitivity and specificity. Am J Clin Pathol. 2007;127:103–13. doi:10.1309/TDP92PQLDE2HLEET
58. Watson MA, Fleming TP. Mammaglobin, a mammary-specific member of the uteroglobin gene family, is overexpressed in human breast cancer. Cancer Res. 1996;56:860–5.
59. Wang Z, Spaulding B, Sienko A, et al. Mammaglobin, a valuable diagnostic marker for metastatic breast carcinoma. Int J Clin Exp Pathol. 2009;2:384–9.
60. Miettinen M, McCue PA, Sarlomo-Rikala M, et al. GATA3: a multispecific but potentially useful marker in surgical pathology: a systematic analysis of 2500 epithelial and nonepithelial tumors. Am J Surg Pathol. 2014;38:13–22. doi:10.1097/PAS.0b013e3182a0218f54
61. Asch-Kendrick R, Cimino-Mathews A. The role of GATA3 in breast carcinomas: a review. Hum Pathol. 2016;48:37–47. doi:10.1016/j.humpath.2

62. Normanno N, De Luca A, Bianco C, et al. Epidermal growth factor receptor (EGFR) signaling in cancer. Gene. 2006;366:2–16. doi:10.1016/j.gene.2005.10.018

63. Abd El-Rehim DM, Pinder SE, Paish CE, et al. Expression and co-expression of the members of the epidermal growth factor receptor (EGFR) family in invasive breast carcinoma. Br J Cancer. 2004;91:1532–42. doi:10.1038/sj.bjc.6602184

64. Masuda H, Zhang D, Bartholomeusz C, et al. Role of epidermal growth factor receptor in breast cancer. Breast Cancer Res Treat. 2012;136:331–45. doi:10.1007/s10549-012-2289-9

65. Vranic S, Frkovic-Grazio S, Lamovec J, et al. Adenoid cystic carcinomas of the breast have low Topo IIα expression but frequently overexpress EGFR protein without EGFR gene amplification. Hum Pathol. 2010;41:1617–23. doi:10.1016/j.humpath.2010.04.013

66. Simon R, Panussis S, Maurer R, et al. KIT (CD117)-positive breast cancers are infrequent and lack KIT gene mutations. Clin Cancer Res. 2004;10:178–83.

67. Azoulay S, Laé M, Fréneaux P, et al. KIT is highly expressed in adenoid cystic carcinoma of the breast, a basal-like carcinoma associated with a favorable outcome. Mod Pathol. 2005;18:1623–31. doi:10.1038/modpathol.3800483

68. Tse GMK, Putti TC, Lui PCW, et al. Increased c-kit (CD117) expression in malignant mammary phyllodes tumors. Mod Pathol. 2004;17:827–31. doi:10.1038/modpathol.3800125

69. Hungermann D, Buerger H, Oehlschlegel C, et al. Adenomyoepithelial tumours and myoepithelial carcinomas of the breast – a spectrum of monophasic and biphasic tumours dominated by immature myoepithelial cells. BMC Cancer. 2005;5:92. doi:10.1186/1471-2407-5-92

70. Kondo K, Kohno N, Yokoyama A, Hiwada K. Decreased MUC1 expression induces E-cadherin-mediated cell adhesion of breast cancer cell lines. Cancer Res. 1998;58:2014–9.

71. Pettinato G, Manivel CJ, Panico L, et al. Invasive micropapillary carcinoma of the breast: clinicopathologic study of 62 cases of a poorly recognized variant with highly aggressive behavior. Am J Clin Pathol. 2004;121:857–66. doi:10.1309/XTJ7-VHB4-9UD7-8X60

72. Kuan SF, Montag AG, Hart J, et al. Differential expression of mucin genes in mammary and extramammary Paget's disease. Am J Surg Pathol. 2001;25:1469–77.

Elena Provenzano and Suet-Feung Chin

Abstract

Breast cancer is not one disease but a heterogeneous group of entities with different clinical outcomes. High-throughput genomic techniques provide new insights into the molecular heterogeneity of breast cancer. This has redefined how we classify breast cancer and offers the potential to revolutionize patient management through more precise determination of prognosis based on tumor biology and the opportunity for targeted treatments directed at the specific molecular aberrations driving tumor growth. This chapter describes models for the molecular classification of breast cancer, current genetic signatures available for predicting prognosis, and future prospects for monitoring disease and response to therapy.

Keywords

Breast cancer • Molecular biology • Gene expression arrays • Molecular prognostic assays

Introduction

Breast cancer represents not a single disease, but a heterogeneous group of entities with very different clinical outcomes [1, 2]. This diversity has long been appreciated at the morphological level, with the recognition of special histological types of breast cancer that have distinct microscopic appearances and clinical behavior; however, 70–80 % of breast cancers fall into the ductal/no special-type category which is heterogeneous with respect to underlying tumor biology and prognosis [3]. The goal in modern oncological practice is to accurately predict tumor behavior in an individual patient, avoiding overtreatment with harmful drugs for good prognosis cancers and identifying poor prognosis cancers that require chemotherapy at the outset [4]. Historically, these decisions were solely based on traditional histological variables such as tumor size, histological grade, nodal status, hormone receptor, and HER2 status, along with patient characteristics such as age and menopausal status [5–9]. These clinic-pathological variables when

E. Provenzano (✉) • S.-F. Chin
University of Cambridge Department of Oncology,
CRUK Cambridge Research Institute,
Li Ka Shing Centre, Cambridge CB2 0RE, UK
e-mail: elena.provenzano@addenbrookes.nhs.uk

© Springer International Publishing Switzerland 2017
S. Shousha (ed.), *Breast Pathology*, DOI 10.1007/978-3-319-28655-6_16

combined in various algorithms such as the Nottingham Prognostic Index (NPI), Predict, and Adjuvant! Online (AOL) show a strong association with survival outcomes [10–16], but are a crude measure of risk in the individual patient. A significant number of women with breast cancer are currently overtreated, with an estimated 85 % of patients deriving no benefit from cytotoxic chemotherapy, while conversely 20 % of women will die despite receiving chemotherapy [17].

Cancer is a genetic disease driven by DNA alterations including chromosomal rearrangements, mutations, and epigenetic changes such as promoter hypermethylation that result in activation of growth-promoting genes (oncogenes) or suppression of growth-inhibiting genes (tumor suppressor genes). In 1992, Kallioniemi et al. revolutionized solid tumor genomics with the development of comparative genomic hybridization (CGH) that enabled quantification of copy number changes across the entire genome and identification of minimal common regions (MCR) of gains or losses, which pinpoint poten-

tial oncogenes and tumor suppressor genes (TSG), respectively [18]. The development of array technology allowed whole genomic/transcriptomic profiling of large numbers of samples revealing the heterogeneity of breast cancer [19]. Next-generation sequencing, or massively parallel sequencing, has the capacity to profile the genome at base pair level providing new insight into intratumoral clonal heterogeneity [20–22].

High-throughput molecular techniques, summarized in Table 16.1, not only have redefined how we classify breast cancer but offer the potential to revolutionize patient management through more precise determination of patient prognosis based on tumor biology and the opportunity for targeted treatment directed at the underlying molecular aberrations driving individual tumor growth [1]. These techniques are currently expensive compared with standard methods such as immunohistochemistry, and the vast amounts of data generated by these experiments require complex bioinformatic analyses limiting their clinical use at the present time.

Table 16.1 Key molecular techniques

Method	Description	Advantages	Disadvantages
qRT-PCR	Amplification using oligonucleotides complementary to target sequences	Specific and sensitive	Limited number of targets compared to expression arrays
		Small amount of RNA required	
		Will work on smaller fragments, e.g., FFPE	
		Does not require complex analysis	
Gene expression arrays	Quantifies whole transcriptome or selected gene panels. Hybridization of fluorescently labeled RNA to complementary oligonucleotides printed onto glass slides	A large number of targets can be profiled in a single hybridization	More background noise
			Needs complex bioinformatics
Comparative genomic hybridization	Quantifies DNA copy number alterations	Entire genome can be examined in a single hybridization	Needs complex bioinformatics
			Currently used for research only
Next-generation sequencing	Quantifies copy number changes, base changes (mutations and single nucleotide variants), and structural alterations for DNA; gene expression, splice variants, and fusion genes for RNA	High-throughput whole-genome screening to base pair level	Expensive. Relatively new technology so still developing data analysis algorithms
		Detects clonal heterogeneity	Needs complex bioinformatics
			Currently used for research only

Molecular Classification of Breast Carcinoma

The seminal paper using gene expression profiling to examine the genetic complexity of breast cancer was published by Perou et al. in 2000 [23]. The authors took a series of 38 invasive breast cancers (36 ductal and 2 lobular), 1 case of DCIS, and 4 benign samples and undertook cDNA microarray analysis followed by hierarchical clustering of differentially expressed genes. This led to the identification of five "intrinsic" subtypes of breast cancer separated primarily by ER status. Follow-up studies showed that these subtypes were associated with differences in survival [24, 25].

Luminal breast cancers are enriched for ER-positive tumors and form a continuous spectrum that can be arbitrarily divided into two subgroups based on the expression of proliferation-related genes [26]:

- Luminal A tumors are typically low grade with an excellent prognosis, characterized by ER and PR positivity and HER2 negativity, with high expression of ER-related genes and low expression of proliferation-related genes [5, 26, 27].
- Luminal B tumors are higher grade, have a worse prognosis, and may be PR negative and/or HER2 positive with high expression of proliferation-related genes [26, 28].

In contrast, ER-negative tumors comprise biologically distinct entities with different drivers that can be divided into three main groups: HER2 enriched, basal-like, and normal-like [26].

- The HER2-enriched group is driven by overexpression of HER2, and genes associated with related pathways or with the HER2 amplicon on chromosome 17q12 and have a poor prognosis. Although the majority of tumors within this subgroup (>80%) show *ERBB2* gene amplification or HER2 protein overexpression on immunohistochemistry, not all clinically defined HER2-positive tumors fall into this subgroup; many ER-positive/

HER2-positive tumors fall into the luminal B group mentioned above [4, 5, 26].

- The basal-like breast cancers are typically high-grade tumors that are ER, PR, and HER2 negative (triple negative) and are characterized by upregulation of genes expressed by basal/myoepithelial cells including high molecular weight cytokeratins (CK5 and CK17), P-cadherin, EGFR, and caveolins [26]. The basal-like group includes diverse histological types of breast cancer including medullary-like cancers with a prominent lymphocytic infiltrate, metaplastic cancers, and rare special-type cancers like adenoid cystic carcinoma which carry a good prognosis [29–34]. Breast cancers arising in *BRCA1* mutation carriers are typically basal-like, and *BRCA1* dysfunction mediated by alternative mechanisms such as methylation has been identified in non-*BRCA1* mutated basal-like tumors [29, 35–37].
- The normal-like group is poorly characterized and clusters with normal breast tissue and is subsequently thought to represent sampling error with overrepresentation by normal breast glands [38].

The existence of these five intrinsic subtypes has been validated by other groups and has changed how we think about the taxonomy of breast cancer [2, 25, 39, 40]. The separation into good and poor prognosis ER-positive groups, HER2-positive, and triple-negative groups is clinically relevant based on current therapeutic regimens centered on hormonal therapy, chemotherapy, and HER2-targeted agents. These molecular signatures have been the basis for many of the multigene assays that are currently available for clinical use.

Classification of cohorts of breast cancers into the five intrinsic subtypes appears robust; however, assignment of individual tumors to a subgroup shows only moderate reproducibility depending upon the array platform used, composition of the entire tumor population, and setting of gene expression thresholds [41–43]. Identification of the basal-like group is most reproducible, with the luminal B and HER2 groups the most poorly reproducible [26, 43, 44].

There have also been attempts to replicate these groups using immunohistochemistry-based panels including ER, PR, HER2, Ki67, and basal cytokeratins; however, concordance between microarray and IHC-defined intrinsic subtypes is modest at best [2, 9, 38, 45].

Triple-Negative Breast Carcinoma

Triple-negative breast cancers have been subdivided into seven subgroups with different molecular drivers, variable clinical outcomes, and response to neoadjuvant chemotherapy [46]. The groups include:

- The luminal androgen receptor group is characterized by high expression of androgen receptor and hormonally regulated pathways with similarities to the molecular apocrine group of breast cancers. They have a good prognosis and show a lower pathological complete response (pCR) rate following neoadjuvant chemotherapy (10%), more akin to ER-positive tumors, and may potentially respond to antiandrogenic agents or PI3K inhibitors [46–48].
- There are two basal-like subgroups, BL1 and BL2, enriched for genes involved in proliferation, DNA damage response (BL1), and growth factor receptor signaling pathways (BL2). The BL1 group shows high pCR rates following neoadjuvant chemotherapy (52%), while the BL2 group shows poor response [48].
- The immune modulatory group is enriched for genes involved in immune cell processes such as B- and T-cell receptor signaling, cytokine signaling, and antigen presentation and shows overlap with the gene profile of medullary-like cancers.
- The mesenchymal (M) and mesenchymal stem-like (MSL) groups show enrichment for genes involved in cell motility, cell differentiation, growth signaling pathways, and extracellular matrix interactions.
- The MSL group shows low expression of proliferation-related genes and high expression of genes associated with stem cells.

The last two groups were associated with worse 5-year distant metastasis-free survival (DMFS) consistent with upregulation of pathways involved in motility and metastasis; the M group showed the poorest DMFS and overall survival (OS) following neoadjuvant chemotherapy [48].

An Alternative Molecular Classification: The Integrative Clusters

Using a combination of gene expression profiling and copy number alterations, Curtis et al. defined a driver-based classification method that divides breast cancer into ten subgroups they termed the integrative clusters (IntClust) [49]. These ten IntClust segregated the above intrinsic subtypes into separate groups with distinct clinical outcomes (Table 16.2) [50]. ER-positive HER2-negative tumors are spread over eight subtypes. IntClust 3, 7, and 8 have a good prognosis and correspond to the luminal A subtypes. IntClust 1, 6, and 9 show an intermediate prognosis and include luminal A and B tumors. IntClust 4 includes ER-positive and ER-negative tumors with upregulation of an immune response signature which is reflected histologically by a lymphocytic infiltrate. IntClust 5 comprises tumors driven by *ERBB2* gene amplification and includes both ER-positive and ER-negative tumors, unlike the intrinsic subtypes that put double-positive tumors into the luminal B group. IntClust 10 includes the majority of triple-negative breast cancers and is characterized by intermediate genetic instability and 5q deletion with associated upregulation of genes involved in cell cycle control, DNA damage repair, and apoptosis. The IntClust provide additional information not only by identifying prognostically significant subgroups of ER-positive breast cancer but by highlighting the molecular drivers of these groups which may provide future options for targeted therapies [1, 50]. The groups also show different response rates to neoadjuvant chemotherapy [1].

Table 16.2 Description of integrative clusters

IntClust	Frequency (%)	Prognosis	Distinguishing molecular features	ER/HER2
1	7	Intermediate	17q23 amplification GATA3 mutations High genomic instability	85% ER+ 15% HER2+
2	4	Poor	11q13/14 amplification (cyclin D1) High genomic instability	96% ER+ 4% HER2+
3	15	Good	Low genomic instability with few copy number changes PIK3CA and CDH1 mutations	96% ER+ 0.3% HER2+
4	17	Good	Low genomic instability Upregulation of immune response genes	70% ER+ 6% HER2 +
5	10	Poor	ERBB2 amplification	42% ER+ 95% HER2+
6	4	Intermediate	8p12 amplification (ZNF703) High genomic instability	100% ER+ 4% HER2+
7	10	Good	16p gain, 16q loss, 8q amplification	98% ER+ 1% HER2+
8	15	Good	1q gain, 16q loss	99% ER+ 0.3% HER2+
9	7	Intermediate	8q gain, 20q amplification High genomic instability	86% ER+ 7% HER2+
10	11	Poor	5q loss, 8q gain, 10p gain, 12p gain	11% ER+ 3% HER2+

Prognostic and Predictive Tests

There are several multigene assays that are currently commercially available based on gene expression signatures that have been identified as predictors of prognosis or response to treatment (Table 16.3). The first generation of multigene prognostic predictors was developed by comparing gene expression profiles from groups of patients who experienced a recurrence with groups of patients who did not [51]. These studies identified proliferation-associated genes and ER-related genes as the most powerful determinants of outcome; as these two cellular processes involve the coordinated expression of multiple pathways and hundreds of genes, a large number of equally strong prognostic signatures with minimal overlap of individual genes can be derived from the same dataset [5, 51–53]. When multiple models are applied to the same patient cohort, they all identify similar low- and high-risk groups with significant differences in outcome; however, there is disagreement in a substantial number of cases at the individual patient level [44, 51, 54–58]. The majority of current gene-based tests are limited to use in ER-positive HER2-negative early breast cancer patients with low nodal burden [5, 44, 52, 59]. Tumor size and nodal status retain independent prognostic value, and some of the assays incorporate these important clinical variables when determining risk [38, 60, 61]. The key molecular tests that are currently available are described below.

Commercial gene expression tests use either quantitative reverse transcriptase-polymerase chain reaction (qRT-PCR) or expression array hybridizations. Array-based tests can measure a higher number of target genes but are confounded by higher positive errors and higher cost and require complex analytical tools to interpret the results [62]. They require high-quality RNA and until recently a major limitation was the requirement for fresh frozen tissue samples. qRT-PCR assays have superior sensitivity and specificity to array-based tests and are suitable for formalin-fixed paraffin-embedded (FFPE) material, but

Table 16.3 Current genomic tests for breast cancer prognosis

Assay name	Company	Material	Assay type	No. of genes	FDA approval
MammaPrint	Agendia	FFPE, FF	Array	70	Yes
MapQuant Dx™ genomic grade test	Ipsogen	FF	Array	97	No
PAM50	University of Utah	FFPE	Array	50	No
Rotterdam signature	Veridex	FFPE, FF	Array	76	No
BreastPRS	Signal Genetics	FFPE, FF	Array	200	No
Prosigna®	NanoString	FFPE, FF	Digital count	50	Yes
Oncotype DX®	Genomic Health	FFPE	qRT-PCR	21	No
EndoPredict®	Sividon Diagnostics	FFPE	qRT-PCR	12	No
Breast Cancer Index℠	Biotheranostics	FFPE	qRT-PCR	11	No

FFPE formalin fixed paraffin embedded, *FF* fresh frozen

can only measure expression of a limited number of genes [62]. Many of the current tests are only performed in central laboratories which ensure reproducibility, but result in higher costs and potential delays in turnaround time. Some of the newer tests are designed to be run in local laboratories which may improve accessibility and reduce costs [63].

MammaPrint

MammaPrint® (Agendia, Amsterdam, Netherlands) was the first gene expression-based signature developed for prognostic use in breast cancer [64]. It is a 70-gene microarray-based test performed in a central laboratory. Initially performed using fresh frozen tissue samples only, it has subsequently been validated on FFPE tissue samples with 97 % success rate and 92 % concordance between sample types [65]. Excellent reproducibility of 96 % has been demonstrated between different laboratories and between different samples from the same tumor. It has FDA approval for use in women under the age of 61 years with pT1-2, lymph node-negative, or 1–3 node-positive breast cancer [26].

The signature was established in a cohort of 78 patients under the age of 55 from the Netherlands Cancer Institute (NKI) with pT1-2, lymph node-negative breast cancer including both ER-positive and ER-negative tumors; 34 had developed distant metastasis and 44 were distant metastasis free at 5 years [64]. Using a supervised clustering approach with gene expression array data on 25,000 genes, a 70-gene classifier was derived that divided patients into good and poor prognosis groups with 83 % accuracy in predicting outcome. The 70-gene panel includes genes related to cell cycle regulation, invasion, metastasis, and angiogenesis. The signature was validated in a 295-patient cohort that included 151 node-negative and 144 node-positive patients and 69 ER-negative patients [66]. One-hundred and fifteen patients fell in the good prognosis group and 180 in the poor prognosis group. The signature showed a correlation with grade (56/75 grade 1 tumors in good prognosis group compared with 14/119 grade 3 tumors; grade 2 tumors were evenly split) and with ER status (66/69 ER-negative tumors in the poor prognosis group) but not with other clinicopathological variables. The signature was shown to be predictive of outcome in node-negative and node-positive subgroups. The signature has been independently validated in 302 node-negative patients from the TRANSBIG series, where it was shown to be independent of clinicopathological variables and outperform the NPI, the AOL, and the St. Gallen criteria [67].

The 70-gene signature is currently being investigated in the prospective randomized MINDACT trial [68]. Patients enrolled into the study have their risk assessed by AOL and MammaPrint®, and discordant patients are randomized to receive therapy according to either the gene test or the AOL results. The outcomes are the number of patients that avoid chemotherapy and non-inferiority in clinical outcomes. The accrual target is 6000 subjects, but recruitment has been slow. A pilot study found 46 % enrolment with 48 % concordant low risk, 25 % concordant high risk, and 27 % discordant (18 % gene test low/AOL high and 9 % gene test high/AOL low) [69]. There was 92 % compliance with the treatment decision. The results are expected soon [51].

In an overview the MammaPrint® signature has been validated in 13 studies, 12 of which showed an association with outcome [59]. This includes studies looking at older patient groups and patients that are heavily node positive [70–73]. However, the results are time dependent with prognostic value for DMFS diminished after 5 years and OS diminished after 10 years [74]. The signature has also been shown to be predictive of chemotherapy benefit, with patients in the high-risk group having a BCSS of 84 % following combined chemotherapy and endocrine therapy compared with 81 % with endocrine therapy alone; the low-risk group had excellent BCSS on endocrine therapy alone (97 % BCSS) with no additional benefit from chemotherapy [75].

Veridex®/Rotterdam Signature

The 76-gene or Rotterdam signature was derived from 22,000 genes using an Affymetrix platform in 115 node-negative breast cancer patients who did not receive adjuvant systemic therapy: 60 genes for ER-positive cancers and 16 genes for ER-negative cancers [76]. Of note, the signature shares no common genes with either Oncotype DX or MammaPrint with an emphasis on proliferation genes. The signature was applied to a 171 patient validation set with 93 % sensitivity and 48 % specificity. The signature was prognostic in pre- and postmenopausal subgroups and was independent of other histological variables. The same group then validated the 76-gene signature in a separate cohort of 180 lymph node-negative patients with 5 years OS of 98 % in the low-risk group compared with 76 % in the high-risk group [77]. Forty percent of patients were spared from adjuvant therapy compared with clinical risk esti-

mates using the St. Gallen criteria. The TRANSBIG group also evaluated the 76-gene signature using 198 patients from the cohort used to validate MammaPrint® [78]. There was 35 % discordance with AOL, and 25 % of ER-negative patients were placed in the low-risk group. Five-year OS was 98 % in the low-risk group and 84 % in the high-risk group. There was a time-dependent effect with reduction in predictive value after 5 years; however, it remained a strong predictor with an HR of 2.55 at 10 years. In a side-by-side comparison, the 70-gene and 76-gene signatures showed 71 % concordance with HR of 10-year DMFS of 7.12 and 3.18, respectively; this difference was not statistically significant [79]. In a comparison study, the 76-gene signature showed the lowest correlation with other gene signatures in predicting risk, although it was the only signature predictive of DMFS in ER-negative patients [44]. The group at the NKI applied the 16-gene ER-negative signature to a group of 71 triple-negative breast cancers and did not find a significant association with survival [80].

PAM50/Prosigna

In the early studies, breast cancer intrinsic subtype was associated with survival outcome [24, 25, 37]. A 50-gene minimized set was derived from a panel of 1906 intrinsic genes to optimize reproducibility in classifying individual samples using a Prediction Analysis of Microarray method resulting in the PAM50 intrinsic classifier [38]. The classifier assigns samples to luminal A, luminal B, HER2-enriched, and basal-like subtypes; 64 % of clinically HER2-positive samples are assigned to the HER2-enriched group and 73 % of ER-positive tumors to the luminal subtypes. The PAM50 gene set was then applied to an untreated cohort of node-negative breast cancers to develop a risk classifier termed the risk of recurrence (ROR) score divided into low-, intermediate-, and high-risk groups. The optimum model included a combination of ROR score and tumor size (ROR-S) and predicted long-term outcome in a heterogeneously treated cohort of

279 patients. The high-risk group was associated with pCR in a separate cohort of patients that received neoadjuvant chemotherapy.

The PAM50 and ROR score have been validated in several clinical trial populations [81–84]. The ROR score added prognostic information to clinical variables in patients treated with endocrine therapy in the ATAC trial in both node-negative and node-positive subgroups and outperformed the RS in the node-negative group with better discrimination of intermediate- and high-risk groups [81]. In a subsequent analysis, ROR was inferior to clinical variables in predicting early outcomes (years 0–5) but added substantial prognostic information for late recurrence in years 5–10 [85]. ROR score also added significant prognostic information in the ABCSG-8 trial comparing tamoxifen versus tamoxifen plus anastrozole with a higher prognostic effect in node-positive compared with node-negative patients [82, 84]. However, in a combined analysis of the two trials looking at node-positive patients, caution was advised in omitting chemotherapy in the two to three node-positive group as although the risk of recurrence was lower (12.5 % ROR low versus 34 % ROR high) it was still substantial [83]. In the single node-positive group, risk of recurrence was 7 % in the low-, 16 % in the intermediate-, and 26 % in the ROR high-risk groups.

PAM50 has also been shown to predict survival outcomes in chemotherapy-treated populations and pCR rates post neoadjuvant chemotherapy [38, 86, 87]. In the ISPY-1 and NOAH neoadjuvant trials, both PAM50 subtype and high ROR score were associated with increased rates of pCR [88, 89]. The NOAH results are particularly interesting as the HER2-enriched tumors showed higher pCR rates following trastuzumab therapy compared with non-HER2-enriched clinically HER2-positive tumors (53 % and 35 %, respectively) [89].

The PAM50 gene set has recently been adapted to the NanoString platform using the nCounter Analysis system in the Prosigna™ (NanoString) assay enabling the test to be performed in decentralized laboratories [90]. NanoString uses bar-coded and fluorescent-tagged pairs of oligonucleotides that hybridize to RNA from either fresh frozen or FFPE tissues.

Genomic Grade Index (MapQuant Dx)

Histological tumor grade is a significant predictor of outcome, but 40–60 % of tumors are grade 2 and clinical decision-making is uncertain in this group [26]. Sotiriou et al. looked at a group of 33 grade 1 and 31 grade 3 ER-positive breast cancers and identified a panel of 97 genes associated with cell cycle and proliferation that were differentially expressed [91]. In a 125-tumor validation set, grade 1 and grade 3 tumors were distinct, with grade 2 tumors showing intermediate characteristics with some showing low-grade and others high-grade profiles. Of note, 23 of the genes identified overlapped with other prognostic gene signatures. This 97-gene genomic grade index (GGI) was then applied to a series of ER-positive tumors, either untreated or treated with tamoxifen, and identified low and high GGI groups with different survival outcomes [92]. The high GGI group had poor survival even with endocrine therapy. The GGI was a better predictor of clinical outcome than histological tumor grade. The GGI was a significant predictor of chemotherapy response in a cohort of 229 patients that included 97 ER-negative cases; 40 % of high GGI tumors showed excellent response (pCR or minimal residual disease) compared with 12 % of low GGI [93]. Despite this, the high GGI group showed worse 5-year survival in the ER-positive group. In the PACS01 trial of adjuvant chemotherapy in node-positive breast cancer, GGI was a stronger predictor of outcome than histological grade or Ki67 index and predicted survival in grade 2 cancers [94].

GGI is available as the MapQuant Dx test (Ipsogen SA, Marseilles, France) and is a microarray-based assay requiring fresh frozen tissue. To overcome this, four genes with highly significant correlation with the GGI were selected and combined with four reference genes in a qRT-PCR-based assay (PCR-GGI) that can be performed on FFPE tissue. The new 8-gene assay showed excellent reproducibility with the 97-gene test on fresh and frozen samples and predicted DRFS in node-negative and node-positive patients treated with tamoxifen [95].

Oncotype DX

Oncotype DX (Genomic Health, Redwood City, CA, USA) is the most commonly used commercially available gene-based test worldwide and is the only test currently included in guidelines for clinical use by ASCO, NCCN, and NICE [26, 59]. It is a qRT-PCR-based assay performed in a central laboratory on FFPE tissue. The test was developed by comparing the expression of 250 candidate genes with known association with cancer biology and prognosis with survival in 447 patients with ER-positive node-negative breast cancer from three clinical trials [96]. The resultant 21-gene panel comprises proliferation genes (*Ki67*, *STK15*, *survivin*, *cyclin B1*, *MYBL2*), ER pathway genes (*ER*, *PR*, *BCL2*, *SCUBE2*), HER2 pathway genes (*HER2*, *GRB7*), invasion genes (*stromelysin 3*, *cathepsin L2*), *GSTM1*, *CD68*, *BAG1*, and five reference genes. The score for each group is entered into an algorithm which gives a recurrence score (RS) from 1 to 100; a score of <18 is classed as low risk, 18–30 as intermediate risk, and 31 or more as high risk. The RS was validated in 668 patients from the tamoxifen arm of the NSABP B-14 trial; 51 % of patients fell in the low-risk, 22 % in the intermediate-risk, and 27 % in the high-risk groups with a 5-year DDFS of 2 %, 9 %, and 22 %, respectively. The RS was the strongest predictor of outcome and was independent of tumor size and patient age and more accurately predicted recurrence than AOL. In a further analysis involving the placebo arm of B-14, it was shown that patients with a low or intermediate RS derived benefit from tamoxifen, whereas patients with a high RS derived no benefit. An analysis of patients from the TransATAC study showed that RS was also predictive of benefit from aromatase inhibitors in both node-positive and node-negative patients; however, in a subsequent study the prognostic strength fell off in years 5–10 [85,

97]. Subsequent studies, including an analysis of the chemotherapy arm of the NSABP B-20 trial, have shown chemotherapy benefit for patients with a high RS but minimal or no benefit with a low RS [98]. For the intermediate group there appears to be no benefit from chemotherapy, but uncertainty estimates could not exclude a clinically significant benefit.

Current recommendation is that patients with low RS be treated with endocrine therapy only, while patients with a high RS receive chemotherapy. The intermediate RS group is the subject of the prospective TAILORx trial, where women with an RS of 11–24 are randomized to chemotherapy or endocrine therapy. The cutoffs were adjusted for the trial with the low-risk group <11, intermediate-risk group 11–24, and high-risk group ≥25; this was to ensure that no patients who might benefit missed out on chemotherapy. Preliminary results of the study have been published [99]. Of 10,253 women enrolled in the study, 16 % were low risk, 67 % intermediate risk, and 17 % high risk. The low-risk women received endocrine therapy alone with a 5-year DMFS of 99 %. Results for the intermediate- and high-risk groups are still awaited.

Oncotype DX has been evaluated in many series including clinical trials and single institution studies [59, 100–102]. Out of 13 studies, 12 showed an association with outcome [59]. In a meta-analysis of 21 studies involving 4156 patients, 49 % had a low RS (36–62 %), 39 % had an intermediate RS (29–47 %), and 12 % had a high RS (7–21 %) [100]. Along with Genomic Health's own data, this suggests a referral bias with clinicians ordering the test in patients with low- or intermediate-risk clinicopathological features.

In eight studies where data was available, there was a 33 % (23–43 %) change in recommended therapy. Interestingly, the test result was more likely to be followed for low-risk than high-risk patients with chemotherapy given in 6 %, 37 %, and 83 % of patients with low, intermediate, and high RS, respectively. It is estimated up to 61 % of patients can be spared from chemotherapy as a result of the test [103].

A major drawback of Oncotype DX is its high cost; however, a review looking at health economic studies of Oncotype DX from Europe, North America, and Asia found it to be cost-effective [104]. Of note in the ATAC trial, the IHC-4 score based on clinical variables and immunohistochemical evaluation of ER, PR, HER2, and Ki67 showed similar prognostic value to the RS at much lower cost [105].

A study comparing the 21-gene and 70-gene signatures found 81 % concordance in outcome prediction when low and intermediate RS groups were combined and compared with the low-risk 70-gene group [56].

EndoPredict

EndoPredict (EP) (Sividon Diagnostics, GmbH, Koln, Germany) is a 12-gene qRT-PCR-based test comprising eight cancer-related genes including genes related to proliferation and ER signaling, three normalization genes, and a gene that measures residual DNA; an EP score from 0 to 15 is derived using an algorithm with <5 indicating low risk and 5 or more indicating high risk of recurrence [60]. The EP score is combined with tumor size and nodal status to give the EPclin score separating patients into low- and high-risk groups with a cutoff of 3.3.

The test was developed in Germany and Austria specifically looking at 964 patients with early-stage ER-positive, HER2-negative breast cancer treated with endocrine therapy only. The test was then validated in 1702 patients from the ABCSG-6 and ABCSG-8 trials treated with tamoxifen or tamoxifen plus anastrozole. Both EP and EPclin scores identified patients with significant differences in 5- and 10-year DRFS independent of other clinicopathological factors including AOL, ER, and Ki67 in both node-negative and node-positive subgroups. The EPclin score showed the best performance in predicting late relapse with low and high groups having DRFS of 98 % and 88 %, respectively; of interest the ER signaling genes were not related to early recurrence but were predictive of recurrence at 5–10 years [106]. In a comparison with the NCCN and St. Gallen clinical guidelines, EPclin reclassified 58–61 % of high-/intermediate-risk patients to low risk; this group had a 10-year DRFS of 95 % [107].

EP score was associated with survival in a cohort of node-positive patients treated with adjuvant chemotherapy [108] and was associated with pCR following neoadjuvant chemotherapy in a separate study (EP low 7 % pCR; EP high 17 % pCR) [109]. There is no current clinical data on its predictive value for chemotherapy benefit.

EP is different from the preceding tests in that it is designed to be performed in decentralized laboratories; a proficiency testing study showed 100 % success rate with a Pearson correlation coefficient of 0.994 and 100 % concordance in assignment to EP risk group [63]. Reproducibility between core biopsy and surgical resection specimens was high (95 %) [110] with robust results in terms of preanalytical variables such as fixation and sample age [111]. Comparison with RS showed moderate concordance of 76 % [57]. In a study of 167 patients, EPclin score resulted in a change in therapy in 37 % of patients, with 25 % switching to endocrine therapy alone [61]. EPclin was cost-effective in an analysis based on the German health-care system [112].

Other Tests

Table 16.3 summarizes the main commercially available molecular tests for breast cancer. The Breast Cancer Index (Biotheranostics, CA, USA) is a qRT-PCR-based assay that includes two independent biomarkers. The HOXB13/ILI7BR ratio was shown to predict outcome in ER-positive breast cancer patients treated with tamoxifen [113]. This was combined with a five-gene molecular grade index composed of proliferation-related genes to predict early and late recurrences following endocrine therapy and identifies patients that may benefit from extended endocrine therapy [51, 114]. The BreastPRS prognostic score is a 200-gene algorithm developed using publically available genomic databases including ER-positive and ER-negative patients [115, 116]. BreastPRS identifies a low-risk group that does not benefit from adjuvant therapy and is unique in that it is an online genomic data analysis platform for laboratories to input gene expression data analyzed locally. In different approaches, gene signatures associated with tumor stroma and hypoxia have also been shown to be associated with outcome [26].

Monitoring Disease: Liquid Biopsies (Circulating Tumor Cells)

New molecular techniques such as next-generation sequencing have given us insight into the genetic complexity of breast cancer. This includes the unraveling of intratumoral heterogeneity, which provides the source for clonal evolution of the tumor over time with emergence of resistant subclones in response to therapy [117]. Liquid biopsies, with analysis of circulating tumor cells (CTCs) or circulating tumor DNA (ctDNA) in blood samples, provide a minimally invasive method for real-time monitoring of response and progression of disease with its associated genetic changes [118, 119].

The presence of tumor cells within the blood has been described as far back as 1869 [119]. CTCs form a rare population of cells within the circulation and detection can be difficult. Cell enrichment using surface antibodies such as epithelial cell adhesion molecule (EpCAM) or the physical properties of the cells is required. The CellSearch system is the only current FDA-approved technology for detection of CTCs and uses EpCAM to enrich for CTCs; however, EpCAM expression may be lost by breast cancer cells that have undergone epithelial-mesenchymal transition limiting the sensitivity of this technique. In early breast cancer when tumor burden is low, CTCs can only be detected in up to 20% of patients with a median of 1 CTC/sample [119].

Detection of CTCs has been associated with reduced survival in both metastatic and early breast cancer. The SWOG S0500 trial looked at CTCs in metastatic breast cancer, with an early switch in therapy in patients with persistent CTCs after 21 days of chemotherapy; there was no improvement in survival following the early switch [120]. Several clinical trials looking at the role of CTCs in therapeutic decisions in breast cancer are currently under way [118, 119]. Elimination of CTCs has potential as an alternative to pCR as a measure of early response in neoadjuvant clinical trials.

Paoletti et al. have developed the CTC-Endocrine Therapy Index (CTC-ETI), a score based on enumeration of CTCs and their expression of ER, bcl2, HER2, and Ki67; the COMETI trial is evaluating the value of the CTC-ETI in identifying women with endocrine refractory metastatic breast cancer [119, 121].

CTCs also provide a valuable research tool with development of cell lines and mouse xenograft models derived from CTCs allowing in vitro and in vivo studies of drug sensitivity. In one study, *ESR1* mutations were identified in three of six CTC-derived cell lines from patients with metastatic breast cancer pretreated with aromatase inhibitors [122]. The *ESR1* mutant cells were resistant to tamoxifen, raloxifene, and fulvestrant. With the advent of individual cell sequencing, CTCs can be used for whole-genome analysis, although there is some uncertainty as to how representative they are at the genetic level with respect to the bulk of the disease [118].

ctDNA is DNA released into the circulation during cell death. As with CTCs it is present at very low levels compared with circulating free DNA from normal cells. ctDNA levels reflect tumor burden so it is more frequently detected in patients with advanced disease, 75% of patients with metastasis compared with up to 50% of patients with early breast cancer [123]. Several studies have shown ctDNA is representative of the tumor genome, and as it is shed from all tumor sites in the body, it reflects tumoral heterogeneity [124, 125]. Genomic profiling of ctDNA can detect mutations with a frequency as low as 0.5%, meaning it has the potential to identify minor subclones with specific mutations associated with resistance. Serial samples can monitor the clonal evolution of the tumor, with loss of sensitive subclones and enrichment of resistant ones, and the emergence of clones with new resistance mutations on therapy.

Serial biopsies cause patient distress and discomfort, so a blood-based means of monitoring tumor genetic changes over time holds huge potential for future applications in personalized medicine. A key role for ctDNA could be as a biomarker used in monitoring disease, either in monitoring response to therapy in the neoadjuvant or metastatic setting or in monitoring patients for relapse. There are two approaches to using ctDNA for tumor monitoring. Primary tumors can be screened for specific mutations, and these mutations can then be detected in ctDNA and followed over time using methods such as digital PCR. Dawson et al. screened 52 patients with metastatic breast cancer and identified suitable mutations in 30; these mutations could be detected in ctDNA in 97 % of women and 82 % of samples [126]. Serial assays reflected response to therapy with changes in ctDNA levels preceding changes on imaging by an average of 5 months. Multiple mutations could be followed; in some patients these showed similar changes over time, while in others there were frequency changes reflecting resistance in a subclone carrying a particular mutation. Garcia-Murillas et al. looked at ctDNA in early breast cancer patients who received neoadjuvant chemotherapy [125]. Persistent ctDNA in postsurgical samples was found in 19 % of cases indicating residual microscopic disease, and this was predictive of relapse with a median of 8-month lead time over clinical relapse. In relapsed patients 50 % had ctDNA detected in a single sample, and 80 % were detected across serial samples. The patient that was negative for ctDNA had a cerebral relapse, suggesting that ctDNA is unable to cross the blood-brain barrier.

The second approach is using whole-genome sequencing or targeted deep sequencing of specified regions; this allows more comprehensive tumor genotyping with identification of therapeutic targets, monitoring of clonal evolution, and development of new mutations with therapy [124]. While results of such studies are exciting, it is still uncertain if diagnosing and treating recurrence at an earlier stage improves survival. Prospective trials to determine the clinical validity and clinical utility of these liquid biopsies are required before they can be introduced into routine practice. Even more controversial is the role of CTCs and ctDNA in cancer screening. These assays have the potential to detect tumors below the resolution of current imaging techniques, and many mutations are not site specific. Given the current controversies regarding overdiagnosis and overtreatment with conventional screening, it is unlikely that even more sensitive techniques with all the inherent uncertainties regarding benefit will be introduced in the foreseeable future.

References

1. Ali HR, Rueda OM, Chin SF, Curtis C, Dunning MJ, Aparicio SA, et al. Genome-driven integrated classification of breast cancer validated in over 7,500 samples. Genome Biol. 2014;15(8):431.
2. Prat A, Pineda E, Adamo B, Galvan P, Fernandez A, Gaba L, et al. Clinical implications of the intrinsic molecular subtypes of breast cancer. Breast. 2015; 24 Suppl 2:S26–35.
3. Lakhani SR, Ellis IO, Schnitt SJ, Tan PH, Van de Vijver MJ, editors. WHO classification of tumours of the breast. 4th ed. Lyon: IARC; 2012.
4. Brenton JD, Carey LA, Ahmed AA, Caldas C. Molecular classification and molecular forecasting of breast cancer: ready for clinical application? J Clin Oncol. 2005;23(29):7350–60.
5. Kittaneh M, Montero AJ, Gluck S. Molecular profiling for breast cancer: a comprehensive review. Biomark Cancer. 2013;5:61–70.
6. Rakha EA, Ellis IO. Modern classification of breast cancer: should we stick with morphology or convert to molecular profile characteristics. Adv Anat Pathol. 2011;18(4):255–67.
7. Rakha EA, Reis-Filho JS, Baehner F, Dabbs DJ, Decker T, Eusebi V, et al. Breast cancer prognostic classification in the molecular era: the role of histological grade. Breast Cancer Res. 2010;12(4):207 [Review].
8. Schnitt SJ. Classification and prognosis of invasive breast cancer: from morphology to molecular taxonomy. Mod Pathol. 2010;23 Suppl 2:S60–4 [Review].
9. Sinn P, Aulmann S, Wirtz R, Schott S, Marme F, Varga Z, et al. Multigene assays for classification, prognosis, and prediction in breast cancer: a critical review on the background and clinical utility. Geburtshilfe Frauenheilkd. 2013;73(9):932–40.
10. Blamey RW, Hornmark-Stenstam B, Ball G, Blichert-Toft M, Cataliotti L, Fourquet A, et al. ONCOPOOL – a European database for 16,944 cases of breast cancer. Eur J Cancer. 2010;46(1):56–71.
11. Haybittle JL, Blamey RW, Elston CW, Johnson J, Doyle PJ, Campbell FC, et al. A prognostic index in primary breast cancer. Br J Cancer. 1982;45(3):361–6.
12. Olivotto IA, Bajdik CD, Ravdin PM, Speers CH, Coldman AJ, Norris BD, et al. Population-based

validation of the prognostic model ADJUVANT! for early breast cancer. J Clin Oncol. 2005;23(12): 2716–25.

13. Ravdin PM. A computer program to assist in making breast cancer adjuvant therapy decisions. Semin Oncol. 1996;23(1 Suppl 2):43–50.

14. Wishart GC, Azzato EM, Greenberg DC, Rashbass J, Kearins O, Lawrence G, et al. PREDICT: a new UK prognostic model that predicts survival following surgery for invasive breast cancer. Breast Cancer Res. 2010;12(1):R1.

15. Wishart GC, Bajdik CD, Dicks E, Provenzano E, Schmidt MK, Sherman M, et al. PREDICT Plus: development and validation of a prognostic model for early breast cancer that includes HER2. Br J Cancer. 2012;107(5):800–7.

16. Wishart GC, Rakha E, Green A, Ellis I, Ali HR, Provenzano E, et al. Inclusion of KI67 significantly improves performance of the PREDICT prognostication and prediction model for early breast cancer. BMC Cancer. 2014;14:908.

17. Peto R, Davies C, Godwin J, Gray R, Pan HC, Clarke M, et al. Comparisons between different polychemotherapy regimens for early breast cancer: meta-analyses of long-term outcome among 100,000 women in 123 randomised trials. Lancet. 2012;379(9814):432–44.

18. Kallioniemi A, Kallioniemi OP, Sudar D, Rutovitz D, Gray JW, Waldman F, et al. Comparative genomic hybridization for molecular cytogenetic analysis of solid tumors. Science. 1992;258(5083):818–21.

19. Cavallaro S, Paratore S, de Snoo F, Salomone E, Villari L, Buscarino C, et al. Genomic analysis: toward a new approach in breast cancer management. Crit Rev Oncol Hematol. 2012;81(3):207–23 [Review].

20. Rizzo JM, Buck MJ. Key principles and clinical applications of "next-generation" DNA sequencing. Cancer Prev Res (Phila). 2012;5(7):887–900.

21. Russnes HG, Navin N, Hicks J, Borresen-Dale AL. Insight into the heterogeneity of breast cancer through next-generation sequencing. J Clin Invest. 2011;121(10):3810–8.

22. Desmedt C, Voet T, Sotiriou C, Campbell PJ. Next-generation sequencing in breast cancer: first take home messages. Curr Opin Oncol. 2012;24(6):597–604.

23. Perou CM, Sorlie T, Eisen MB, van de Rijn M, Jeffrey SS, Rees CA, et al. Molecular portraits of human breast tumours. Nature. 2000;406(6797):747–52.

24. Sorlie T, Perou CM, Tibshirani R, Aas T, Geisler S, Johnsen H, et al. Gene expression patterns of breast carcinomas distinguish tumor subclasses with clinical implications. Proc Natl Acad Sci U S A. 2001;98(19):10869–74.

25. Sotiriou C, Neo SY, McShane LM, Korn EL, Long PM, Jazaeri A, et al. Breast cancer classification and prognosis based on gene expression profiles from a population-based study. Proc Natl Acad Sci U S A. 2003;100(18):10393–8.

26. Weigelt B, Baehner FL, Reis-Filho JS. The contribution of gene expression profiling to breast cancer classification, prognostication and prediction: a retrospective of the last decade. J Pathol. 2010;220(2):263–80.

27. Prat A, Cheang MC, Martin M, Parker JS, Carrasco E, Caballero R, et al. Prognostic significance of progesterone receptor-positive tumor cells within immunohistochemically defined luminal A breast cancer. J Clin Oncol. 2013;31(2):203–9.

28. Cheang MC, Chia SK, Voduc D, Gao D, Leung S, Snider J, et al. Ki67 index, HER2 status, and prognosis of patients with luminal B breast cancer. J Natl Cancer Inst. 2009;101(10):736–50.

29. Badve S, Dabbs DJ, Schnitt SJ, Baehner FL, Decker T, Eusebi V, et al. Basal-like and triple-negative breast cancers: a critical review with an emphasis on the implications for pathologists and oncologists. Mod Pathol. 2011;24(2):157–67 [Review].

30. Geyer FC, Lambros MB, Natrajan R, Mehta R, Mackay A, Savage K, et al. Genomic and immunohistochemical analysis of adenosquamous carcinoma of the breast. Mod Pathol. 2010;23(7):951–60.

31. Jacquemier J, Padovani L, Rabayrol L, Lakhani SR, Penault-Llorca F, Denoux Y, et al. Typical medullary breast carcinomas have a basal/myoepithelial phenotype. J Pathol. 2005;207(3):260–8.

32. Weigelt B, Kreike B, Reis-Filho JS. Metaplastic breast carcinomas are basal-like breast cancers: a genomic profiling analysis. Breast Cancer Res Treat. 2009;117(2):273–80.

33. Wetterskog D, Lopez-Garcia MA, Lambros MB, A'Hern R, Geyer FC, Milanezi F, et al. Adenoid cystic carcinomas constitute a genomically distinct subgroup of triple-negative and basal-like breast cancers. J Pathol. 2012;226(1):84–96.

34. Sabatier R, Finetti P, Cervera N, Lambaudie E, Esterni B, Mamessier E, et al. A gene expression signature identifies two prognostic subgroups of basal breast cancer. Breast Cancer Res Treat. 2011;126(2):407–20.

35. Foulkes WD, Stefansson IM, Chappuis PO, Begin LR, Goffin JR, Wong N, et al. Germline BRCA1 mutations and a basal epithelial phenotype in breast cancer. J Natl Cancer Inst. 2003;95(19):1482–5.

36. Severson TM, Peeters J, Majewski I, Michaut M, Bosma A, Schouten PC, et al. BRCA1-like signature in triple negative breast cancer: molecular and clinical characterization reveals subgroups with therapeutic potential. Mol Oncol. 2015;9(8):1528–38.

37. Sorlie T, Tibshirani R, Parker J, Hastie T, Marron JS, Nobel A, et al. Repeated observation of breast tumor subtypes in independent gene expression data sets. Proc Natl Acad Sci U S A. 2003;100(14):8418–23.

38. Parker JS, Mullins M, Cheang MC, Leung S, Voduc D, Vickery T, et al. Supervised risk predictor of breast cancer based on intrinsic subtypes. J Clin Oncol. 2009;27(8):1160–7.

39. Hu Z, Fan C, Oh DS, Marron JS, He X, Qaqish BF, et al. The molecular portraits of breast tumors are

conserved across microarray platforms. BMC Genomics. 2006;7:96.

40. Comprehensive molecular portraits of human breast tumours. Nature. 2012;490(7418):61–70.

41. Mackay A, Weigelt B, Grigoriadis A, Kreike B, Natrajan R, A'Hern R, et al. Microarray-based class discovery for molecular classification of breast cancer: analysis of interobserver agreement. J Natl Cancer Inst. 2011;103(8):662–73.

42. Pusztai L, Mazouni C, Anderson K, Wu Y, Symmans WF. Molecular classification of breast cancer: limitations and potential. Oncologist. 2006;11(8):868–77.

43. Weigelt B, Mackay A, A'Hern R, Natrajan R, Tan DS, Dowsett M, et al. Breast cancer molecular profiling with single sample predictors: a retrospective analysis. Lancet Oncol. 2010;11(4):339–49.

44. Zhao X, Rodland EA, Sorlie T, Vollan HK, Russnes HG, Kristensen VN, et al. Systematic assessment of prognostic gene signatures for breast cancer shows distinct influence of time and ER status. BMC Cancer. 2014;14:211.

45. Prat A, Perou CM. Deconstructing the molecular portraits of breast cancer. Mol Oncol. 2011;5(1):5–23.

46. Lehmann BD, Bauer JA, Chen X, Sanders ME, Chakravarthy AB, Shyr Y, et al. Identification of human triple-negative breast cancer subtypes and preclinical models for selection of targeted therapies. J Clin Invest. 2011;121(7):2750–67.

47. Lehmann BD, Bauer JA, Schafer JM, Pendleton CS, Tang L, Johnson KC, et al. PIK3CA mutations in androgen receptor-positive triple negative breast cancer confer sensitivity to the combination of PI3K and androgen receptor inhibitors. Breast Cancer Res. 2014;16(4):406.

48. Masuda H, Baggerly KA, Wang Y, Zhang Y, Gonzalez-Angulo AM, Meric-Bernstam F, et al. Differential response to neoadjuvant chemotherapy among 7 triple-negative breast cancer molecular subtypes. Clin Cancer Res. 2013;19(19):5533–40.

49. Curtis C, Shah SP, Chin SF, Turashvili G, Rueda OM, Dunning MJ, et al. The genomic and transcriptomic architecture of 2,000 breast tumours reveals novel subgroups. Nature. 2012;486(7403):346–52.

50. Dawson SJ, Rueda OM, Aparicio S, Caldas C. A new genome-driven integrated classification of breast cancer and its implications. Embo J. 2013;32(5):617–28 [Review].

51. Gyorffy B, Hatzis C, Sanft T, Hofstatter E, Aktas B, Pusztai L. Multigene prognostic tests in breast cancer: past, present, future. Breast Cancer Res. 2015;17:11.

52. Desmedt C, Haibe-Kains B, Wirapati P, Buyse M, Larsimont D, Bontempi G, et al. Biological processes associated with breast cancer clinical outcome depend on the molecular subtypes. Clin Cancer Res. 2008;14(16):5158–65.

53. Wirapati P, Sotiriou C, Kunkel S, Farmer P, Pradervand S, Haibe-Kains B, et al. Meta-analysis of gene expression profiles in breast cancer: toward a unified understanding of breast cancer subtyping and prognosis signatures. Breast Cancer Res. 2008;10(4):R65.

54. Kelly CM, Bernard PS, Krishnamurthy S, Wang B, Ebbert MT, Bastien RR, et al. Agreement in risk prediction between the 21-gene recurrence score assay (Oncotype DX(R)) and the PAM50 breast cancer intrinsic Classifier in early-stage estrogen receptor-positive breast cancer. Oncologist. 2012;17(4):492–8.

55. Prat A, Parker JS, Fan C, Cheang MC, Miller LD, Bergh J, et al. Concordance among gene expression-based predictors for ER-positive breast cancer treated with adjuvant tamoxifen. Ann Oncol. 2012;23(11):2866–73.

56. Fan C, Oh DS, Wessels L, Weigelt B, Nuyten DS, Nobel AB, et al. Concordance among gene-expression-based predictors for breast cancer. N Engl J Med. 2006;355(6):560–9.

57. Varga Z, Sinn P, Fritzsche F, von Hochstetter A, Noske A, Schraml P, et al. Comparison of EndoPredict and Oncotype DX test results in hormone receptor positive invasive breast cancer. PLoS ONE. 2013;8(3):e58483.

58. Ebbert MT, Bastien RR, Boucher KM, Martin M, Carrasco E, Caballero R, et al. Characterization of uncertainty in the classification of multivariate assays: application to PAM50 centroid-based genomic predictors for breast cancer treatment plans. J Clin Bioinforma. 2011;1:37.

59. Azim Jr HA, Michiels S, Zagouri F, Delaloge S, Filipits M, Namer M, et al. Utility of prognostic genomic tests in breast cancer practice: the IMPAKT 2012 Working Group Consensus Statement. Ann Oncol. 2013;24(3):647–54.

60. Filipits M, Rudas M, Jakesz R, Dubsky P, Fitzal F, Singer CF, et al. A new molecular predictor of distant recurrence in ER-positive, HER2-negative breast cancer adds independent information to conventional clinical risk factors. Clin Cancer Res. 2011;17(18):6012–20.

61. Muller BM, Keil E, Lehmann A, Winzer KJ, Richter-Ehrenstein C, Prinzler J, et al. The EndoPredict gene-expression assay in clinical practice – performance and impact on clinical decisions. PLoS ONE. 2013;8(6):e68252.

62. Marchionni L, Wilson RF, Marinopoulos SS, Wolff AC, Parmigiani G, Bass EB, et al. Impact of gene expression profiling tests on breast cancer outcomes. Evid Rep Technol Assess (Full Rep). [Review]. 2007;(160):1–105.

63. Denkert C, Kronenwett R, Schlake W, Bohmann K, Penzel R, Weber KE, et al. Decentral gene expression analysis for ER+/Her2- breast cancer: results of a proficiency testing program for the EndoPredict assay. Virchows Arch. 2012;460(3):251–9.

64. van 't Veer LJ, Dai H, van de Vijver MJ, He YD, Hart AA, Mao M, et al. Gene expression profiling predicts clinical outcome of breast cancer. Nature. 2002;415(6871):530–6.

65. Sapino A, Roepman P, Linn SC, Snel MH, Delahaye LJ, van den Akker J, et al. MammaPrint molecular diagnostics on formalin-fixed, paraffin-embedded tissue. J Mol Diagn. 2014;16(2):190–7.

66. van de Vijver MJ, He YD, van't Veer LJ, Dai H, Hart AA, Voskuil DW, et al. A gene-expression signature as a predictor of survival in breast cancer. N Engl J Med. 2002;347(25):1999–2009.

67. Cardoso F, Van't Veer L, Rutgers E, Loi S, Mook S, Piccart-Gebhart MJ. Clinical application of the 70-gene profile: the MINDACT trial. J Clin Oncol. 2008;26(5):729–35.

68. Bogaerts J, Cardoso F, Buyse M, Braga S, Loi S, Harrison JA, et al. Gene signature evaluation as a prognostic tool: challenges in the design of the MINDACT trial. Nat Clin Pract Oncol. 2006;3(10):540–51 [Review].

69. Rutgers E, Piccart-Gebhart MJ, Bogaerts J, Delaloge S, Veer LV, Rubio IT, et al. The EORTC 10041/BIG 03-04 MINDACT trial is feasible: results of the pilot phase. Eur J Cancer. 2011;47(18):2742–9.

70. Saghatchian M, Mook S, Pruneri G, Viale G, Glas AM, Guerin S, et al. Additional prognostic value of the 70-gene signature (MammaPrint((R))) among breast cancer patients with 4–9 positive lymph nodes. Breast. 2013;22(5):682–90.

71. Bueno-de-Mesquita JM, Linn SC, Keijzer R, Wesseling J, Nuyten DS, van Krimpen C, et al. Validation of 70-gene prognosis signature in node-negative breast cancer. Breast Cancer Res Treat. 2009;117(3):483–95.

72. Wittner BS, Sgroi DC, Ryan PD, Bruinsma TJ, Glas AM, Male A, et al. Analysis of the MammaPrint breast cancer assay in a predominantly postmenopausal cohort. Clin Cancer Res. 2008;14(10):2988–93.

73. Hartmann S, Gerber B, Elling D, Heintze K, Reimer T. The 70-gene signature as prognostic factor for elderly women with hormone receptor-positive, HER2-negative breast cancer. Breast Care (Basel). 2012;7(1):19–24.

74. Drukker CA, van Tinteren H, Schmidt MK, Rutgers EJ, Bernards R, van de Vijver MJ, et al. Long-term impact of the 70-gene signature on breast cancer outcome. Breast Cancer Res Treat. 2014;143(3):587–92.

75. Knauer M, Mook S, Rutgers EJ, Bender RA, Hauptmann M, van de Vijver MJ, et al. The predictive value of the 70-gene signature for adjuvant chemotherapy in early breast cancer. Breast Cancer Res Treat. 2010;120(3):655–61.

76. Wang Y, Klijn JG, Zhang Y, Sieuwerts AM, Look MP, Yang F, et al. Gene-expression profiles to predict distant metastasis of lymph-node-negative primary breast cancer. Lancet. 2005;365(9460):671–9.

77. Foekens JA, Atkins D, Zhang Y, Sweep FC, Harbeck N, Paradiso A, et al. Multicenter validation of a gene expression-based prognostic signature in lymph node-negative primary breast cancer. J Clin Oncol. 2006;24(11):1665–71.

78. Desmedt C, Piette F, Loi S, Wang Y, Lallemand F, Haibe-Kains B, et al. Strong time dependence of the 76-gene prognostic signature for node-negative breast cancer patients in the TRANSBIG multicenter independent validation series. Clin Cancer Res. 2007;13(11):3207–14.

79. Haibe-Kains B, Desmedt C, Piette F, Buyse M, Cardoso F, Van't Veer L, et al. Comparison of prognostic gene expression signatures for breast cancer. BMC Genomics. 2008;9:394.

80. Kreike B, van Kouwenhove M, Horlings H, Weigelt B, Peterse H, Bartelink H, et al. Gene expression profiling and histopathological characterization of triple-negative/basal-like breast carcinomas. Breast Cancer Res. 2007;9(5):R65.

81. Dowsett M, Sestak I, Lopez-Knowles E, Sidhu K, Dunbier AK, Cowens JW, et al. Comparison of PAM50 risk of recurrence score with oncotype DX and IHC4 for predicting risk of distant recurrence after endocrine therapy. J Clin Oncol. 2013;31(22):2783–90.

82. Gnant M, Filipits M, Greil R, Stoeger H, Rudas M, Bago-Horvath Z, et al. Predicting distant recurrence in receptor-positive breast cancer patients with limited clinicopathological risk: using the PAM50 Risk of Recurrence score in 1478 postmenopausal patients of the ABCSG-8 trial treated with adjuvant endocrine therapy alone. Ann Oncol. 2014;25(2):339–45.

83. Gnant M, Sestak I, Filipits M, Dowsett M, Balic M, Lopez-Knowles E, et al. Identifying clinically relevant prognostic subgroups of postmenopausal women with node-positive hormone receptor-positive early-stage breast cancer treated with endocrine therapy: a combined analysis of ABCSG-8 and ATAC using the PAM50 risk of recurrence score and intrinsic subtype. Ann Oncol. 2015;26(8):1685–91.

84. Filipits M, Nielsen TO, Rudas M, Greil R, Stoger H, Jakesz R, et al. The PAM50 risk-of-recurrence score predicts risk for late distant recurrence after endocrine therapy in postmenopausal women with endocrine-responsive early breast cancer. Clin Cancer Res. 2014;20(5):1298–305.

85. Sestak I, Dowsett M, Zabaglo L, Lopez-Knowles E, Ferree S, Cowens JW, et al. Factors predicting late recurrence for estrogen receptor-positive breast cancer. J Natl Cancer Inst. 2013;105(19):1504–11.

86. Cheang MC, Voduc KD, Tu D, Jiang S, Leung S, Chia SK, et al. Responsiveness of intrinsic subtypes to adjuvant anthracycline substitution in the NCIC. CTG MA.5 randomized trial. Clin Cancer Res. 2012;18(8):2402–12.

87. Martin M, Prat A, Rodriguez-Lescure A, Caballero R, Ebbert MT, Munarriz B, et al. PAM50 proliferation score as a predictor of weekly paclitaxel benefit in breast cancer. Breast Cancer Res Treat. 2013;138(2):457–66.

88. Esserman LJ, Berry DA, Cheang MC, Yau C, Perou CM, Carey L, et al. Chemotherapy response and recurrence-free survival in neoadjuvant breast cancer depends on biomarker profiles: results from the I-SPY 1 TRIAL (CALGB 150007/150012; ACRIN 6657). Breast Cancer Res Treat. 2012;132(3):1049–62.

89. Prat A, Bianchini G, Thomas M, Belousov A, Cheang MC, Koehler A, et al. Research-based PAM50 subtype predictor identifies higher responses and improved survival outcomes in HER2-positive

breast cancer in the NOAH study. Clin Cancer Res. 2014;20(2):511–21.

90. Wallden B, Storhoff J, Nielsen T, Dowidar N, Schaper C, Ferree S, et al. Development and verification of the PAM50-based Prosigna breast cancer gene signature assay. BMC Med Genomics. 2015;8:54.

91. Sotiriou C, Wirapati P, Loi S, Harris A, Fox S, Smeds J, et al. Gene expression profiling in breast cancer: understanding the molecular basis of histologic grade to improve prognosis. J Natl Cancer Inst. 2006;98(4):262–72.

92. Loi S, Haibe-Kains B, Desmedt C, Lallemand F, Tutt AM, Gillet C, et al. Definition of clinically distinct molecular subtypes in estrogen receptor-positive breast carcinomas through genomic grade. J Clin Oncol. 2007;25(10):1239–46.

93. Liedtke C, Hatzis C, Symmans WF, Desmedt C, Haibe-Kains B, Valero V, et al. Genomic grade index is associated with response to chemotherapy in patients with breast cancer. J Clin Oncol. 2009;27(19):3185–91.

94. Bertucci F, Finetti P, Roche H, Le Doussal JM, Marisa L, Martin AL, et al. Comparison of the prognostic value of genomic grade index, Ki67 expression and mitotic activity index in early node-positive breast cancer patients. Ann Oncol. 2013;24(3):625–32.

95. Toussaint J, Sieuwerts AM, Haibe-Kains B, Desmedt C, Rouas G, Harris AL, et al. Improvement of the clinical applicability of the Genomic Grade Index through a qRT-PCR test performed on frozen and formalin-fixed paraffin-embedded tissues. BMC Genomics. 2009;10:424.

96. Paik S, Shak S, Tang G, Kim C, Baker J, Cronin M, et al. A multigene assay to predict recurrence of tamoxifen-treated, node-negative breast cancer. N Engl J Med. 2004;351(27):2817–26.

97. Dowsett M, Cuzick J, Wale C, Forbes J, Mallon EA, Salter J, et al. Prediction of risk of distant recurrence using the 21-gene recurrence score in node-negative and node-positive postmenopausal patients with breast cancer treated with anastrozole or tamoxifen: a TransATAC study. J Clin Oncol. 2010;28(11):1829–34.

98. Paik S, Tang G, Shak S, Kim C, Baker J, Kim W, et al. Gene expression and benefit of chemotherapy in women with node-negative, estrogen receptor-positive breast cancer. J Clin Oncol. 2006;24(23):3726–34.

99. Sparano JA, Gray RJ, Makower DF, Pritchard KI, Albain KS, Hayes DF, et al. Prospective validation of a 21-gene expression assay in breast cancer. N Engl J Med. 2015;373(21):2005–14.

100. Carlson JJ, Roth JA. The impact of the Oncotype Dx breast cancer assay in clinical practice: a systematic review and meta-analysis. Breast Cancer Res Treat. 2013;141(1):13–22.

101. Sparano JA, Paik S. Development of the 21-gene assay and its application in clinical practice and clinical trials. J Clin Oncol. 2008;26(5):721–8 [Review].

102. Habel LA, Shak S, Jacobs MK, Capra A, Alexander C, Pho M, et al. A population-based study of tumor gene expression and risk of breast cancer death among lymph node-negative patients. Breast Cancer Res. 2006;8(3):R25.

103. Gligorov J, Pivot XB, Jacot W, Naman HL, Spaeth D, Misset JL, et al. Prospective clinical utility study of the use of the 21-gene assay in adjuvant clinical decision making in women with estrogen receptor-positive early invasive breast cancer: results from the SWITCH study. Oncologist. 2015;20(8):873–9.

104. Rouzier R, Pronzato P, Chereau E, Carlson J, Hunt B, Valentine WJ. Multigene assays and molecular markers in breast cancer: systematic review of health economic analyses. Breast Cancer Res Treat. 2013;139(3):621–37.

105. Cuzick J, Dowsett M, Pineda S, Wale C, Salter J, Quinn E, et al. Prognostic value of a combined estrogen receptor, progesterone receptor, Ki-67, and human epidermal growth factor receptor 2 immunohistochemical score and comparison with the Genomic Health recurrence score in early breast cancer. J Clin Oncol. 2011;29(32):4273–8.

106. Dubsky P, Brase JC, Jakesz R, Rudas M, Singer CF, Greil R, et al. The EndoPredict score provides prognostic information on late distant metastases in ER+/HER2- breast cancer patients. Br J Cancer. 2013;109(12):2959–64.

107. Dubsky P, Filipits M, Jakesz R, Rudas M, Singer CF, Greil R, et al. EndoPredict improves the prognostic classification derived from common clinical guidelines in ER-positive, HER2-negative early breast cancer. Ann Oncol. 2013;24(3):640–7.

108. Martin M, Brase JC, Calvo L, Krappmann K, Ruiz-Borrego M, Fisch K, et al. Clinical validation of the EndoPredict test in node-positive, chemotherapy-treated ER+/HER2- breast cancer patients: results from the GEICAM 9906 trial. Breast Cancer Res. 2014;16(2):R38.

109. Bertucci F, Finetti P, Viens P, Birnbaum D. EndoPredict predicts for the response to neoadjuvant chemotherapy in ER-positive, HER2-negative breast cancer. Cancer Lett. 2014;355(1):70–5.

110. Muller BM, Brase JC, Haufe F, Weber KE, Budzies J, Petry C, et al. Comparison of the RNA-based EndoPredict multigene test between core biopsies and corresponding surgical breast cancer sections. J Clin Pathol. 2012;65(7):660–2.

111. Poremba C, Uhlendorff J, Pfitzner BM, Hennig G, Bohmann K, Bojar H, et al. Preanalytical variables and performance of diagnostic RNA-based gene expression analysis in breast cancer. Virchows Arch. 2014;465(4):409–17.

112. Blank PR, Filipits M, Dubsky P, Gutzwiller F, Lux MP, Brase JC, et al. Cost-effectiveness analysis of prognostic gene expression signature-based stratification of early breast cancer patients. Pharmacoeconomics. 2015;33(2):179–90.

113. Ma XJ, Wang Z, Ryan PD, Isakoff SJ, Barmettler A, Fuller A, et al. A two-gene expression ratio predicts

clinical outcome in breast cancer patients treated with tamoxifen. Cancer Cell. 2004;5(6):607–16.

114. Sgroi DC, Sestak I, Cuzick J, Zhang Y, Schnabel CA, Schroeder B, et al. Prediction of late distant recurrence in patients with oestrogen-receptor-positive breast cancer: a prospective comparison of the breast-cancer index (BCI) assay, 21-gene recurrence score, and IHC4 in the TransATAC study population. Lancet Oncol. 2013;14(11):1067–76.

115. D'Alfonso TM, van Laar RK, Vahdat LT, Hussain W, Flinchum R, Brown N, et al. BreastPRS is a gene expression assay that stratifies intermediate-risk Oncotype DX patients into high- or low-risk for disease recurrence. Breast Cancer Res Treat. 2013;139(3):705–15.

116. Van Laar RK. Design and multiseries validation of a web-based gene expression assay for predicting breast cancer recurrence and patient survival. J Mol Diagn. 2011;13(3):297–304.

117. Yates LR, Gerstung M, Knappskog S, Desmedt C, Gundem G, Van Loo P, et al. Subclonal diversification of primary breast cancer revealed by multiregion sequencing. Nat Med. 2015;21(7):751–9.

118. Gingras I, Salgado R, Ignatiadis M. Liquid biopsy: will it be the 'magic tool' for monitoring response of solid tumors to anticancer therapies? Curr Opin Oncol. 2015;27(6):560–7.

119. Ignatiadis M, Dawson SJ. Circulating tumor cells and circulating tumor DNA for precision medicine: dream or reality? Ann Oncol. 2014;25(12):2304–13.

120. Smerage JB, Barlow WE, Hortobagyi GN, Winer EP, Leyland-Jones B, Srkalovic G, et al. Circulating tumor cells and response to chemotherapy in metastatic breast cancer: SWOG S0500. J Clin Oncol. 2014;32(31):3483–9.

121. Paoletti C, Muniz MC, Thomas DG, Griffith KA, Kidwell KM, Tokudome N, et al. Development of circulating tumor cell-endocrine therapy index in patients with hormone receptor-positive breast cancer. Clin Cancer Res. 2015;21(11):2487–98.

122. Yu M, Bardia A, Aceto N, Bersani F, Madden MW, Donaldson MC, et al. Cancer therapy. Ex vivo culture of circulating breast tumor cells for individualized testing of drug susceptibility. Science. 2014;345(6193):216–20.

123. Bettegowda C, Sausen M, Leary RJ, Kinde I, Wang Y, Agrawal N, et al. Detection of circulating tumor DNA in early- and late-stage human malignancies. Sci Transl Med. 2014;6(224):224ra24.

124. De Mattos-Arruda L, Weigelt B, Cortes J, Won HH, Ng CK, Nuciforo P, et al. Capturing intra-tumor genetic heterogeneity by de novo mutation profiling of circulating cell-free tumor DNA: a proof-of-principle. Ann Oncol. 2014;25(9):1729–35.

125. Garcia-Murillas I, Schiavon G, Weigelt B, Ng C, Hrebien S, Cutts RJ, et al. Mutation tracking in circulating tumor DNA predicts relapse in early breast cancer. Sci Transl Med. 2015;7(302):302ra133.

126. Dawson SJ, Tsui DW, Murtaza M, Biggs H, Rueda OM, Chin SF, et al. Analysis of circulating tumor DNA to monitor metastatic breast cancer. N Engl J Med. 2013;368(13):1199–209. Comparative Study.

Uncommon Benign Breast Lesions

17

Sami Shousha

Abstract

This chapter deals with some of the uncommon breast lesions that can be encountered during routine daily practice and need differentiating from malignant lesions.

Keywords

Microglandular adenosis • Adenomyoepithelioma • Collagenous spherulosis • Pleomorphic adenoma • Ductal adenoma • Nipple adenoma • Adenosis tumor • Syringomatous adenoma • Hidradenoma • Granulomatous mastitis

Introduction

Uncommon benign lesions have always been encountered in the breast, but their incidence seems to have increased since the introduction of regular mammographic breast screening. In addition to the well-characterized lesions like microglandular adenosis, pleomorphic adenoma, and collagenous spherulosis, which will be dealt with here in detail, there are other lesions which are occasionally seen, mostly as a result of an abnormal radiological investigation, and that are commonly seen in other organs or represent unusual

forms of calcification. These will be listed and some illustrated at the end of this chapter.

Microglandular Adenosis

This is a benign proliferative lesion that can mimic tubular carcinoma clinically and histologically, first described in 1983 almost simultaneously by Azzopardi [1], Rosen [2], and Tavassoli and Norris [3]. Patients affected vary in age between 28 and 82 years, with most patients being 45–55 years old. The lesions vary widely in size and may occasionally present as a palpable mass.

Microscopically, the lesion characteristically consists of small uniform-rounded glands lined by a single layer of cuboidal epithelium and having well-defined lumina containing a drop of eosinophilic secretion that is Periodic acid-Shciff positive (Fig. 17.1a, b). Like tubular carcinoma,

S. Shousha
Department of Histopathology, Charing Cross Hospital & Imperial College, Fulham Palace Road, London W6 8RF, UK
e-mail: s.shousha@imperial.ac.uk

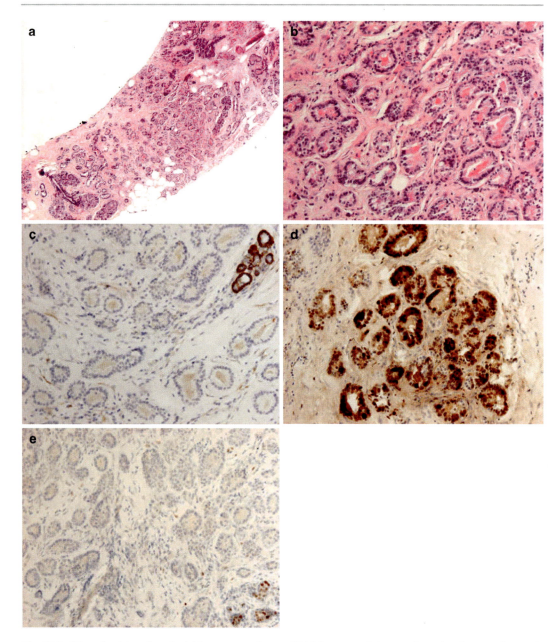

Fig. 17.1 Microglandular adenosis. (**a**) Low power view of a core biopsy with microglandular adenosis involving the middle two thirds of the biopsy showing the characteristic small uniform-rounded glands. (**b**) High power view of the same case showing the uniform glands in more details with the luminal eosinophilic secretion (H&E). (**c**) CD10 immunostaining confirms the absence of myoepithelial layer around the glands. Note the presence of a few positively stained normal ducts in the right upper corner. (**d**) The cells are S100 strongly positive and (**e**) ER negative. A few positively stained normal ducts are present in the right lower corner

these proliferating glands have no myoepithelial layer; hence myoepithelial markers like p63, smooth muscle actin, and CD10 are always negative (Fig. 17.1c). However, unlike tubular carcinoma, the cells are S100 strongly positive (Fig. 17.1d) and Estrogen Receptors negative (Fig. 17.1e). Also, unlike tubular carcinoma, the stroma is bland with no evidence of desmoplasia.

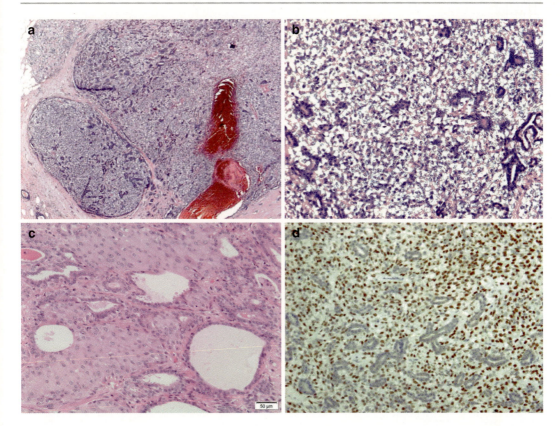

Fig. 17.2 Adenomyoepithelioma. (**a**) Low power view showing a lobulated well-demarcated lesion. (**b**) High power view showing the compressed ducts surrounded with abundant myoepithelial cells with clear cytoplasm. (**c**) Another case where the myoepithelium is apocrine-like with abundant eosinophilic cytoplasm. (**d**) p63 immunostaining of the case seen in a and b, demonstrating the positively stained myoepithelial nuclei and negative compressed ducts

The glands are scattered haphazardly in the stroma and adjacent fat, and the borders of the lesion can be irregular.

The main differential diagnosis is invasive tubular carcinoma. In addition to the immunohistochemical differences mentioned above, the glands in tubular carcinoma are irregular and have tapering ends, and the lining cells usually have prominent cytoplasmic snouts protruding into the lumen.

Various histological types of breast carcinoma have been described in association with microglandular adenosis, and the condition may be precancerous [4, 5]; hence it is usually given a B3 when seen in a core biopsy. The subject is dealt with in more details in Chap. 18.

Adenomyoepithelioma

This is an uncommon benign, usually solitary and centrally located breast lesion in which there is a prominent proliferation of myoepithelial cells associated with glandular structures. The proliferating myoepithelial cells can be spindle shaped or cuboidal with clear (Fig. 17.2a, b) or eosinophilic, apocrine-like (Fig. 17.2c) cytoplasm, staining positively with myoepithelial markers (Fig. 17.2d). They surround normal-looking or compressed ducts (Fig. 17.2). The ratio of ducts to myoepithelial cells is variable, but the latter usually compose more than 20 % of the lesion.

In a report of 27 cases, the size range was 1–7 cm and 22 cases were sharply demarcated or lobulated [6]. Radiologically, they may resemble fibroadenomas. Malignant transformation can occur [7]; hence it is advisable to give the lesion a B3 score when seen in a core biopsy. Malignant adenomyoepithelioma is discussed in Chap. 18.

Collagenous Spherulosis

An uncommon benign intraductal lesion characterized by the presence of epithelial/myoepithelial proliferation (Fig. 17.3a). The estimated incidence is 1 % in excision biopsies [8]. The lesion is characterized by the presence of eosinophilic collagen and laminin-rich spherules (Fig. 17.3b) closely surrounded by myoepithelial (Fig. 17.3c) and epithelial cells. The lesions can be multifocal and are usually of small size varying between 1–11 m [9], but may very rarely present as a mass [10]. Microcalcification may be present. There is no evidence that the lesion is precancerous, but it has been reported to be frequently associated with LCIS [8, 9], as well as other benign and malignant lesions [9]. In a review of 81 cases referred to the Armed Forces Institute of Pathology, Washington, DC, the lesion was correctly diagnosed in 15 % of cases and was misdiagnosed as atypical ductal hyperplasia in 17 % and as DCIS or invasive carcinoma in 11 % of cases [9].

The main differential diagnoses are cribriform DCIS and adenoid cystic carcinoma. Immunostaining for ER and CD10 can differentiate between the three lesions. ER is strongly and diffusely positive in cribriform DCIS, negative in adenoid cystic carcinoma, and heterogeneously positive in collagenous spherulosis

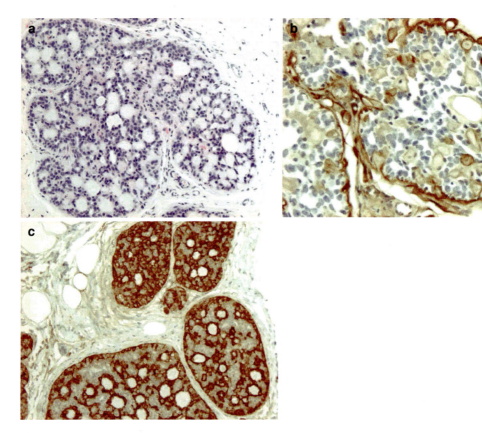

Fig. 17.3 Collagenous spherulosis. (**a**) H&E-stained section showing the cribriform pattern. (**b**) Positive immunostaining for laminin within the spherules. (**c**) Positive immunostaining for CD10 of the myoepithelial cells surrounding the spherules

(Fig. 18.1d). CD10 is negative in DCIS (except for the surrounding myoepithelium), mostly negative in adenoid cystic carcinoma, and shows a characteristic positive staining around the spherules in collagenous spherulosis (Fig. 17.3c).

Pleomorphic Adenoma

A rare well-circumscribed lesion that can be mistaken radiologically for a fibroadenoma [11] and histologically as a carcinoma particularly in a core biopsy [12]. It has been described in male as well as female patients, mostly in the peri-areolar region suggesting an origin from large ducts [13]. It usually presents as a single lesion, but multiple lesions have been described, and cases associated with carcinoma have been reported [13]. Sizes vary between 0.6 and 5.0 cm [13, 14].

Microscopically, there is an admixture of benign glandular epithelial and myoepithelial elements that can be arranged in glands, small solid groups, or cords, together with cartilaginous or myxoid areas and sometimes bone (Fig. 17.4). A transition between different morphological elements may be present. There may be pseudo-capsules around the lesion, but this may be penetrated by tongues of the tumor. The diagnosis is usually clinched, particularly in a core biopsy, by immunohistochemistry which will demonstrate the presence of a mixture of benign epithelial and myoepithelial cells as demonstrated by markers for both elements like p63, S100, smooth muscle actin, and ER, all showing a mixture of negative and positive

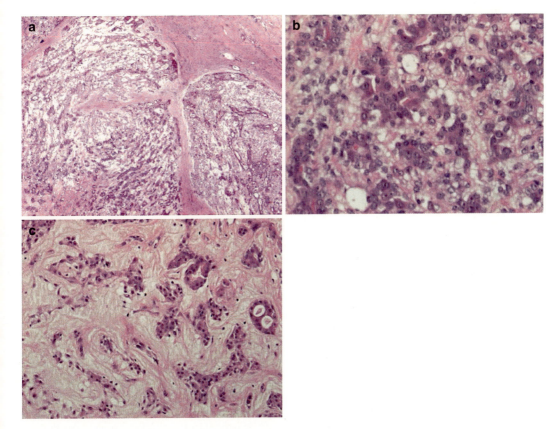

Fig. 17.4 Pleomorphic adenoma. (a) The lesion is well circumscribed and consists of disorderly arranged epithelial and myoepithelial elements in a fibromyxomatous stroma. (b) Part of the lesion showing an admixture of darkly stained epithelial cells and myoepithelial cells with clear cytoplasm. (c) Another part of the lesion composed of epithelial cells arranged in cords, solid groups, and glandular structures

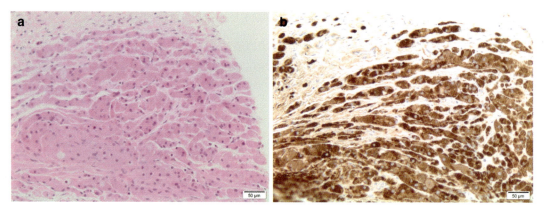

Fig. 17.5 Granular cell tumor. (**a**) The tumor consists of closely packed sheets and nests of large polygonal cells with faintly stained granular cytoplasm and small rounded nuclei. (**b**) The tumor cells are S100 strongly positive

cells. Recurrence is unusual, but has been described [15].

Granular Cell Tumor

An uncommon benign tumor that has been described in male as well as female patients. It is usually a solitary lesion but can be multiple [16]. In a series of 17 cases from New York, the age range was 17–68 years [16], but a case diagnosed in a 14-year-old girl has also been described [17]. It can vary in size between 1 and 6 cm and has a firm consistency. Grossly the lesion appears circumscribed, but may have infiltrative borders. Microscopically, it consists of closely packed sheets and nests of large polygonal cells with faintly stained granular cytoplasm and small rounded nuclei (Fig. 17.5a). Mitosis and nuclear pleomorphism are not usually seen. The cytoplasmic granules are PAS positive, diastase resistant. Immunohistochemically, the cells are strongly positive for S100 (Fig. 17.5b) and sometimes for CD68. The cells are cytokeratin and ER negative. Most lesions are benign, but incomplete excision may result in recurrence. Malignant granular cell tumors have been described, in organs other than the breast; hence it is advisable to give the lesion a score of B3 when seen in a core biopsy with a recommendation for excision.

Ductal Adenoma

This probably is a variant of intraductal papilloma, where the epithelial proliferation is more solid or cribriform, rather than papillary, and the ductal lumen is totally or almost totally obliterated (Fig. 17.6a). It is usually solid and can be clinically confused with carcinoma. Microscopically, the lesion is well circumscribed. Myoepithelial cells, as demonstrated by immunohistochemistry, are seen mixed with epithelial cells. Calcification may be present (Fig. 17.6b) and occasional atypical cells may be seen [18–20]. The lesion is probably the benign equivalent of solid papillary carcinoma.

Adenosis Tumor

This is a benign lesion composed of closely packed nodules of sclerosing adenosis that remain relatively well defined (Fig. 17.7a, b). It usually presents as a hard lump which can be clinically highly suspicious of malignancy. Patients are mostly under the age of 45 years [21]. The lesion is grossly firm, well defined, and pale gray in color. Microscopically the borders can be irregular (Fig. 17.7a). The nodules consist of glandular structures of variable sizes, some can be cystic (Fig. 17.7a, b), surrounded by intact layer of myoepithelium (Fig. 17.7c). Apocrine

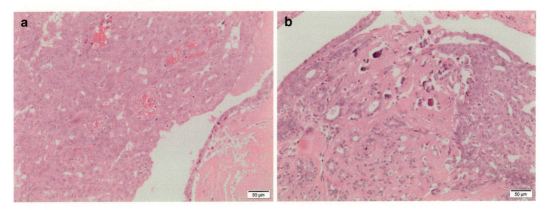

Fig. 17.6 Ductal adenoma. (**a**) The lesion is well circumscribed, mostly solid or cribriform, and consists of a mixture of benign epithelial and myoepithelial cells. Note the presence of part of a lumen at the *right* hand side of the picture, but this is sometimes completely obliterated. (**b**) Microcalcification seen in part of the lesion

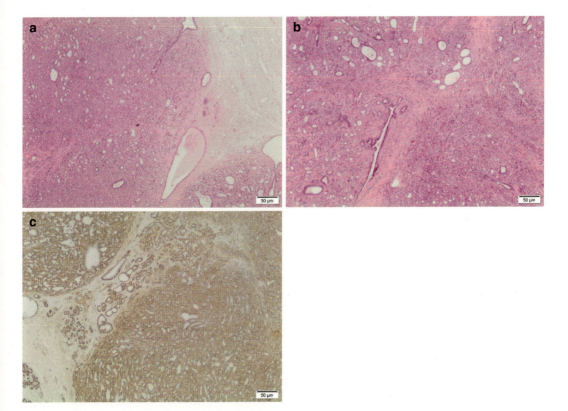

Fig. 17.7 Benign adenosis tumor. (**a**) The lesion has irregular but well-defined borders and consists of large closely packed nodules of sclerosing adenosis. (**b**) Scattered cysts may be present. (**c**) All glands are surrounded by intact myoepithelial cell layer as demonstrated here by positive staining for smooth muscle actin

metaplasia and nuclear atypia are sometimes seen. No recurrences were noted in 27 surgically excised cases that were followed up for 1–9 years (mean 3.75 years) [21].

Nipple Adenoma (Florid Papillomatosis of the Nipple)

A benign lesion of the nipple that usually shows florid usual type hyperplasia with solid or cribriform areas [22]. It may be associated with erosion and ulceration of the nipple, thus mimicking Paget's disease clinically (Fig. 17.8a). The center of the lesion may become sclerosed entrapping small ducts, giving an appearance suspicious of tubular carcinoma. The benign nature of the lesion is confirmed by CK5 immunostaining which will show a mixture of positive (basal/myoepithelial) and negative (epithelial) stained cells demonstrating the presence of mixed epithelial and myoepithelial cells (Fig. 17.8b).

Syringomatous Adenoma of the Nipple

A benign locally infiltrating lesion that is histologically similar to syringoma of the skin. The age range is 28–74 years. Microscopically, it consists of tubular duct-like structures, cell nests,

and keratinizing cysts embedded in fibrous tissue (Fig. 17.9a). In a core biopsy, the lesion can be easily confused with invasive tubular carcinoma (Fig. 17.9b). The site of the lesion near the nipple, the variability of size and shape of the glands, the presence of keratin cysts, and the absence of a desmoplastic stroma should help in pointing to the correct diagnosis. However, the diagnosis in most cases will only be established by immunohistochemistry as the lesion, unlike tubular carcinoma, is ER negative (Fig. 17.9c) and p63 positive (Fig. 17.9d). The lesion is also positive for CK5 (Fig. 17.9e) and CK7 (Fig. 17.9f). The tumor does not metastasize but can recur [23–26]. Similar tumors have been described within the breast parenchyma away from the skin and nipple [27].

Hidradenoma

Skin-type hidradenoma can rarely arise in the nipple/areola region of the breast [28]. Microscopically, the lesion is well circumscribed and consists of cystic space containing proliferating epithelial and myoepithelial cells which may be arranged in papillary structures (hidradenoma papilliferum) or solid masses (nodular hidradenoma, Fig. 17.10). Sometimes the lesion consists almost entirely of clear, presumably myoepithelial, cells (clear cell hidradenoma).

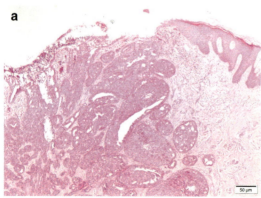
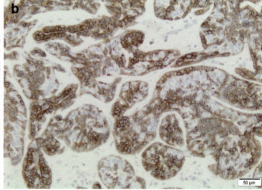

Fig. 17.8 Nipple adenoma. (**a**) The lesion consists of solid and glandular proliferation of epithelial and myoepithelial cells that has caused ulceration of the nipple. (**b**) CK5 immunostaining shows a benign mosaic pattern of negative and positive cells

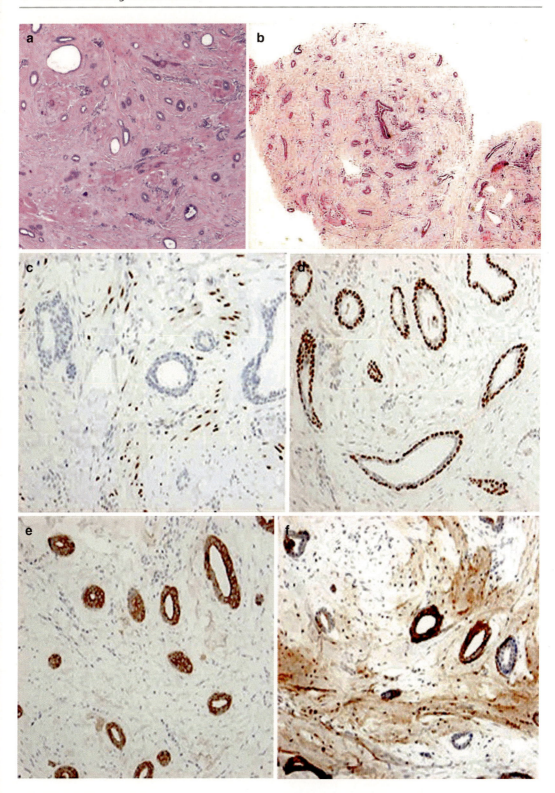

Fig. 17.9 Syringomatous adenoma of the nipple. (**a**) The tumor consists of glandular structures of variable size and shape embedded in a bland stroma. (**b**) Core biopsy showing an appearance that can be easily confused with tubular carcinoma, but the glands are (**c**) ER negative and (**d**) p63 positive. The glands are also positive for (**e**) CK5 and (**f**) CK7

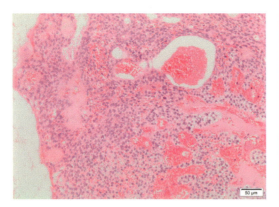

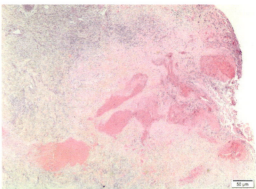

Fig. 17.10 Nodular hidradenoma of the breast. The lesion was partly cystic and partly solid composed of a mixture of epithelial and myoepithelial cells, some having clear cytoplasm

Fig. 17.11 Mondor's disease. A biopsy of a long-standing ulcerated lesion showing thrombosed blood vessel surrounded by heavy inflammatory cell infiltrate

Mondor's Disease

An uncommon benign condition characterized by acute superficial thrombophlebitis of the breast and chest wall. Clinically it presents as a suddenly appearing painful subcutaneous cord-like structure that can measure up to 10 cm. The condition usually develops spontaneously but has been reported as a rare complication of breast core or sentinel node biopsy. The lesion is usually self-limiting, easily diagnosed clinically with no need for biopsy. In a rare case that was biopsied because of its long standing, the sections showed ulcerated skin with underlying wedge-shaped area of inflammation and mild small blood vessel proliferation surrounding a thrombosed blood vessel that ran from the base of the wedge to the ulcerated surface (Fig. 17.11) [29].

Granulomatous Lobular Mastitis

An uncommon inflammatory condition occurring mainly in women of reproductive age (17–42) and often associated with a recent history of childbirth [30]. It presents as a distinct firm mass at the periphery of the breast. Microscopically, the lesions are lobulocentric, composed of heavy inflammatory cell infiltrate, partly or completely replacing mammary lobules (Fig. 17.12a). There may be a central collection of neutrophils sur-

rounded by lymphocytes, plasma cells, histiocytes, and multinucleated giant cells (Fig. 17.12b). Well-defined noncaseating granulomas are commonly present. The intervening stroma is also involved, to a lesser extent, by the inflammation. Stains for microorganisms and fungi are negative. The differential diagnosis includes other granulomatous inflammations particularly tuberculosis and sarcoidosis.

Cases with cysts surrounded by neutrophils as illustrated in Fig 17.12 have been recently separated from cases of granulomatous mastitis without such cysts and labelled 'Cystic neutrophilic granulomatous mastitis' [31–33]. Gram positive bacilli are sometimes seen in these cysts which in some cases were consistent with Corynebacterium species [32, 33.]

Other Benign Screen-Detected Lesions

Calcified fibroadenomas (Fig. 17.13a) are now relatively more commonly seen and biopsied as a result of mammographic screening. Less commonly seen are foci of dystrophic calcification within fat (Fig. 17.13b) and foci of benign intraductal calcification (Fig. 17.13c). Coarse calcification is sometimes seen in core biopsies, surrounded by fibrosis and heavy lymphocytic infiltration with no detectable epithelial elements in spite of multiple sectioning. As there is a pos-

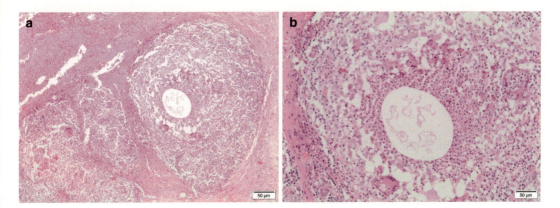

Fig. 17.12 Granulomatous mastitis. (**a**) Low power view of the lobulocentric lesion. (**b**) High power view of one of the lobules which is completely replaced by inflammatory reaction with central necrotic cavity surrounded by neutrophils followed by chronic inflammatory cells including foreign body giant cells

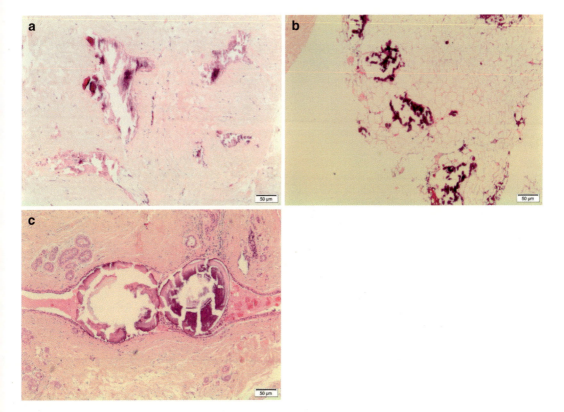

Fig. 17.13 Unusual screen-detected benign microcalcification. (**a**) Calcified fibroadenoma. (**b**) Dystrophic calcification within fat. (**c**) Intraductal calcification

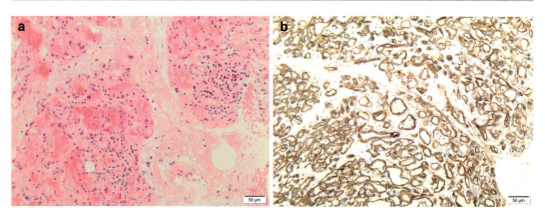

Fig. 17.14 Screen-detected capillary hemangioma. (**a**) Core biopsy showing closely packed small blood vessels (**b**) that are positive with CD34

sibility that these may represent "burnt out" foci of DCIS, we usually give them a score of B4 with a recommendation of re-biopsy or excision. Other benign lesions that may cause radiologic deformity necessitating biopsy include intramammary lymph nodes, lipomas, hemangiomas (Fig. 17.14a, b), leiomyomas, neurofibromas, and schwannomas.

References

1. Clement PB, Azzopardi JG. Microglandular adenosis of the breast- a lesion simulating tubular carcinoma. Histopathology. 1983;7:169–80.
2. Rosen PP. Microglandular adenosis. A benign lesion simulating invasive mammary carcinoma. Am J Surg Pathol. 1983;7:137–44.
3. Tavassoli FA, Norris HI. Microglandular adenosis of the breast. A clinicopathologic study of 11 cases with ultrastructural observations. Am J Surg Pathol. 1983;7:731–7.
4. Rosenblum MK, Purrazzella R, Rosen PP. Is microglandular adenosis a precancerous disease? A study of carcinoma arising therein. Am J Surg Pathol. 1986;10:237–47.
5. Khalifeh IM, Albarracin C, Diaz LK, Symmans FW, Edgerton ME, Hwang RF, Sneige N. Clinical, histopathologic and immunohistochemical features of microglandular adenosis and transition into in situ and invasive carcinoma. Am J Surg Pathol. 2008;32:544–52.
6. Tavassoli FA. Myoepithelial lesions of the breast. Myoepitheliosis, adenomyoepithelioma, and myoepithelial carcinoma. Am J Surg Pathol. 1991;15:554–68.
7. Hayes MM. Adenomyoepithelioma of the breast: a review stressing its propensity for malignancy transformation. J Clin Pathol. 2011;64:477–84.
8. Resetkova E, Albarracin C, Sneig N. Collagenous spherulosis of breast. Morphologic study of 59 cases and review of the literature. Am J Surg Pathol. 2006;30:20–7.
9. Mooney EE, Kayani N, Tavassoli FA. Spherulosis of the breast. A spectrum of mucinous and collagenous lesions. Arch Pathol Lab Med. 1999;123:626–30.
10. Devaris DXG, Smith S, Leask D, Troster M, O'Malley FP. Complex collagenous spherulosis of the breast presenting as a palpable mass. A case report with immunohistochemical and ultrastructural studies. Breast J. 2000;6:199–203.
11. Ginter PS, Scognamiglio T, Touchi-Nishi P, Antonio LB, Hoda SA. Pleomorphic adenoma of the breast: a radiological and pathological study of a common tumor in an uncommon location. Case Reorts Pathol. 2015;ID172750.
12. Djakovic A, Engel JB, Geisinger A, Honig A, Tschammler A, Dietl J. Pleomorphic adenoma of the breast initially misdiagnosed as metaplastic carcinoma in preoperative stereotactic biopsy. Eur J Gynaecol Oncol. 2011;32:427–30.
13. Diaz NM, McDivitt RW, Wick MR. Pleomorphic adenoma of the breast: a clinicopathologic and immunohistochemical study of 10 cases. Hum Pathol. 1991;14:1206–14.
14. Moran CA, Suster S, Carter D. Benign mixed tumours (pleomorphic adenoma) of the breast. Am J Surg Pathol. 1990;14:913–21.
15. Soreide A, Anda O, Eriksen L, Holter J, Kjellevold KH. Pleomorphic adenoma of the human breast with local recurrence. Cancer. 1988;61:997–1001.
16. Adeniran A, Al-Ahmadi H, Mahoney MC. Granular cell tumour of the breast: a series of 17 cases and a review of the literature. Breast J. 2004;10:528–31.

17. De Simone N, Aggon A, Christy C. Granular cell tumour of the breast: clinical and pathologic characteristics of a rare case in a 14-year-old girl. J Clin Oncol. 2011;29:e656–7.
18. Azzopardi JG, Salm B. Ductal adenoma of the breast: a lesion which can mimic carcinoma. J Pathol. 1984;144:15–23.
19. Gusterson BA, Sloane JP, Midwood C, Gazet JC, Trott P, Taylor-papadimitrious J, Bartek J. Ductal adenoma of the breast- a lesion exhibiting a myoepithelial/epithelial phenotype. Histopathology. 1987;11:103–10.
20. Lammie GA, Millis RR. Ductal adenoma of the breast- a review of fifteen cases. Hum Pathol. 1989;20:903–8.
21. Nielsen BB. Adenosis tumour of the breast- a clinicpathological investigations of 27 cases. Histopathology. 1987;11:1259–75.
22. Diaz NM, Palmer JO, Wick MR. Erosive adenomatosis of the nipple: histology, immunohistology and differential diagnosis. Mod Pathol. 1992;5:179–83.
23. Rosen PP. Syringomatous adenoma of the nipple. Am J Surg Pathol. 1983;7:745–59.
24. Jones MW, Norris HJ, Snyder RC. Infiltrating syringomatous adenoma of the nipple. Am J Surg Pathol. 1989;13:197–201.
25. Ward BE, Cooper PH, Subramony G. Syringomatous tumor of the nipple. Am J Clin Pathol. 1989;92:692–6.
26. Slaughter MS, Pomerantz RA, Murad T, Hines JR. Infiltrating syringomatous adenoma of the nipple. Surgery. 1992;111:711–13.
27. Suster S, Moran CA, Hurt MA. Syringomatous squamous tumors of the breast. Cancer. 1991;67:2350–5.
28. Kazakov DV, Vanecek T, Belousova IE, Mukensnabl P, Kollertova D, Michal M. Skin-type hidradenoma of the breast parenchyma with t(11;9) translocation: hidradenoma of the breast. Am J Dermatopathol. 2007;5:457–61.
29. Shousha S, Chun J. Ulcerated Mondor's disease of the breast. Histopathology. 2007;52:395–6.
30. Going JJ, Anderson TJ, Wilkinson S, Chetty U. Granulomatous lobular mastitis. J Clin Pathol. 1987;40:535–40.
31. Renshaw AA, Derhagopian RP, Gould EW. Cystic neutrophilic granulomatous mastitis. An underappreciated pattern strongly associated with Gram-Positive bacilli. Am J Clin Pathol 2011;136:424–7
32. D'Alfonso TM, Moo T-A, Arleo EK, Cheng E, Antonio LB, Hoda SA. Cystic neutrophilic granulomatous mastitis. Further characterization of a distinctive histopathologic entity not always demonstrabley attributable to corynebacterium infection. Am J Surg Pathol 2015;39:1440–7
33. Troxell ML, Gordon NT, Stone Dogett J, Ballard M, Vetto JT, Pommier RF, Naik AM. Cystic neutrophilic granulomatous mastitis. Association with Gram-positive bacilli and Corynebacterium. Am J Clin Pathol 2016;145:635–45

Uncommon Malignant Lesions

18

Sami Shousha

Abstract

Twelve selected rare types of malignant breast lesions are presented, described, and illustrated.

Keywords

Adenoid cystic carcinoma • Acininc cell carcinoma • Secretory carcinoma • Malignant adenomyoepithelioma • Pleomorphic invasive ductal carcinoma • Neuroendocrine tumors

Salivary Gland-Type Malignant Lesions

These include four triple-negative tumors: adenoid cystic, secretory, acinic cell, and epithelial-myoepithelial carcinomas. Although they all belong to the basal-like molecular class of breast carcinomas, they usually have good prognosis unlike the rest of the members of this class.

Adenoid Cystic Carcinoma

This is a triple-negative, slow-growing tumor with good prognosis which may recur but rarely metastasize [1–3]. The tumor cells are usu-

ally monomorphic with small low-grade nuclei, showing minimal mitotic activity. The cells are arranged in variable-sized groups mostly exhibiting a cribriform pattern (Fig. 18.1a). Solid areas may be present (Fig. 18.1b), and the prognosis seems to be inversely related to the amount of solid areas present in the tumor [4, 5]. Immunohistochemically, a mixture of cells expressing epithelial (e.g.,CK7, CK18) and myoepithelial (e.g., SMA and p63) markers is present, and 83–100 % of cases express c-kit (CD117) to a variable degree in the cell membrane or the cytoplasm [2, 6, 7].

When the tumor shows predominantly a cribriform pattern, it can be confused, particularly in a core biopsy, with two other cribriform breast lesions, namely, in situ or invasive cribriform carcinoma and secretory carcinoma. The three lesions can be differentiated from each other by staining for ER and S100. ER is positive in cribriform carcinoma and negative in adenoid cystic and secretory carcinomas. S100 is negative in

S. Shousha
Department of Histopathology, Charing Cross Hospital & Imperial College,
Fulham Palace Road, London W6 8RF, UK
e-mail: s.shousha@imperial.ac.uk

© Springer International Publishing Switzerland 2017
S. Shousha (ed.), *Breast Pathology*, DOI 10.1007/978-3-319-28655-6_18

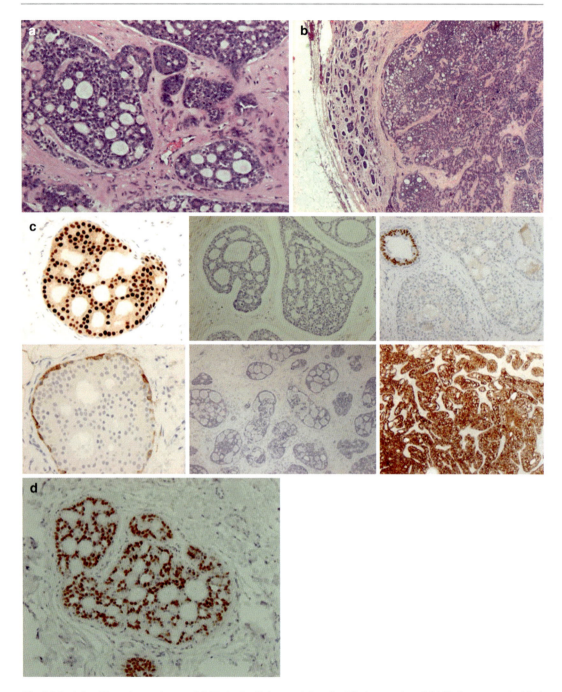

Fig. 18.1 Adenoid cystic carcinoma. (**a**) Typical cribriform pattern. (**b**) Mixed cribriform and solid patterns. (**c**) Differentiating cribriform DCIS (*left*) from adenoid cystic carcinoma (*middle*) and secretory carcinoma (*right*) by staining for ER (*top* raw) and S100 (*bottom* raw). (**d**) A focus of collagenous spherulosis showing heterogeneous staining for ER

cribriform carcinoma (except for the surrounding myoepithelium in cribriform DCIS) and adenoid cystic carcinoma (except for an occasional positive cell) and strongly positive in secretory carcinoma (Fig. 18.1c).

Collagenous spherulosis is a benign cribriform lesion that can be confused with the other malignant cribriform lesions described above particularly in a small core biopsy. However, collagenous spherulosis is usually a small lesion, and staining for ER will show a heterogeneous pattern of staining (Fig. 18.1d) which is not seen in the three malignant lesions described above (Fig. 18.1c). The lesion is described in more details in Chap. 17.

Secretory Carcinoma

Secretory carcinoma is a rare triple-negative low-grade breast carcinoma first described by McDivitt and Stewart in 1966 as children's breast cancer [8]. Later, it was realized that it occurs also in young women and occasionally in older ones [9–12]. The median age of reported cases is 25 years. Rare cases have been described in young boys [10], in adult men [10, 11], and in axillary ectopic breast tissue [13].

The tumor is usually present as a well-defined subareolar mass (Fig. 18.2a). The neoplastic cells have low-grade nuclei and granular to vacuolated cytoplasm which may contain eosinophilic secretion. Mitotic activity is minimal. The cells are arranged in cribriform patterns with the spaces also containing eosinophilic secretion (Fig. 18.2b). Microcysts and tubular structures containing secretion may be present. Typically, the cells are ER negative (Fig. 18.2c) and S100 strongly positive (Fig. 18.2d) [12, 14]. The cells express basal cytokeratins, thus belonging to the basal-like molecular group of breast carcinoma [15]. In the latter study, all six cases studied expressed CK8/18, 83 % expressed CK5/6 and S100, 50 % expressed EGFR, and 33 % expressed CK14. Weak c-kit staining was seen in 66 % and all cases were negative for p63.

Prognosis is favorable and is thought to be better in children than in adults. Local recurrences, if developed, are late. Lymph node metastases are uncommon and distal metastasis are exceedingly rare. Death is unusual but has been reported.

Genetically, the tumor is characterized by the presence of a chromosomal translocation (12:15) (p13:q25) which results in the formation of *ETV6-NTRK3* fusion gene [15, 16].

Acinic Cell Carcinoma

Acinic cell carcinoma is a breast carcinoma similar to that seen in the parotid gland, first described by Roncaroli et al. in 1996 [17]. Patients vary in age between 35 and 80 years [18]. The tumor presents as a palpable mass measuring between 1 and 5 cm. Grossly, the tumor can be well defined with a fibrous pseudocapsule or can have infiltrative borders. Microscopically, the tumor cells are arranged in microglandular, microcystic, nest, or solid patterns (Fig. 18.3a, b). Central comedo-like necrosis may be present [17]. The cells have abundant cytoplasm with eosinophilic zymogen-type granules and monomorphic rounded or ovoid nuclei. The granules can be coarse, bright red in color resembling Paneth cell granules (Fig. 18.3c). Cells with clear cytoplasm are common. Prominent mitotic activity is sometimes seen. Immunohistochemically, the cells are positive for alpha-1-chymotrypsin, lysozyme, EMA, and S100 and can be positive for GCDFP-15. The tumor is negative for ER, PgR, and HER2. Prognosis is good, but lymph node metastasis can occur [18].

Epithelial-Myoepithelial Carcinoma

This is a rare low-grade triple-negative breast carcinoma similar to that described in salivary glands and the upper aerodigestive tract [19] and lung [20], characterized by the presence of a biphasic tubular histology. In my opinion it is different from malignant adenomyoepithelioma which is described below. On low-power view, the tumor consists of deceptively benign-looking relatively well-formed glandular structures of

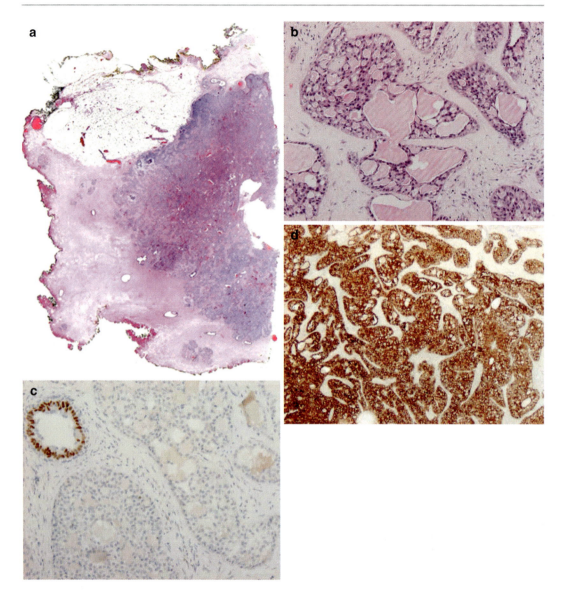

Fig. 18.2 Secretory carcinoma. (**a**) Low-power view showing the well-circumscribed tumor border (H&E). (**b**) High-power view showing the tumor cells arranged in a cribriform pattern with the spaces between the cells con-taining eosinophilic secretion. (**c**) The tumor cells are negative for ER (a normal duct at the *left*-hand corner acts as an internal control) and (**d**) strongly positive for S100

variable sizes (Fig. 18.4a). Branching and papillary proliferations are present, and the cells on high-power view show a moderate degree of nuclear pleomorphism (Fig. 18.4b). The tumor has an infiltrative margin (Fig. 18.4c). It is ER negative (Fig.18.4d), which differentiates it from tubular carcinoma, and S100 negative, except for a few scattered positive cells (Fig. 18.4e), which differentiates it from microglandular adenosis. The characteristic feature is the presence of an intact myoepithelial layer around almost all the neoplastic glands (Fig. 18.4f). The tumor is also PgR and HER2 negative and E-cadherin positive (Fig. 18.4c). Judged by the outcome reported for similar tumors in other organs [19], the prognosis should be favorable.

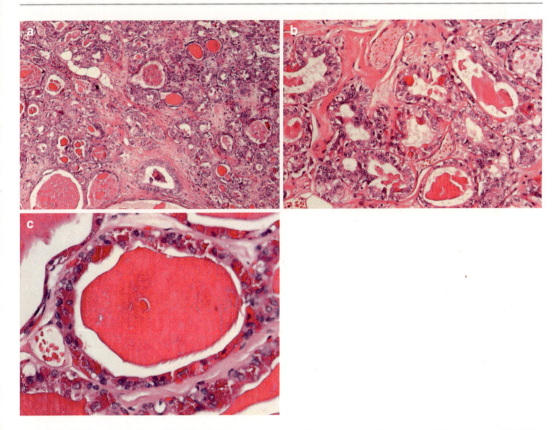

Fig. 18.3 Acinic cell carcinoma. (**a**) Glandular structures and microcysts containing eosinophilic secretion. (**b**) High-power view of the same tumor. (**c**) Glands containing coarse, *bright red* zymogen granules

Malignant Adenomyoepithelioma

This is the malignant counterpart of benign ade-nomyoepithelioma, and it is not uncommon to see part of the lesion still showing benign ade-nomyoepithelioma features in continuity, sug-gesting that malignant transformation has developed in the benign lesion [21, 22]. Commonly, but not always, the patient presents with a large lump with a history of a long-stand-ing stable breast mass that has recently started to grow rapidly. Grossly part of the lesion may be cystic or necrotic, but it has infiltrative borders.

Microscopically, part of the lesion may still consists of benign adenomyoepithelioma com-posed of well-defined glands surrounded by abundant myoepithelial cells, both elements showing no or minimal atypical features (Fig. 18.5a, b). The infiltrative part of the lesion

can consist of epithelial or myoepithelial ele-ments or a mixture of the two, one or both of which showing malignant features (Fig. 18.5c, d). The tumor is ER negative (Fig. 18.5e) and CK14 positive (Fig. 18.5f). Lymph node metastases are uncommon and can express a mixture of luminal and myoepithelial markers [22] (Fig. 18.5g). Distal metastases have been reported in up to 40 % of cases in several organs including the liver, bone, thyroid gland, and brain [21–24].

Carcinoma Arising in Association with Microglandular Adenosis

These have been first reported by Rosen et al. in 1983 who described four cases (31 %) among a total of 13 cases of microglandular adenosis [25]. Rosen and his colleagues later reported

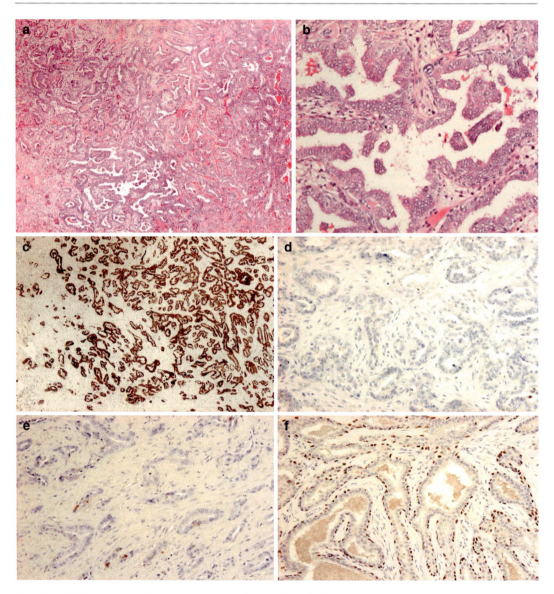

Fig. 18.4 Epithelial-myoepithelial carcinoma. (**a**) Low-power view showing relatively well-formed glandular structures. (**b**) High-power view showing intraductal papillary proliferation and a moderate degree of nuclear pleomorphism. (**c**) Low-power view of the tumor stained for E-cadherin to show the glandular pattern and infiltrative border. (**d**) The tumor is ER negative and (**e**) S100 almost totally negative. (**f**) Staining for p63 shows an intact layer of positive myoepithelial cells around all neoplastic glands

more cases and suggested that microglandular adenosis may be a precancerous lesion [26]. This is supported by the presence of transition forms [26, 27], by the immunohistochemical similarity of the two lesions when they coexist [27–31] and by the presence of shared molecular changes [30, 31] (Fig. 18.6a–g). Reported histological types of breast carcinoma associated with microglandular adenosis included ductal (Fig. 18.6a–c), lobular, adenoid cystic, metaplastic (Fig. 18.6d, e), and acinic cell [32]. We have also recently seen a case of encapsulated papillary carcinoma associated with microglandular adenosis (Fig. 18.6f, g). The tumors, like the associated microglandular adenosis, are triple negative and S100 positive.

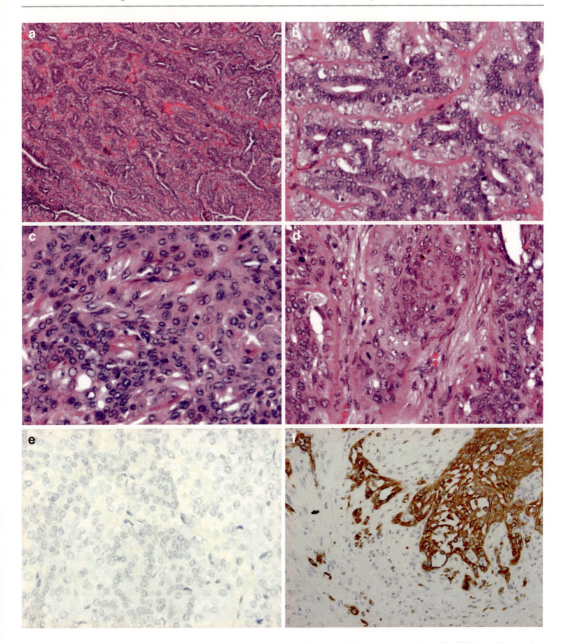

Fig. 18.5 Malignant adenomyoepithelioma. (**a**) Benign part of the lesion composed of a mixture of glands and abundant vacuolated myoepithelial cells. (**b**) High-power view of the same area showing the mixed two elements. (**c**) Malignant part of the lesion composed of solid sheets of polyhedral and (**d**) spindle-shaped myoepithelial cells. (**e**) Negative ER immunostaining. (**f**) CK14-positive staining of the malignant elements, note the infiltrative margin. (**g**) Lymph node metastasis of the same case stained with CK19. The metastasis also stained with smooth muscle antigen indicating the presence of luminal and myoepithelial elements [22]

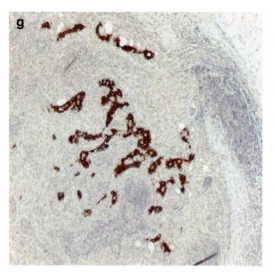

Fig. 18.5 (Continued)

Pleomorphic Invasive Ductal Carcinoma

This is an invasive ductal carcinoma of the breast that is characterized by two features [33, 34]:

- The presence of marked nuclear pleomorphism more than sixfold variation in nuclear size in more than 50 % of the tumor cells
- The presence of multinucleated tumor giant cells

In a series of 37 cases [34], the age incidence was 23–78 years. The tumors varied in size between 1.2 and 11.6 cm and 61 % were well circumscribed. Necrosis was present in 76 % of cases, focal spindle cell component in 38 %, and typical invasive ductal elements in 22 %. Associated DCIS was present in 38 % of cases.

Axillary node metastases occurred in 52 % of patients. Immunohistochemically, ER and PgR were negative in 94–100 %, HER2 negative in 40–84 %, p53 positive in 60–71 %, S100 positive in 40 %, and p63 positive in 20 % (spindle cell elements), and Ki67 was highly expressed in all tumors [33–35]. Five-year survival was reported as 38 % if there are spindle cell elements and 89 % in the absence of spindle cells [34]. We have seen a case developing in a patient with Huntington's disease who died within 15 months of presentation. Spindle cell elements were present (Fig. 18.7) [36].

Carcinomas Associated with Cytoplasmic Inclusions

These include carcinomas with neuroendocrine granules, glycogen-rich carcinoma, lipid-rich carcinoma, as well as signet ring cell carcinoma which was discussed with mucinous lesions in Chap. 9.

Breast Carcinoma with Neuroendocrine Features

Neuroendocrine granules, as demonstrated by immunohistochemistry for chromogranin, synaptophysin, or neuron-specific enolase, are present in variable amounts in around 20 % of invasive breast carcinomas [37, 38]. They are particularly more prevalent in mucinous and solid papillary carcinomas. Apart from these two tumors, breast carcinoma with neuroendocrine features is classified into three groups; all are usually ER positive and HER2 negative [38]:

Fig. 18.6 Carcinoma arising in association with microglandular adenosis. (**a**) Invasive ductal carcinoma (*left*) arising in association with microglandular adenosis (*right*). (**b**) Transition zone between the two lesions seen in (**a**). Note a degree of atypia in the form of multilayering of the epithelium and nuclear enlargement. (**c**) Both benign microglandular elements (most of the field) and invasive ductal carcinoma (*lower left corner*) staining strongly for S100. (**d**) Metaplastic breast carcinoma (matrix producing) arising in association with microglandular adenosis. (**e**) Same tumor seen in (**d**) stained for ER. Both microglandular element (*upper left*) and metaplastic carcinoma (*lower*) are ER negative. Normal ducts seen on the *right* are ER positive. (**f**) Encapsulated papillary carcinoma arising in association with microglandular adenosis (Courtesy of Dr Sussan Gharaie, Kingston Hospital, UK). (**g**) Same tumor seen in (**f**) staining positively for S100

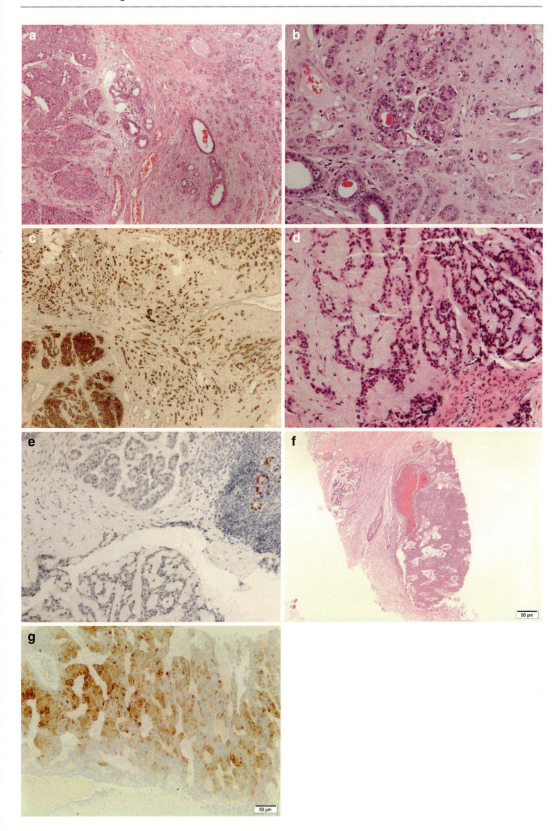

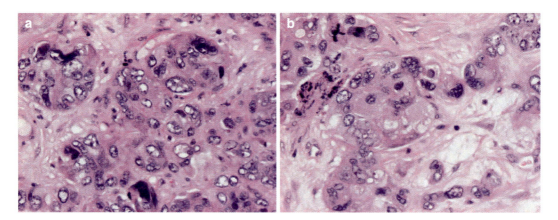

Fig. 18.7 Pleomorphic invasive ductal carcinoma. (**a**) Note the presence of marked nuclear pleomorphism and huge multinucleated tumor giant cells. (**b**) Same case showing abnormal mitotic figures and more tumor giant cells (H&E)

- *Neuroendocrine tumor, well differentiated.* These are carcinoid-like, similar to carcinoid tumors of the gastrointestinal tract and lung. The cells are polyhedral or spindle with low-grade nuclei. They are strongly positive for chromogranin A and synaptophysin as well as ER and CK7. When seen in the breast, the possibility of metastasis from the lung or GI tract has to be excluded. They have good prognosis.
- *Neuroendocrine tumor, poorly differentiated.* These have a morphology similar to that of small-cell anaplastic carcinoma of the lung and may express TTF1, as well as neuroendocrine markers; hence radiological investigations are essential to exclude the possibility of being a metastasis from a lung primary. The cells can be spindle with high-grade fusiform hyperchromatic nuclei. They are aggressive tumors with frequent lymphatic invasion.
- *Invasive breast carcinoma with neuroendocrine differentiation.* These are mostly invasive ductal carcinomas that express neuroendocrine markers. There used to be a requirement of at least 50 % of the tumor cells expressing such markers to be included in this category, but this threshold has been abandoned in the new WHO classification of breast tumors [38]. The histology may be difficult to differentiate from the usual cases of ductal carcinomas, but careful microscopic examination may identify focal "car-

cinoid" features (Fig. 18.8a), leading to further immunohistochemical tests to investigate the possibility of neuroendocrine differentiation. Chromogranin (Fig. 18.8b) and synaptophysin are the two neuroendocrine markers recommended as they are more specific although less sensitive than neuron-specific enolase and CD56. The tumors are ER strongly positive (Fig. 18.8c) and HER2 negative. They are E-cadherin positive (Fig. 18.8d), which differentiates them from the alveolar variant of invasive lobular carcinoma, and p63 negative (Fig. 18.8e), differentiating them from closely packed foci of solid DCIS. The presence of neuroendocrine differentiation does not seem to alter the prognosis in these cases [38].

Glycogen-Rich Clear Cell Carcinoma

These are rare breast tumors composed mostly (more than 90 %) of cells with clear cytoplasm that contains abundant glycogen that is PAS positive and diastase-PAS negative (Fig. 18.9a–d). The cells are polygonal with sharply defined borders and hyperchromatic small monomorphic nuclei. The cells are CD10 negative (Fig. 18.9e) which differentiates them from clear cell metastatic renal carcinoma which is usually CD10 positive. ER is positive in around 60 % of cases [39] (Fig. 18.9f), which, if positive, would also

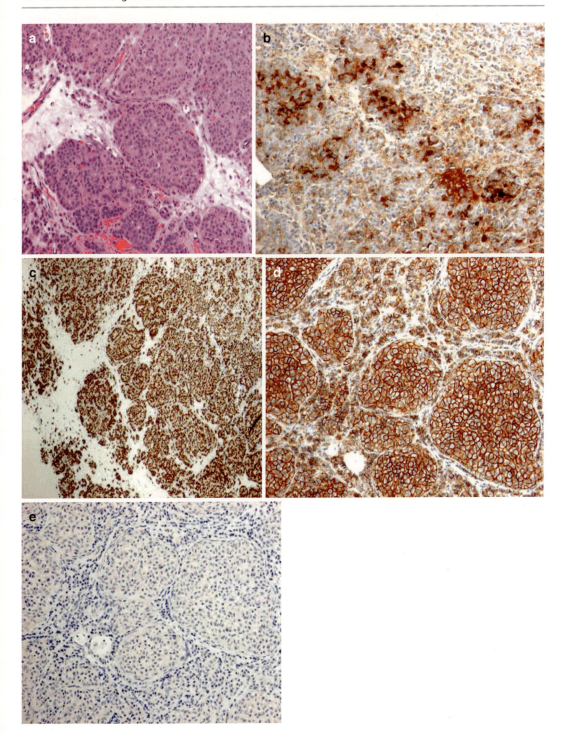

Fig. 18.8 Invasive breast carcinoma with neuroendocrine differentiation. (**a**) Focal areas suggestive of "carcinoid" differentiation in the form of relatively well-defined arrangement of the tumor cells in alveolar patterns. (**b**) The tumor cells are chromogranin positive, (**c**) ER strongly positive, (**d**) E-cadherin positive, and (**e**) p63 negative

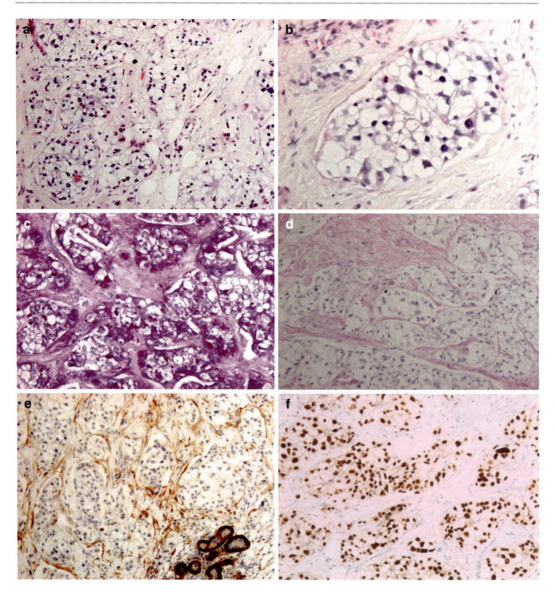

Fig. 18.9 Glycogen-rich clear cell carcinoma. (**a**) The tumor cells have clear cytoplasm and small monomorphic nuclei. The cells in this case are arranged in alveolar pattern. (**b**) High-power view showing the sharp defined borders of the tumor cells. (**c**) Tumor cells are rich in glycogen as demonstrated by positive PAS staining and (**d**) negative diastase-PAS staining. (**e**) The tumor cells are CD10 negative and (**f**) ER strongly positive

help in excluding the possibility of metastatic renal cell carcinoma. The tumor cells can be arranged in alveolar patterns, and CD10 staining will also help in differentiating these cases from clear cell DCIS which would have a CD10 positively stained myoepithelial layer (Fig. 18.9e). However, foci of clear cell DCIS may occur in association with the invasive tumor [40]. Other growth patterns described include cords and sheets. Because of these patterns, the tumors are usually grade 2 or 3.

A study of 28 cases [39] showed an age range of 31–81 years and a tumor size varying between 0.8 and 7.5 cm. The tumors were HER2 positive in

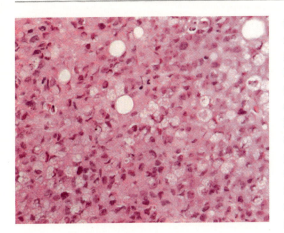

Fig.18.10 Lipid-rich carcinoma. The tumor consisted of sheets of polygonal cells with foamy cytoplasm

12% and p53 positive in 45%. Lymph node metastases were present in 46%, but the disease-free and overall survival were not different from matched cases of invasive ductal carcinoma [39, 40].

Lipid-Rich Carcinoma

These are rare invasive breast carcinomas composed of relatively large cells, 90% of which have abundant foamy or clear cytoplasm containing lipids (Fig. 18.10) [41]. The latter can be demonstrated by staining frozen sections with Sudan III. PAS stain for glycogen is negative. The tumor cells are arranged in nests, cords, and solid sheets. In a study of 17 cases, all tumors were negative for ER, CK5/6, CK14, S100, and p63 and positive for HER2 [41]. One was positive for PgR. In another report of five cases, all were negative for ER and PgR [42]. However, weak ER staining was demonstrated in a reported case [43].

Lymphoepithelioma-Like Carcinoma

Lymphoepithelioma-like carcinoma is a breast carcinoma that microscopically resembles nasopharyngeal lymphoepithelioma [44, 45]. The tumor consists of relatively small groups of markedly pleomorphic cytokeratin-positive malignant cells present as islands within a heavy lymphocytic infiltrate. The latter can be sometimes so heavy that it obscures the presence of the carcinoma cells [46, 47] (Fig. 18.11a–e). We have seen core biopsies from such a lesion which consisted entirely of lymphocytes, raising the possibility of lymphoma. The lymphocytes, however, lacked any atypical features and had an immunoprofile which was interpreted as reactive rather than neoplastic. Further biopsies demonstrated small islands of carcinoma within the heavy lymphocytic infiltrate. It is therefore advisable to carry out cytokeratin stains in any core biopsy with a heavy lymphocytic infiltrate and no obvious epithelial elements to confirm the presence or absence of any hidden malignant epithelial elements. If the latter are absent, lymphoma markers have to be carried out.

Patients affected varied in age between 42 and 69 years and the reported cases varied in size between 10 and 40 mm. The tumors are usually grade 3 and are EBV and HPV negative. ER and HER2 can be positive or negative. BRCA1 mutation was present in one case [44]. The prognosis is similar to that of invasive ductal carcinoma of similar grade and stage.

The main differential diagnosis is medullary carcinoma which can be also heavily infiltrated with lymphocytes but not to that extent. The other main differences are the well-circumscribed borders seen in medullary carcinoma which also usually show more marked nuclear pleomorphism and higher mitotic activity.

Lymphoma

Lymphomas of the breast are rare accounting for less than 0.5% of breast neoplasms. They can arise as a primary tumor of the breast or involve the breast in a setting of disseminated lymphoma. Between 30 and 50% are primary involving only the breast or at most ipsilateral axillary lymph nodes. There are no

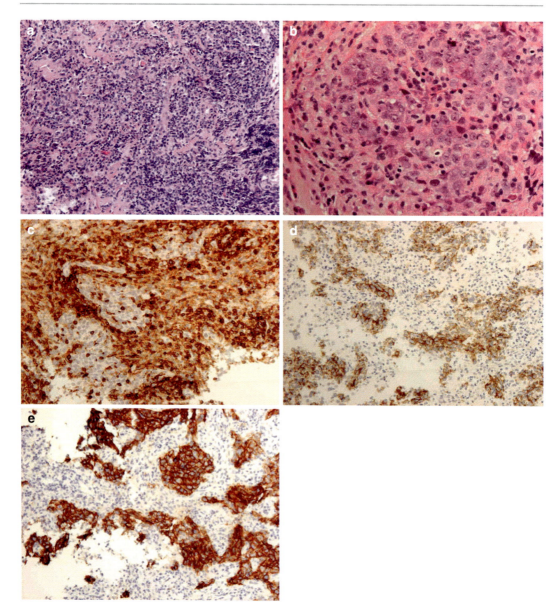

Fig. 18.11 Lymphoepithelioma-like carcinoma. (**a**) Low-power view showing abundant lymphocytes and no obvious carcinoma cells. (**b**) High-power view suggesting the presence of larger epithelial cells, in some areas, within the lymphocytic infiltrate. (**c**) Immunostaining for CD45 demonstrating the abundant lymphocytes, with small islands devoid of staining. (**d**) Immunostaining for CK19 and (**e**) for E-cadherin, both demonstrating the presence of islands of carcinoma within the heavy lymphocytic infiltrate seen in some areas of the biopsy

morphological differences between primary and secondary cases [48, 49]. The majority are B cell lymphomas mostly of diffuse large cell type [50], but other types have been described including MALT and Burkitt-like lymphomas, follicle center lymphoma, marginal zone lymphoma, as well as T cell lymphoma and Hodgkin's disease

[51]. Rare cases have been described in association with breast implants usually anaplastic large cell lymphomas [52].

They commonly present as a unilateral painless breast lump. The age range is 17–87 years and 97 % are female patients. The diagnosis is usually made by a breast core biopsy which

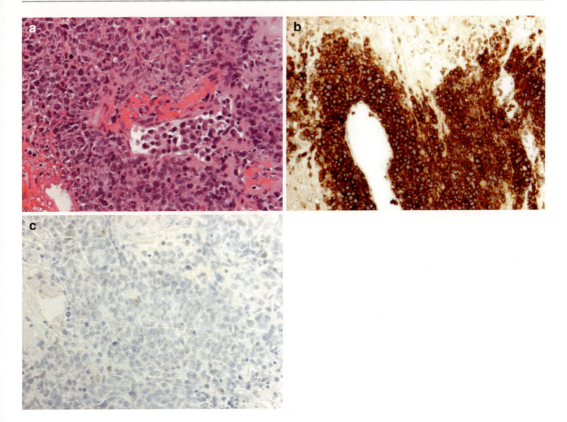

Fig. 18.12 Breast lymphoma. (**a**) A core biopsy showing anaplastic cells, (**b**) positive for CD45 and (**c**) negative for ER

shows neoplastic cells positive for CD45 and negative for cytokeratins and ER (Fig. 18.12a–c). The prognosis is similar to that of nodal lymphomas of similar histological type and stage.

References

1. Trendell-Smith NJ, Peston D, Shousha S. Adenoid cystic carcinoma of the breast: a tumour commonly devoid of oestrogen receptors and related proteins. Histopathology. 1999;35:241–8.
2. Azoulay S, Lee M, Frenaux P, Merls S, Al Ghuzian A, Chnecker C, et al. KIT is highly expressed in adenoid cystic carcinoma of the breast, a basal-like carcinoma associated with a favorable outcome. Mod Pathol. 2005;18:1623–31.
3. Ghabach B, Anderson WF, Curtis RE, Huycke MM, Lavigne JA, Doris GM. Adenoid cystic carcinoma of the breast in the United States (1977–2006): a population-based cohort study. Breast Cancer Res. 2010;12:R54.
4. Ro JY, Silva EG, Gallager HS. Adenoid cystic carcinoma of the breast. Hum Pathol. 1987;18:1276–81.
5. Shin SJ, Rosen PP. Solid variant of mammary adenoid cystic carcinoma with basaloid features: a study of nine cases. Am J Surg Pathol. 2002;26:413–20.
6. Crisi GM, Marconi-Judson G, Goulart RA. Expression of c-kit in adenoid cystic carcinoma of the breast. Am J Clin Pathol. 2005;124:733–9.
7. Mastropasqua MG, Maiorano E, Pruneri G, Orvieto E, Mazzarol G, Vento AR, Viale G. Immunoreactivity for c-kit and p63 as an adjunct in the diagnosis of adenoid cystic carcinoma of the breast. Mod Pathol. 2005;18:1277–82.
8. McDivitt RW, Stewart FW. Breast carcinoma in children. JAMA. 1966;195:388–90.
9. Oberman HA. Secretory carcinoma of the breast in adults. Am J Surg Pathol. 1980;4:465–70.
10. Tavassoli FA, Norris HJ. Secretory carcinoma of the breast. Cancer. 1980;45:2404–13.
11. Krausz T, Jenkins D, Grontoft O, Pollock DJ, Azzopardi JG. Secretory carcinoma of the breast in adults: emphasis on late recurrence and metastasis. Histopathology. 1989;14:25–36.
12. Rosen PP, Granor ML. Secretory carcinoma of the breast. Arch Pathol Lab Med. 1991;115:141–4.
13. Shin SJ, Sheikh FS, Allenby PA, Rosen PP. Invasive secretory (juvenile) carcinoma arising in ectopic breast tissue of the axilla. Arch Pathol Lab Med. 2001;125:1372–4.

14. Lamovec J, Bracho M. Secretory carcinoma of the breast: light microscopical, immunohistochemical and flow cytometric study. Mod Pathol. 1994;7:475–9.

15. Lae M, Freneaux P, Sastre-Garau X, Chouchane O, Sigal-Zafrani B, Vincent-Salomon A. Secretory breast carcinoma with *ETV6-NTRK3* fusion gene belong to the basal-like carcinoma spectrum. Mod Pathol. 2009;22:291–8.

16. Tognon C, Knezevich SR, Hntsman D, Roskelley CD, Melnyk N, Mathers JA, et al. Expression of the *ETV6-NTRK3* gene fusion as a primary event in human secretory breast carcinoma. Cancer Cell. 2002;2:367–76.

17. Roncaroli F, Eusebi V, Lamovec J, Zidar A. Acinic cell-like carcinoma of the breast. Virchows Arch. 1996;429:69–74.

18. Damiani S, Pasquinelli G, Lamovec J, Peteres L, Eusebi V. Acinic cell carcinoma of the breast: an immunohistochemical and ultrastructural study. Virchows Arch. 2000;437:74–81.

19. Seethala RR, Barnes EL, Hunt JL. Epithelial-myoepithelial carcinoma: a review of the clinic-pathologic spectrum and immunophenotypic characteristics in 61 tumors of the salivary glands and upper aerodigestive tract. Am J Surg Pathol. 2007;31:44–57.

20. Nguyen CV, Suster S, Moran CA. Pulmonary epithelial-myoepithelial carcinoma: a clinic-pathologic and immunohistochemical study of 5 cases. Hum Pathol. 2009;40:366–73.

21. Hayes MM. Adenomyoepithelioma of the breast: a review stressing its propensity for malignancy transformation. J Clin Pathol. 2011;64:477–84.

22. Awamleh AA, Gudi M, Shousha S. Malignant adenomyoepithelioma of the breast with lymph node metastasis. A detailed immunohistochemical study. Case Rep Pathol. 2012;2012:Article ID 305858.

23. Bult P, Verwiel JMM, Wobbes T, Kooy-Smits MM, Biert J, Holland R. Malignant adenomyoepithelioma of the breast with metastasis in the thyroid gland 12 years after excision of the primary tumour. Virchows Arch. 2000;436:158–66.

24. Jones C, Tooze R, Lakhani SR. Malignant adenomyoepithelioma of the breast metastasizing to the liver. Virchows Arch. 2003;442:504–6.

25. Rosen PP. Microglandular adenosis. A benign lesion simulating invasive mammary carcinoma. Am J Surg Pathol. 1983;7:137–44.

26. Rosenblum MK, Purrazzella R, Rosen PP. Is microglandular adenosis a precancerous disease? A study of carcinoma arising therein. Am J Surg Pathol. 1986;10:237–47.

27. Acs G, Simpson JF, Bleiweiss IJ, Hugh J, Reynolds C, Olson S, Page DL. Microglandular adenosis with transition into adenoid cystic carcinoma of the breast. Am J Surg Pathol. 2003;27:1052–60.

28. Khalifeh IM, Albarracin C, Diaz LK, Symmans FW, Edgerton ME, Hwang RF, Sneige N. Clinical, histopathologic and immunohistochemical features of microglandular adenosis and transition into in situ and invasive carcinoma. Am J Surg Pathol. 2008;32:544–52.

29. Salarieh A, Sneige N. Breast carcinoma arising in microglandular adenosis. A review of the literature. Arch Pathol Lab Med. 2007;131:1397–9.

30. Shin SI, Simpson PT, Da Silva L, Jayanthan J, Reid L, Lakhani SR, Rosen PP. Molecular evidence for progression of microglandular adenosis to invasive carcinoma. Am J Surg Pathol. 2009;33:496–504.

31. Geyer FC, Lacroix-Triki M, Colombo P-E, Patani N, Gauthier A, Natrajan R, et al. Molecular evidence in support of the neoplastic and precursor nature of microglandular adenosis. Histopathology. 2012;60:E115–30.

32. Felleti J, Coletti G, Rispoli E, Scarabeo F, Cervasio M, Tornillo L, et al. Acinic cell carcinoma of the breast arising in microglandular adenosis. Case Rep Pathol. 2013;2013;Article ID 736048.

33. Silver SA, Tavassoli FA. Pleomorphic carcinoma of the breast: clinicopathological analysis of 25 cases of an unusual high-grade phenotype of ductal carcinoma. Histopathology. 2000;36:505–14.

34. Nguyen CV, Falco-Escobedo R, Hunt KK, Nayeemuddin KM, Lester TR, Harrell RK, et al. Pleomorphic ductal carcinoma of the breast. Predictors of decreased overall survival. Am J Surg Pathol. 2010;34:486–93.

35. Zhao J, Lang R, Guo X, Chen L, Gu F, Fan Y, et al. Clinicopathologic characteristics of pleomorphic carcinoma of the breast. Virchows Arch. 2010;60(456):31–7.

36. Shousha S. Pleomorphic invasive ductal carcinoma of the breast in a patient with Huntington's disease. Case Rep Pathol. 2014;Article ID 979137.

37. Makretsov N, Gilks B, Coldman AJ, Hayes M, Huntsman D. Tissue microarray analysis of neuroendocrine differentiation and its prognostic significance in breast cancer. Hum Pathol. 2003;34:1001–8.

38. Tan PH, Schnitt SJ, van de Vijver MJ, Ellis IO, Lakhani SR. Papillary and neuroendocrine breast lesions: the WHO stance. Histopathology. 2015;66:761–70.

39. Ma X, Han Y, Fan Y, Cao X, Wang X. Clinicopathologic characteristics and prognosis of glycogen-rich clear cell carcinoma of the breast. Breast J. 2014;20:166–73.

40. Hayes MMM, Seidman JD, Ashton MA. Glycogen-rich clear cell carcinoma of the breast. A clinicopathologic study of 21 cases. Am J Surg Pathol. 1995;19:904–11.

41. Guan B, Wang H, Cao S, Wang Y, Zhu Y, Shi Q, et al. Lipid-rich carcinoma of the breast: clinicopathologic analysis of 17 cases. Ann Diagn Pathol. 2011;15:225–32.

42. Wrba F, Ellinger A, Reiner G, Spona I, Holzner IH. Ultrastructural and immunohistochemical characteristics of lipid-rich carcinoma of the breast. Virchows Arch A Pathol Anat Histopathol. 1988;413:381–5.

43. Reis-Filho JS, Fulford LG, Lakhani SR, Schmitt FC. Pathologic quiz case. A 62-year-old woman with a 4.5-cm nodule in the right breast. Arch Pathol Lab Med. 2003;127:e396–8.
44. Ddmanesh F, Peterse JL, Sapino A, Fonelli A, Eusebi V. Lymphoepithelioma-like carcinoma of the breast: lack of evidence of Epstein-Barr virus infection. Histopathology. 2001;38:54–61.
45. Naidoo P, Chetty R. Lymphoepithelioma-like carcinoma of the breast with associated sclerosing lymphocytic lobulitis. Arch Pathol Lab Med. 2001;125:669–72.
46. Sanati S, Ayala AG, Middleton LP. Lymphoepithelioma-like carcinoma of the breast: report of a case mimicking lymphoma. Ann Diagn Pathol. 2004;8:309–15.
47. Saleh R, DaCamara P, Radhi J, Boutross-Tadross O. Lymphoepithelioma-like carcinoma of the breast mimicking nodular sclerosing Hodgkin's lymphoma. Breast J. 2005;11:353–4.
48. Mattia AR, Ferry JA, Harris NL. Breast lymphoma. A B-cell spectrum including the low grade B-cell lymphoma of mucosa associated lymphoid tissue. Am J Surg Pathol. 1993;17:574–87.
49. Topalovski M, Crisan D, Mattson JC. Lymphoma of the breast. A clinicopathologic study of primary and secondary cases. Arch Pathol Lab Med. 1999;123:1208–18.
50. Radkani P, Joshi D, Paramo JC, Mesko TW. Primary breast lymphoma. 30 years of experience with diagnosis and treatment at a single medical center. JAMA Surg. 2014;149:91–3.
51. Hoimes CJ, Selbst MK, Shafi NQ, Rose MG, Rosado MF. Hodgkin's lymphoma of the breast. J Clin Oncol. 2010;28:e11–3.
52. Miranda RN, Aladily TN, Prince HM, Kanagal-Shamanna R, de Jong D, Fayad LE, et al. Breast implant-associated anaplastic large cell lymphoma: long-term follow-up of 60 patients. J Clin Oncol. 2013;28(32):114–20.

Abeer Shaaban

Abstract

This chapter deals mainly with the two most important causes of enlargement of the male breast, namely, gynecomastia and breast cancer. Gynecomastia is the commonest cause of male breast lump. Most of the lesions are idiopathic, but enlargement due to various physiological and pathological causes may occur. The lesions histologically show florid epithelial proliferation within a cellular stroma in the early (active) phase and fibrosis with minimal epithelial proliferation in the late (fibrous) phase. Male breast cancer is a rare disease, but the incidence has been increasing worldwide. Several factors have been implicated including BRCA2 mutations, old age, liver cirrhosis, and testicular disorders. Many predisposing factors are related to increased estrogen levels relative to androgen. Male breast cancer is commonly of the ductal no special type with a high proportion of papillary carcinoma. Lobular carcinoma is extremely rare in the male breast. Management strategies are similar to and derived from the female disease.

Keywords

Male breast • Gynecomastia • Male breast cancer

Abbreviations

CI   Confidence interval
DCIS   Ductal carcinoma in situ

ER   Estrogen receptor
FMC   Female breast cancer
LCIS   Lobular carcinoma in situ
MBC   Male breast cancer
NST   No special type
PASH   Pseudoangiomatous stromal hyperplasia
PLCIS   Pleomorphic lobular carcinoma in situ
PR   Progesterone receptor
RR   Relative risk

A. Shaaban
Department of Histopathology, Queen Elizabeth Hospital Birmingham and University of Birmingham, Mindelsohn Way, Edgbaston, Birmingham, West Midlands B15 2GW, UK
e-mail: a.shaaban@bham.ac.uk

© Springer International Publishing Switzerland 2017
S. Shousha (ed.), *Breast Pathology*, DOI 10.1007/978-3-319-28655-6_19

Introduction

There are several causes for male breast enlargement/lumps, many of which are shared with the female breast [1]. The commonest cause of male breast enlargement is gynecomastia. Here, we provide an overview of the diagnosis and management of male breast lesions with emphasis on the commonest entities, namely, gynecomastia and male breast cancer.

Embryology and Normal Male Breast

Similar to the female breast, the male breast develops from ectodermal ridges, called mammary lines in the fourth to sixth weeks in utero. Most of these ridges undergo atrophy leaving only mammary buds. At birth, the male and female breasts have similar histological appearances comprising few lactiferous ducts. At puberty and during pregnancy and lactation, the female breast undergoes ductal, glandular, and stromal proliferation under the effect of estrogen and progesterone. The normal male breast, therefore, comprises few mammary ducts in a predominant fibrofatty stroma [2, 3].

Gynecomastia

Gynecomastia refers to a non-neoplastic proliferation of mammary tissue in men. It is the commonest abnormality in male breast accounting for approximately 85% of male breast lumps. Pseudogynecomastia is a term used to describe increased adipose tissue within the male breast due to fatty hypertrophy or obesity. Based on the duration of the disease, gynecomastia is classified into an early (active), intermediate, and late (fibrous) phase [4]. There is no proven link between gynecomastia and the risk of male breast cancer.

Etiology

The precise etiology is unknown and most cases are regarded as idiopathic. However, hormonal imbalances leading to relative excess of estrogen to androgen are thought to play an important role [5]. Physiological gynecomastia occurs in neonates (transient gynecomastia), adolescence, and men over 50 years of age. Pathological gynecomastia, due to an underlying disease, may occur secondary to alcoholic liver cirrhosis, endocrine disorders as hyperthyroidism, Klinefelter's syndrome [6], and testicular cancer [1]. Various drugs, such as spironolactone, medications used for hormonal treatment of prostate cancer, cocaine, and anabolic steroids, can contribute to the development of gynecomastia [7, 8]

Microscopic Features

Pseudogynecomastia shows excess fat deposition with no ductal elements. The early (active) phase of true gynecomastia is characterized by an intraductal cell proliferation which can be very florid and often shows a micropapillary pattern with fingerlike projections (Fig. 19.1a, b). In those florid cases, the hyperplastic ducts may mimic micropapillary DCIS. Squamous metaplasia may occur (Fig. 19.1c). The stroma is often cellular, edematous, and/or myxoid and may show pseudoangiomatous stromal hyperplasia (PASH, Fig. 19.1b). The edema is more prominent around the mammary ducts and becomes more fibrous further away.

In the late (fibrous) phase, there is minimal epithelial proliferation, and the stroma becomes densely fibrous and acellular (Fig. 19.1d). A combination of the two phases may be present simultaneously.

While mammary lobules are known to be absent/poorly developed in the male breast, in the author's experience, lobules can be encountered in some examples of gynecomastia particularly in those patients with current or past history of drug intake such as anabolic steroids (Fig. 19.1e).

In the current climate of financial constrictions, the routine histological analysis of all specimens removed as gynecomastia has been challenged. Agostini et al. analyzed the unexpected cancer and atypia reported in the literature in those specimens and recommended histological analysis in the presence of unilateral

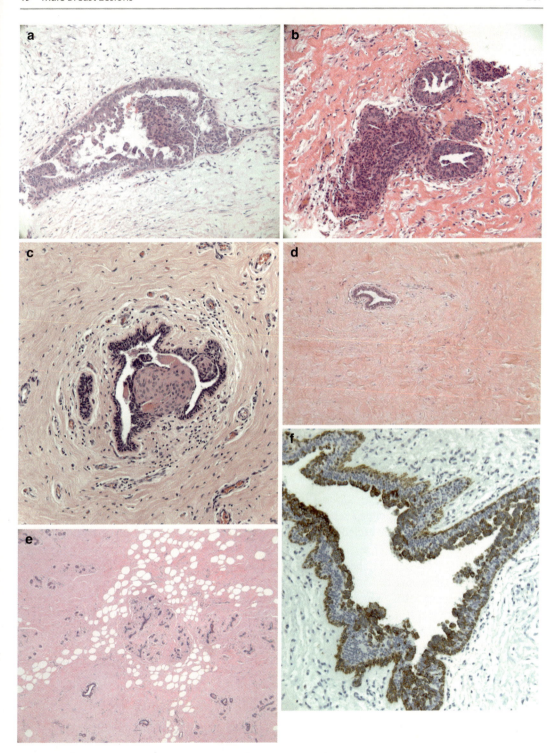

Fig. 19.1 Histological features and immunohistochemical profile of gynecomastia. (**a**) Florid epithelial hyperplasia in active gynecomastia. (**b**) Gynecomastoid hyperplasia with stromal pseudoangiomatous stromal hyperplasia (PASH) in active gynecomastia. (**c**) Squamous metaplasia of the lining epithelium of a male mammary duct. (**d**) Late-phase gynecomastia; dense fibrous stroma without associated epithelial proliferation. (**e**) An example of well-developed mammary lobules in male breast related to drug intake. (**f**) Typical pattern of CK5 immunohistochemistry in a male mammary duct showing two layers of positive epithelium and myoepithelium enclosing a negative layer

gynecomastia, family history of breast tumor, estrogen/steroid therapy, marijuana use, and obesity [9].

Differential Diagnosis

Clinically, pathological causes of gynecomastia should be excluded by careful history taking, clinical examination, and blood investigations [1].

Microscopically, florid gynecomastoid hyperplasia may mimic micropapillary DCIS. However, they lack the bulbous ends characteristic of micropapillary DCIS and also lack cytological atypia. A mixed pattern of positive and negative ER and basal cytokeratin expression may be helpful in supporting the diagnosis of hyperplasia (Fig. 19.1f). It is to be noted, however, that the pattern of basal cytokeratin expression in male mammary ducts is distinct from that in the female ducts [10]. Basal cytokeratin markers are expressed within the inner epithelium and outer myoepithelium enclosing a negative middle layer giving a tri-layered pattern (Fig. 19.1f). This immunohistochemical pattern should not be mistaken for atypia.

Management

Physiological gynecomastia is often a self-limiting disease. Careful investigations to exclude an underlying pathological cause for breast enlargement such as testicular tumors should be performed.

In idiopathic gynecomastia, hormonal treatment is used for active (early) gynecomastia with 30 % response rate and hence the importance of distinguishing this phase microscopically. Surgical treatment including liposuction or surgical excision is offered for late or unresponsive cases. A detailed algorithm for gynecomastia workup and management has been published [1].

Uncommon Benign Lesions

Many lesions that occur in the female breast are shared with men [3]. These include apocrine metaplasia (Fig. 19.2a), cysts (Fig. 19.2b), fibroadenoma (Fig. 19.2c), lipoma, nipple adenoma [11], fat necrosis, chronic inflammation, and abscesses. A recent publication suggested that columnar cell lesions do not occur in men [12]. In the author's experience and others [13], however, columnar cell lesions can be seen microscopically in the male breast (Fig. 19.2d).

Male Breast Cancer

Incidence

Male breast cancer (MBC) is rare representing less than 1 % of all newly diagnosed breast cancers. It is estimated that one MBC is diagnosed for every 200 female breast cancers (FBCs). The American Cancer Society estimated approximately 2350 male breast cancers will be diagnosed in the USA in 2015 and about 440 men will die from the disease [14, 15]. While FBC has a bimodal age distribution, MBC is unimodal with a peak at the age of 71 [16].

Over the last few decades, the incidence of male breast cancer has been rising [17]. This trend was observed in the USA, Canada, Europe, and Australia. In the UK, the incidence increased from 0.86 to 1.08 per 100,000 in the general population between 1973 and 1998 with currently around 350 new cases diagnosed every year [18]. For men, the lifetime risk of developing breast cancer is about 1 in 1000.

The increase in MBC incidence has likely occurred due to several factors including increased longevity, alcohol-related liver disease, obesity, inactive lifestyle, radiation exposure, and others (see section "Risk Factors" below).

Ethnicity

Male breast cancer is more common in black men than whites [16]. The highest incidence has been reported in Israelis [19]. California Cancer Registry data of 606 MBC patients showed differences in survival by race/ethnic group in all patients and also in hormone receptor-positive

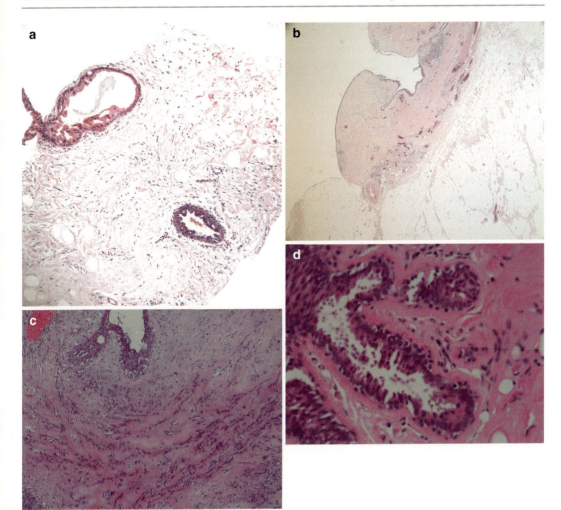

Fig. 19.2 Uncommon benign lesions of the male breast. (a) Apocrine metaplasia with mild apocrine papillary hyperplasia in a core biopsy. (b) Single apocrine cyst in a male breast presenting as a symptomatic lump. Note the bland epithelial lining, fibrous cyst wall, and associated chronic inflammation. (c) Fibroadenoma presenting as a well-circumscribed mobile lump. The lesion comprises benign compressed ductal structures with surrounding loose fibrous stroma. (d) An example of columnar cell change in the male breast. Note the regular polarized columnar epithelium lining mammary ducts with apical snouts

tumors. Non-Hispanic men had poorer outcome [20]. Poor access to health care and insurance also affects MBC outcome [21].

Risk Factors

Several well-established, and other possible, risk factors have been implicated in MBC development, some of which are shared with the female counterpart. For systematic review, see Ruddy et al. [22].

Age

Similar to FBC, older age is associated with an increased risk for MBC. At presentation, men are approximately 5–10 years older than the female patients worldwide as reported in the USA [15], the UK [23], Scandinavia [24], Africa [25], and the Far East [26, 27].

Familial and Genetic Factors

A family history of breast cancer incurs an increased risk in MBC. An affected first-degree relative confers ×2 risk which increases to ×5 with number of affected relatives and young age at diagnosis [28]. BRCA2 carriers have 6% estimated cumulative risk by 70 years which is 100-fold higher than the general male population.

Cancer susceptibility genes for MBC with high, moderate, or low penetrance have been identified [19]. Of the high susceptibility genes, BRCA1 and BRCA2 mutations are the most important with BRCA2 mutations occurring much more commonly in men. BRCA2 mutations are estimated to account for 60–76% of familial MBC compared with 10–16% for BRCA1 [29].

Other moderate penetrance genes conferring a lower risk include the CHEK2 1100delC mutation and PALPB2. CHEK2 1100delC mutation has been shown to confer approximately a tenfold increase of breast cancer risk in men who do not have BRCA1/BRCA2 mutations [19].

Other genetic factors that have been linked to MBC include Klinefelter's syndrome (50-fold risk) [6], Cowden syndrome, ataxia telangiectasia (PTEN, ATM germline mutations), and androgen receptor mutation [22]. These conditions lead to a high estradiol to androgen ratio, thus increasing the MBC risk.

Hormonal Factors

Factors that lead to an increase in estradiol relative to androgen have been associated with an increased risk. More recently, the male breast cancer pooling project consortium showed that circulating estradiol levels, but not androgen levels or estradiol/androgen ratio, were strongly associated with MBC risk. This was independent of age or body mass index [30].

Alcohol
Alcohol-induced liver damage/cirrhosis with associated impaired function and increased estradiol levels has been linked to male breast cancer [31]. Other studies, however, have shown no link between alcohol consumption, tobacco, smoking, and MBC [32].

Obesity
Lifestyle trends, particularly over the last decades, have led to unprecedented rates of obesity across the world. The association between obesity and various cancers, including breast cancer, has been highlighted and MBC is no exception [33, 34].

Testicular Disorders
Men with testicular disorders such as orchiectomy, cryptorchidism, and congenital inguinal hernia are at an increased risk [22].

Radiation Exposure
Male breast cancer has been shown to increase in the Japanese atomic bomb survivors [35].

Gynecomastia
There is no established link between gynecomastia and the development of MBC. However, one study reported an increased relative risk in men with gynecomastia (RR = 5.08, CI: 3.21–8.03 [34].

Clinical Presentation

Approximately two thirds of MBC present with a painless lump often eccentric to the nipple [36, 37]. Due to lack of awareness of the disease, MBC usually presents with a larger tumor at a higher stage compared with FBC. Frequent involvement of the overlying skin, nodal metastasis, and lymphovascular invasion have, therefore, been reported [38].

Macroscopic Features

The specimen is often a mastectomy showing a large grayish-white tumor (Fig. 19.3a, b) with or without nodal metastasis. Sentinel lymph node biopsy is performed for clinically node-negative patients. The macroscopic findings are similar to those in women and sampling and assessment are done following the same guidelines for handling and reporting of female breast cancer.

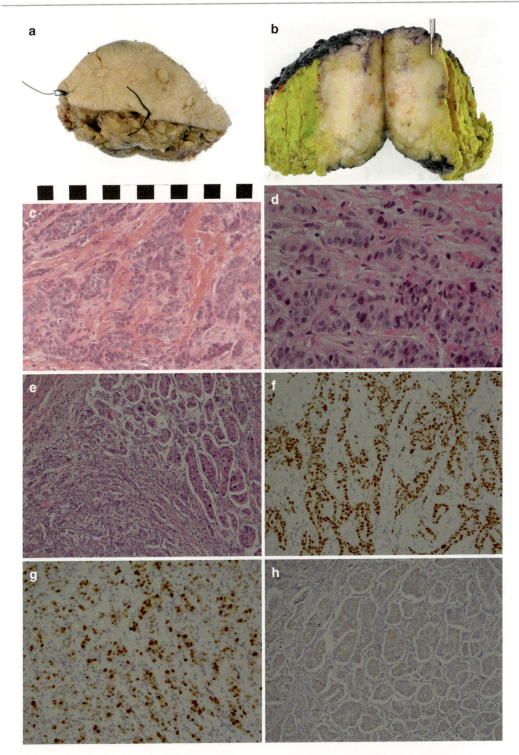

Fig. 19.3 Gross and microscopic features of male breast cancer. (**a**) Macroscopic appearance of an intact mastectomy specimen. (**b**) Slicing shows a large, *grayish-white*, well-circumscribed tumor against a fatty background. (**c**, **d**) The commonest microscopic type is ductal carcinoma of no special type (NST). (**e**) Invasive mammary carcinoma showing a mixture of micropapillary pattern (*right*) and ductal NST pattern (*left*). (**f**–**h**) The commonest molecular profile of male breast carcinoma is ER positive (**f**), PR positive (**g**), and HER2 negative (**h**)

Microscopic Features

In Situ Carcinoma

DCIS represented 9.4 % of all MBC in the SEER data of the period between 1973 and 2001. The incidence of DCIS in men rose by 123 % over the same period. The median age at diagnosis for DCIS was 62 years which is significantly higher than that reported for DCIS in women (median age 58 years). In men, papillary DCIS was the commonest architectural type. The DCIS was often of the low-grade, ER-/PR-positive phenotype [39]. A rare example of DCIS arising on top of nipple adenoma has been reported [11].

LCIS in the male breast is very rare. There has been only one case report of pleomorphic LCIS (PLCIS) in the male breast [40]. Paget's disease of the nipple is also known to occur in men [41]

Invasive Carcinoma

The commonest histological type of MBC is the ductal no special type (NST) which represents around 90 % of cases (Fig. 19.3c, d). This is followed by papillary carcinoma which is two times more likely in men compared with women (Fig. 19.3e), then mucinous carcinoma. Invasive lobular carcinoma of the male breast is extremely rare [23, 42].

The majority (~90 %) of male breast carcinomas express estrogen receptor, and ~70 % are progesterone receptor positive [23, 43], (Fig. 19.3f, g). Earlier studies suggested a high incidence of HER2 positivity. However, recent studies with standardized protocols for immunohistochemical staining and interpretation suggest that the incidence of HER2-positive tumors in men is low [23] (Fig. 19.3h).

Differential Diagnosis

DCIS in male breast should be distinguished from florid gynecomastoid hyperplasia in active gynecomastia. The latter should exhibit no cytological atypia. Immunohistochemistry for basal cytokeratin, e.g., cytokeratin 5 or 14, and ER can be helpful, taking into consideration the pattern of CK5 and CK14 staining in male ducts (Fig. 19.1f).

Invasive carcinoma should be differentiated from metastases to male breast. Clinicopathological correlation, history of previous cancer, and histological comparison are important in this setting. Histologically, the identification of DCIS is a helpful clue to confirming a mammary origin. A panel of immunohistochemical markers to identify the likely primary origin can be helpful.

Management of Male Breast Cancer

Due to the rarity of the disease, no randomized controlled trials on male breast cancer were done, and treatment options are currently derived from the extensive data on female patients [44]. Treatment is generally similar to female breast cancer [45], although mastectomy is the most likely surgical option due to the small amount of breast tissue in men. Conservative surgery, if applicable, must be followed by radiotherapy.

The majority of male breast cancers are hormone receptor positive, and tamoxifen has been shown to be effective in the management of male breast cancer in both the adjuvant and metastatic settings. A significant proportion of men (1:4), however, experience symptoms related to treatment such as hot flushes and sexual dysfunction and therefore discontinue treatment. Antiandrogen therapy has been used in the treatment of metastatic cancer of male breast [46].

References

1. Rahmani S, Turton P, Shaaban A, Dall B. Overview of gynecomastia in the modern era and the Leeds Gynaecomastia Investigation algorithm. Breast J. 2011;17:246–55.
2. Johnson RE, Murad MH. Gynecomastia: pathophysiology, evaluation, and management. Mayo Clin Proc. 2009;84:1010–5.
3. Ng AM, Dissanayake D, Metcalf C, Wylie E. Clinical and imaging features of male breast disease, with pathological correlation: a pictorial essay. J Med Imag Radiat Oncol. 2014;58:189–98.

4. Bannayan GA, Hajdu SI. Gynecomastia: clinicopathologic study of 351 cases. Am J Clin Pathol. 1972;57:431–7.

5. Abaci A, Buyukgebiz A. Gynecomastia: review. Pediatr Endocrinol Rev: PER. 2007;5:489–99.

6. Hultborn R, Hanson C, Kopf I, et al. Prevalence of Klinefelter's syndrome in male breast cancer patients. Anticancer Res. 1997;17:4293–7.

7. O'Sullivan AJ, Kennedy MC, Casey JH, et al. Anabolic-androgenic steroids: medical assessment of present, past and potential users. Med J Aust. 2000;173:323–7.

8. Gardette V, Vezzosi D, Maiza JC, Montastruc JL, Olivier P. Gynecomastia associated with fenofibrate. Ann Pharmacother. 2007;41:508–10.

9. Agostini T, Perello R, Famiglietti M, Quattrini LA. Six factors justify the pathologic analysis of subcutaneous mastectomy specimens in patients with gynaecomastia. J Plast Reconstr Aesthet Surg. 2014;67:1760–1.

10. Kornegoor R, Verschuur-Maes AH, Buerger H, van Diest PJ. The 3-layered ductal epithelium in gynecomastia. Am J Surg Pathol. 2012;36:762–8.

11. Rao P, Shousha S. Male nipple adenoma with DCIS followed 9 years later by invasive carcinoma. Breast J. 2010;16:317–8.

12. Verschuur-Maes AH, Kornegoor R, de Bruin PC, Oudejans JJ, van Diest PJ. Do columnar cell lesions exist in the male breast? Histopathology. 2014;64:818–25.

13. Ni YB, Mujtaba S, Shao MM, et al. Columnar cell-like changes in the male breast. J Clin Pathol. 2014;67:45–8.

14. Society. AC. American Cancer Society: cancer facts and figures 2015. Atlanta: American Cancer Society; 2015. Last accessed Sept 2015. http://www.cancer.org/cancer/breastcancerinmen/.

15. Siegel RL, Miller KD, Jemal A. Cancer statistics, 2015. CA Cancer J Clin. 2015;65:5–29.

16. Anderson WF, Althuis MD, Brinton LA, Devesa SS. Is male breast cancer similar or different than female breast cancer? Breast Cancer Res Treat. 2004;83:77–86.

17. Speirs V, Shaaban AM. The rising incidence of male breast cancer. Breast Cancer Res Treat. 2009;115:429–30.

18. UK. CR. http://www.cancerresearchuk.org/health-professional/cancer-statistics/incidence.

19. Rizzolo P, Silvestri V, Tommasi S, et al. Male breast cancer: genetics, epigenetics, and ethical aspects. Ann Oncol. 2013;24 Suppl 8:viii75–82.

20. Chavez-Macgregor M, Clarke CA, Lichtensztajn D, Hortobagyi GN, Giordano SH. Male breast cancer according to tumor subtype and race: a population-based study. Cancer. 2013;119:1611–7.

21. Sineshaw HM, Freedman RA, Ward EM, Flanders WD, Jemal A. Black/white disparities in receipt of treatment and survival among men with early-stage breast cancer. J Clin Oncol. 2015;33:2337–44.

22. Ruddy KJ, Winer EP. Male breast cancer: risk factors, biology, diagnosis, treatment, and survivorship. Ann Oncol. 2013;24:1434–43.

23. Shaaban AM, Ball GR, Brannan RA, et al. A comparative biomarker study of 514 matched cases of male and female breast cancer reveals gender-specific biological differences. Breast Cancer Res Treat. 2012;133:949–58.

24. Miao H, Verkooijen HM, Chia KS, et al. Incidence and outcome of male breast cancer: an international population-based study. J Clin Oncol. 2011;29:4381–6.

25. Ndom P, Um G, Bell EM, et al. A meta-analysis of male breast cancer in Africa. Breast. 2012;21:237–41.

26. Kuroishi T, Hirose K, Tajima K, Tominaga S. Descriptive epidemiology of male breast cancer in Japan. Breast Cancer. 1997;4:77–83.

27. Park S, Kim JH, Koo J, Park BW, Lee KS. Clinicopathological characteristics of male breast cancer. Yonsei Med J. 2008;49:978–86.

28. Thompson D, Easton D. The genetic epidemiology of breast cancer genes. J Mammary Gland Biol Neoplasia. 2004;9:221–36.

29. Frank TS, Deffenbaugh AM, Reid JE, et al. Clinical characteristics of individuals with germline mutations in BRCA1 and BRCA2: analysis of 10,000 individuals. J Clin Oncol. 2002;20:1480–90.

30. Brinton LA, Key TJ, Kolonel LN, et al. Prediagnostic sex steroid hormones in relation to male breast cancer risk. J Clin Oncol. 2015;33:2041–50.

31. Misra SP, Misra V, Dwivedi M. Cancer of the breast in a male cirrhotic: is there an association between the two? Am J Gastroenterol. 1996;91:380–2.

32. Cook MB, Guenel P, Gapstur SM, et al. Tobacco and alcohol in relation to male breast cancer: an analysis of the male breast cancer pooling project consortium. Cancer Epidemiol Biomarkers Prev. 2015;24:520–31.

33. Humphries MP, Jordan VC, Speirs V. Obesity and male breast cancer: provocative parallels? BMC Med. 2015;13:134.

34. Brinton LA, Carreon JD, Gierach GL, McGlynn KA, Gridley G. Etiologic factors for male breast cancer in the U.S. Veterans Affairs medical care system database. Breast Cancer Res Treat. 2010;119:185–92.

35. Ron E, Ikeda T, Preston DL, Tokuoka S. Male breast cancer incidence among atomic bomb survivors. J Natl Cancer Inst. 2005;97:603–5.

36. Jamal S, Mamoon N, Mushtaq S, Luqman M. Carcinoma of the male breast: a study of 141 cases from northern Pakistan. Asian Pac J Cancer Prev: APJCP. 2006;7:119–21.

37. Alali L, Honarpisheh H, Shaaban A, Speirs V. Conditions of the male breast: gynaecomastia and male breast cancer (review). Mol Med Rep. 2010;3:21–6.

38. Joshi MG, Lee AK, Loda M, et al. Male breast carcinoma: an evaluation of prognostic factors contributing to a poorer outcome. Cancer. 1996;77:490–8.

39. Anderson WF, Devesa SS. In situ male breast carcinoma in the Surveillance, Epidemiology, and End Results database of the National Cancer Institute. Cancer. 2005;104:1733–41.

40. Ishida M, Mori T, Umeda T, et al. Pleomorphic lobular carcinoma in a male breast: a case report with review of the literature. Int J Clin Exp Pathol. 2013;6:1441–4.
41. Sandoval-Leon AC, Drews-Elger K, Gomez-Fernandez CR, Yepes MM, Lipman ME. Paget's disease of the nipple. Breast Cancer Res Treat. 2013;141(1):1–12.
42. Burga AM, Fadare O, Lininger RA, Tavassoli FA. Invasive carcinomas of the male breast: a morphologic study of the distribution of histologic subtypes and metastatic patterns in 778 cases. Virchows Arch. 2006;449:507–12.
43. Giordano SH, Valero V, Buzdar AU, Hortobagyi GN. Efficacy of anastrozole in male breast cancer. Am J Clin Oncol. 2002;25:235–7.
44. Speirs V, Pollock S, Shaaban AM, Hanby AM. Problems (and solutions) in the study of male breast cancer. Rare Tumors. 2010;2, e28.
45. PDQ(R) Adult Treatment Editorial Board. PDQ male Breast Cancer Treatment. Bethesda, MD; National Cancer Institute. Updated 02/12/2016. Available at. http://www.cancer.gov/types/breast/hp/male-breast-treatment-pdq. Accessed 08/09/2016. [PMID: 26389234].
46. Di Lauro L, Vici P, Barba M, et al. Antiandrogen therapy in metastatic male breast cancer: results from an updated analysis in an expanded case series. Breast Cancer Res Treat. 2014; 148:73–80.

Index

A

Acinic cell carcinoma, 249, 251
Actin, 126
Adenoid cystic carcinoma, 236
    collagenous spherulosis, 248, 249
    cribriform pattern, 247, 248
    H&E of, 200
    solid patterns, 247, 248
Adenomyoepithelioma, 235, 236
    benign, 251
    malignant, 253
    myoepithelial cells, 235
Adenosis tumor, 238–240
Adenosquamous carcinoma, 153, 155
    high-grade, 156
    low-grade, 156, 159–160
AE1/AE3, 124, 157, 176–179, 181
Alcian blue/PAS stain, 110
Alpha-1-chymotrypsin, 249
Alveolar variant of invasive lobular
    carcinoma, 256
Anaplastic lymphoma kinase (ALK), 130
Androgen and estrogen receptors, 126
Angiosarcoma, 130, 132–134, 208, 209
Antoni A, 129, 131
Antoni B, 129, 131
Apocrine cysts, 110, 269
Apocrine DCIS, 69–71, 81
Apocrine lesions, 54, 71
Apocrine metaplasia, 138, 139, 143
    with acceptable nuclear variation, 71
    and atypia DCIS, 70
    with mild apocrine papillary hyperplasia, 269
Atypical ductal hyperplasia (ADH), 139, 236
    differential diagnosis of, 36
    qualitative assessment, 35
    quantitative assessment, 36
Atypical intraductal epithelial proliferation (AIDEPs),
    51–52, 54, 62
Atypical lobular hyperplasia (ALH), 33, 38, 51, 53,
    77–79
Atypical vascular lesions (AVLs), 208
Audit grade distribution, 90
Axillary lymph node biopsies, 175–176
    core biopsies (*see* Core biopsies)

CUP, 182–185
    dissection, 182
    non-sentinel nodes, 182
    sentinel lymph nodes (*see* Sentinel lymph node
        (SLN))
Axillary sampling, 182

B

B1 (normal tissue), 46–47
B2 (benign), 47
B3, lesion of uncertain malignant potential, 50–51
B4 suspicious diagnosis, 58–59
B5 (malignant), 47
    B5a (in situ), 47–48
    B5b (invasive), 48–49
    B5c (not assessable), 47
Basal cytokeratins, 35, 43, 52, 55–57, 83, 196–199, 268
Bed biopsies, 3, 5
Benign breast inclusions, 181
Benign breast lesions, 47, 110
    adenomyoepithelioma, 235–236
    adenosis tumor, 238–240
    benign intraductal calcification, 242, 243
    calcified fibroadenomas, 242, 243
    collagenous spherulosis, 236–237
    core biopsy, 244
    ductal adenoma, 238, 239
    dystrophic calcification within fat, 242, 243
    granular cell tumor, 238
    granulomatous lobular mastitis, 242, 243
    hidradenoma, 240, 242
    microglandular adenosis, 233–235
    Mondor's disease, 242
    nipple adenoma, 240
    pleomorphic adenoma, 237, 238
    syringomatous adenoma of the nipple, 240, 241
Benign inclusions in lymph nodes, 181
Benign intraductal calcification, 242, 243
Benign phyllodes tumor, 10, 100–101, 103, 105
Beta-catenin (β-catenin), 48, 57, 83, 125, 129, 131, 202,
    210
Biomarker, 44, 49, 50, 89, 93, 161, 162, 193, 224, 226
Block sampling, invasive carcinoma, 90
BRCA1 mutation, 217, 259, 270

© Springer International Publishing Switzerland 2017
S. Shousha (ed.), *Breast Pathology*, DOI 10.1007/978-3-319-28655-6

BRCA2 mutation, 270
Breast cancer
    IHC (*see* Immunohistochemistry (IHC))
    management, 141
    MBC (*see* Metaplastic breast carcinomas (MBCs))
    molecular classification
        basal-like group, 217
        Breast Cancer Index, 224
        BreastPRS prognostic score, 224
        EndoPredict (EP), 224
        ER-negative tumors, 217
        genomic grade index (MapQuant Dx), 222–223
        HER2-enriched group, 217
        HOXB13/IL17BR ratio, 224
        integrative clusters, 218–219
        liquid biopsies, 225–226
        luminal A tumors, 217
        luminal B tumors, 217
        MammaPrint®, 220–221
        molecular techniques, 216
        normal-like group, 217
        Oncotype DX, 223–224
        PAM50/Prosigna, 221–222
        prognostic and predictive tests, 219–220
        triple-negative breast carcinoma, 218
        tumor biology, 216
        Veridex®/Rotterdam signature, 221
    neoadjuvant chemotherapy for, 24
    papillary carcinomas (*see* Papillary carcinomas)
    triple-negative breast carcinoma, 218
Breast implants, 125, 260

C
C125, 183
CA19.9, 169
CA125, 119, 120, 169, 170, 172, 185
Calcification
    and adjacent columnar cell change, 79
    and comedo necrosis, 80
    dystrophic, 58, 242, 243
    fibroadenomas, 242, 243
    intraductal, 243
    luminal, 110
    radiological, 38, 45
Calponin, 81, 132, 150
Cam 5.2, 38, 124
Capsular metastasis, 179
Carcinoma of unknown primary (CUP)
    immunohistochemistry, 183–185
    molecular studies, 184
    morphology, 182–183
Carney's syndrome, 98
CD10, 132, 133, 183, 258
CD31, 134, 161, 208, 209
CD34, 57, 209, 244
    absence of, 132
    phyllodes tumors, 99
CD45, 50, 169, 183, 260, 261
CD56, 204, 205, 256
CD68, 17, 126, 238

CD117, 247
CDX2, 161, 169, 173
Chest wall sarcomas, 134, 135
Chromogranin, 72, 146, 169, 183, 204, 205, 254, 256, 257
Chromosomal translocation (12:15), 249
Circulating tumor cells (CTCs), 225–226
Circulating tumor DNA (ctDNA), 225, 226
C-kit, 247, 249
CKs. *See* Cytokeratins (CKs)
Clear cell metastatic renal carcinoma, 256
Clear cell ovarian carcinoma, 169, 170, 172
Collagenous spherulosis, 120, 236–237, 248, 249
Colonic adenocarcinoma, 169–171
Columnar cell change, 33, 38–39, 53, 79, 198, 269
Columnar cell hyperplasia (CCH)
    AB/PAS, 113
    and columnar cell change, 38–40
    H&E, 68
Columnar cell lesions, 33, 38, 71, 72, 74, 268
Comparative genomic hybridization (CGH), 104, 216
Complex sclerosing lesion (CSL), 34, 49, 55–56, 125
Concentric shrinking, chemotherapy, 18, 19
Conservative surgery, 2, 9, 182, 272
Core biopsies, 1, 2, 110, 169, 175, 176, 244
    anaplastic cells, 261
    apocrine lesions, 54
    atypical intraductal epithelial proliferation, 51–52
    B1 category, 46–47
    B2 category, 47
    B3, lesion of uncertain malignant potential, 50–51
    B4 suspicious diagnosis, 58–59
    B5 category, 47
    B5a category, 47–48
    B5b category, 48–49
    cystic lesion, 170
    diagnosis of MBC, 162–163
    flat epithelial atypia, 53–54
    frozen sections, 5, 176, 180, 259
    lobular neoplasia, 52–53
    macroscopic specimen handling, 44–46
    microbubble contrast-enhanced axillary sentinel node, 176–177
    moderately differentiated adenocarcinoma, 171
    mucocele-like lesions, 57
    papillary lesions, 54–55
    phyllodes tumor, 56–57
    problematic malignant lesions, 49–59
    prognostic and predictive factors assessment, 49
    radial scar, 55–56
    spindle cell lesions, 57, 123–124, 173
    ultrasound-guided axillary node, 176
Cribriform carcinoma, 142, 206, 247, 249
CTC-Endocrine Therapy Index (CTC-ETI), 225
CUP origin. *See* Carcinoma of unknown primary (CUP)
Cystic hypersecretory DCIS, 116, 117
Cystic pseudolactation, 110
Cytokeratins (CKs), 17, 249, 259, 261
    CK5, 35, 37, 52, 81, 198–201, 217, 267, 272
    CK5/6, 35, 74, 75, 161, 249, 259
    CK7, 118, 120, 157, 161, 169–171, 200, 247, 256

CK8, 249
CK14, 35, 37, 52, 81, 124, 132, 157, 158, 160, 161,
    199, 200, 249, 251, 253
CK18, 160, 200, 247, 249
CK19, 197, 253, 260
CK20, 118, 120, 169, 171, 183
    diagnostic utility, antibodies of, 194
    general/broad-spectrum, 194–197
    high molecular weight (basal), 161, 197, 217
        adenoid cystic carcinoma, 197, 200
        adenomyoepithelial tumor, 198, 200
        DCIS, 198, 199, 201
        metaplastic carcinoma, 197, 199
        positive staining, 197, 198
        usefulness of, 196, 197
    low molecular weight (luminal), 199, 201
Cytoplasmic inclusions, 254

D
DCIS. *See* Ductal carcinoma in situ (DCIS)
Desmin, 57, 125, 126, 129–132, 173
Diabetes mellitus, 126
Diabetic mastopathy, 126–128
Distant metastases, 106, 141, 142, 148, 160, 218, 220
Distant metastasis-free survival (DMFS), 218, 221, 223
Ductal adenoma, 238, 239
Ductal breast lesions
    atypical ductal hyperplasia, 35–36
    ductal carcinoma in situ, 37
    epithelial proliferation, 37–38
    Paget's disease of the nipple, 38
    usual epithelial hyperplasia, 34–35
Ductal carcinoma in situ (DCIS), 8, 37, 203–206, 208
    apocrine, 70–71
    "burnt out" foci of, 244
    clear cell, 72, 258
    columnar cell lesions, 71–72
    cribriform, 236
    cystic hypersecretory, 116, 117
    diagnostic and therapeutic excision specimens, 63
    diagnostic approaches, 64–65
    diagnostic core biopsies, 62
    disease extent in excision specimens, 64
    high-grade, 18, 68–69
    high molecular weight cytokeratins, 198, 199, 201
    immunohistochemistry, 73–75
    intermediate-grade, 67–68
    low-grade, 66–68, 74
    mastectomy specimens, 63–64
    MBC, 272
    microinvasion and invasion in, 73
    micropapillary pattern, 69–70
    mucinous, 114–117, 120
    neoadjuvant systemic therapy, 72–73
    papillary, 142–143
    problems in grading, 69
    re-excisions, 63
    solid, 256
    specimen handling, 61–64
    therapeutic mammoplasties, 63

Dystrophic calcification, 242, 243

E
E-cadherin, 256, 257, 260
    EMA, 210
    immunohistochemistry, 81–83, 203
    immunophenotyping, 48
    membrane expression of, 48
    signet ring cell carcinoma, 118, 119
    staining for, 204
Ectopic breast tissue, carcinoma in, 183, 249
EGFR. *See* Epidermal growth factor receptor (EGFR)
EMA. *See* Epithelial membrane antigen (EMA)
Encapsulated papillary carcinoma (EPC), 137–139,
    147–149, 252
    diagnostic features, 143
    gross examination, 143
    high-grade lesions, 144
    incidence of, 143
    molecular studies, 145
    peripheral myoepithelial cells, 145
    postoperative radiation and endocrine therapy, 148
    risk of recurrence, 148
    vs. SPC, 140
    tumor nodules of, 145
    whole tumor size, assessment of, 146
Endosalpingiosis, 181, 197
EPC. *See* Encapsulated papillary carcinoma (EPC)
Epidermal growth factor receptor (EGFR), 104, 210, 249
Epithelial hyperplasia
    absence of, 103
    in active gynecomastia, 267
    usual, 34–35, 37, 74
Epithelial membrane antigen (EMA), 50, 124, 159, 161,
    210–211, 249
Epithelial-mesenchymal transition (EMT), 164, 225
Epithelial-myoepithelial carcinoma, 210, 247, 249
    ER negative, 250, 252
    glandular structures, 249, 252
    infiltrative margin, 250, 252
    nuclear pleomorphism, 250, 252
    p63, 252
    S100, 250, 252
EQA. *See* External quality assurance (EQA)
Estrogen receptor (ER), 205–207, 252
    GGI, 222
    LCIS lesions, 83
    metaplastic squamous cell carcinoma, 156
    metastatic colonic adenocarcinoma, 171
    metastatic lobular carcinoma, 206
    metastatic parotid adenocarcinoma, 171
    metastatic renal cell carcinoma, 172
    mucinous carcinomas, 117
    secretory carcinoma, 268
    signet ring cell tumors, 120
ETV6-NTRK3 fusion gene, 249
Excision margin status, 5, 7–8
External quality assurance (EQA),
    92, 193, 204, 207, 211
Extracapsular metastasis, 179

F

Female breast cancer (FBC), 268–270, 272
Fibroadenoma, 268, 269
  vs. benign phyllodes tumor, 100–101
  bizarre multinucleate giant cells, 98
  calcified, 242, 243
  juvenile, 98
  low-power architecture, 98
  MED12 mutations, 104
  PASH in, 126, 127
  polyclonal stromal and epithelial components, 104
  TERT mutations, 104
Fibroepithelial lesions, 51, 52, 56
  core biopsy diagnosis, 101–104
  fibroadenoma (*see* Fibroadenoma)
Fibromatosis, 124–126, 153, 157–160
Fibrosarcoma, 124–126, 130–132, 158
Fibrosarcoma-malignant fibrous histiocytoma,
      130–132
Fine-needle aspiration (FNA), 12, 125, 175, 176
Fine-needle aspiration cytology (FNAC),
      34, 43, 44, 47, 57
Flat epithelial atypia (FEA), 39–40, 53–54, 110, 113
  columnar cell hyperplasia, 38
  hematoxylin and eosin, 54
  superimposed architectural atypia, 37
Florid papillomatosis of the nipple, 240
Formalin-fixed paraffin-embedded (FFPE),
      219, 220, 222, 223

G

GATA3, 119, 120, 169, 170, 172, 173, 183, 208, 209
GCDFP-15, 143, 249
Gene expression arrays, 216, 220
Gene expression profiling,
      93, 184, 190, 193, 202, 204, 217, 218
Genomic grade index (GGI), 222–223
Giant cell tumor of soft tissue, 134, 135
Globoid cells, 143
Glycogen-rich clear cell carcinoma, 256, 258, 259
Grading system
  DCIS
    College of American Pathologists' guidelines,
        66, 67
    high-grade, 68–69
    intermediate-grade, 67–68
    low-grade, 66–67
    objectives, 65
    problems in, 69
    UK NHSBSP guidelines, 66, 67
  invasive carcinoma
    histological grade, 92–93
    methodology, 90–93
    mitotic counting, 90–92
    numerical scoring system, 90
    principles, 89–90
Granular cell tumor, 238
Granulomatous lobular mastitis, 242, 243

Gross cystic disease fluid protein (GCDFP),
      206, 208, 209
Gynecomastia, 98, 161, 266
  definition, 266
  dense fibrous stroma, 266, 267
  differential diagnosis, 267, 268
  etiology, 266
  florid epithelial hyperplasia, 266, 267
  mammary lobules, 266, 267
  management, 268
  squamous metaplasia, 266, 267
  stromal pseudoangiomatous stromal hyperplasia,
      266, 267

H

H&E. *See* Hematoxylin and eosin (H&E)
Hemangiomas, 244
Hematoxylin and eosin (H&E), 57
  adenocarcinoma, 184
  adenoid cystic carcinoma, 200
  adenomyoepithelial tumor, 200
  apocrine cysts, 110, 111
  axillary sentinel node, 197
  clear cell DCIS, 72
  columnar cell hyperplasia, architectural atypia, 68
  cribriform pattern, 236
  invasive mucinous carcinoma, 117
  low-volume metastatic disease, 196
  lymph node, 179–181, 184
  metaplastic (spindle cell) carcinoma, 199
  micropapillary hyperplasia, 70
  morphology, 149
  mucocele-like lesion, core biopsy, 112
  papillary pattern, 183
  sclerosing adenosis, 75
  signet ring cell carcinoma, 119
HepPar-1, 120
HER2. *See* Human epidermal growth factor receptor 2
      (HER2)
Hidradenoma, 240, 242
High-quality tissue processing, 89
Histological grade, invasive carcinoma
  molecular genetics, 93
  reproducibility of, 92–93
  semiquantitative method, 90
Human epidermal growth factor receptor 2 (HER2),
      81, 217, 254
  core biopsy, 193
  IHC, 207
  loss of, 27
  SPC, 146
Huntington's disease, 254

I

Immunohistochemistry (IHC), 37, 80–84, 89
  audit, 193
  automated immunostainers, 192

basal-like markers, 202
basic principles, 190
breast differentiation, markers of, 208–210
CD10, 82
CKs (*see* Cytokeratins (CKs))
CUP, 183–185
DCIS, 73–75
E-cadherin, 81–83
EGFR, 210
EMA, 210–211
estrogen receptor, 205–207
factors, 191
fixation issues, 190, 192
HER2, 207
Ki67, 208
KIT (CD117), 210
laboratory procedures, 192–193
lobular neoplasia, markers of, 202–204
myoepithelial markers, 49, 202
negative control, 192
neuroendocrine markers, 204–205
of papillary lesions, 149–150
pathologist performance, 193
positive control, 192, 193
progesterone receptor, 205–207
proliferation markers, 204
quality assurance, 193
reporting, 193
SLN, 178, 179
tissue processing, 192
validated antibodies, 192
vascular markers, 207–209
Imprint cytology, 180
Infiltrating lobular carcinomas (ILC), 194, 195, 202–204
Inflammatory myofibroblastic tumor, 129–130, 162
In situ carcinoma with mixed ductal and lobular features, 81, 82
In situ lobular neoplasia, 38, 78, 79, 81, 84
Integrative clusters (IntClust), 218–219
Intermediate-grade DCIS, 34, 67–68, 73–74, 145
International Ki67 Breast Cancer Working Group, 204
Intraductal calcification, 242, 243
Intraductal papilloma, 37, 137–139, 143, 238
Intramammary lymph nodes, 244
Intramammary postoperative scar, 125
Intraoperative assessment, of sentinel nodes, 180
Intraoperative molecular assessment
    benign epithelial inclusions, 181
    cytokeratin 19, 180
    OSNA system, 180, 181
Invasive ductal carcinoma (IDC), 57, 155, 163, 203, 254, 256, 259
Invasive lobular carcinoma (ILC), 4, 50, 90, 118, 178, 256, 272
    core biopsies, 49
    and LCIS, 78
Invasive mammary carcinoma, 87, 154, 161, 271, 272
Invasive micropapillary carcinoma, 138, 149, 210, 211

Invasive mucinous carcinoma, 57, 109, 110, 114, 117–118
Invasive papillary carcinoma, 137, 139, 141, 142, 148
    microscopic features, 149
    prognosis of, 149
Isolated tumor cells (ITCs), 22, 178–180, 196

J
Juvenile fibroadenoma, 98

K
Kalmar prognostic index, 88
Ki67, 26, 204, 208, 209, 222–225, 254

L
LCIS. *See* Lobular carcinoma in situ (LCIS)
Leiomyomas, 128–129, 162, 206, 244
Leiomyosarcoma, 130, 168–170, 173
Lipid-rich carcinoma, 254, 259
Lipomas, 46, 126, 162, 244, 268
Liposarcoma, 99, 100, 130, 134
Lobular breast lesions, 38–40
Lobular carcinoma in situ (LCIS), 38, 47, 202–204, 206
    classical, 78
    with comedo necrosis, 81–83
    differential diagnosis, 84
    immunoprofile, 83
    incidence, 77–78
    management, 84–85
    molecular profile, 84
    PALCIS, 81
    pleomorphic, 78–81
Lobular neoplasia, 33, 38, 40, 48, 52–53, 77.
        See also Lobular carcinoma in situ (LCIS)
    markers of, 202–204
    variants, 80
Low-grade metaplastic carcinomas, 159
Low-grade mucoepidermoid carcinoma, 160
Low molecular weight cytokeratins, 50, 143, 157, 160, 199, 201, 202
Lumpectomy specimens, 8
Lung metastases, 173
Lymph node metastasis, 26, 163, 171, 176, 249, 251, 253–254
Lymphocytic infiltrate, 18, 128, 217, 218, 259, 260
Lymphoepithelioma-like carcinoma, 259, 260
Lymphoma, 47, 50, 130, 167, 169, 181, 183, 259–261
Lymphovascular invasion (LVI), 20, 142, 150, 163, 207, 208, 270
Lysozyme, 249

M
Macrometastasis, 23, 177, 178, 180

Male breast cancer (MBC)
    age factor, 269
    alcohol-induced liver damage/cirrhosis, 270
    clinical presentation, 270
    differential diagnosis, 272
    ethnicity, 268, 269
    familial and genetic factors, 269–270
    and gynecomastia, 270
    incidence, 268
    in situ carcinoma, 272
    invasive carcinoma, 271, 272
    macroscopic features, 270, 271
    management, 272
    obesity, 270
    radiation exposure, 270
    testicular disorders, 270
Male breast lesions
    apocrine metaplasia, 268, 269
    columnar cell lesions, 268, 269
    embryology, 266
    fibroadenoma, 268, 269
    gynecomastia, 266–268, 270, 272
    MBC (see Male breast cancer (MBC))
    single apocrine cyst, 268, 269
Malignant adenomyoepithelioma, 236
    CK14-positive staining, 251, 253
    glands and abundant myoepithelial cells, 251, 253
    lymph node metastasis, 251, 253–254
    negative ER immunostaining, 251, 253
    spindle-shaped myoepithelial cells, 251, 253
Malignant lesions, 162
    acinic cell carcinoma, 249, 251
    adenoid cystic carcinoma, 247–249
    cytoplasmic inclusions, 254
    epithelial-myoepithelial carcinoma, 249, 250, 252
    epithelium in, 139
    glycogen-rich clear cell carcinoma, 256, 258, 259
    lipid-rich carcinoma, 259
    lymphoepithelioma-like carcinoma, 259, 260
    lymphoma, 259–261
    malignant adenomyoepithelioma, 251, 253–254
    microglandular adenosis, 251, 252, 254–255
    neuroendocrine features, 254, 256, 257
    pleomorphic invasive ductal carcinoma, 254, 256
    problematic, 49–59
    secretory carcinoma, 249, 250
Malignant melanoma, 50, 167–169
Malignant phyllodes tumors, 98, 104–106, 210
    with liposarcoma, 99, 100
    nuclear pleomorphism and mitoses, 98, 99
MammaPrint®, 220–221
Mammary sarcoma with CD10 expression, 130, 133
Mammographic screening, 78, 110, 133, 242
Mastectomies, 8, 9, 13, 66, 142, 148, 172, 190
    ductal carcinoma in situ, 63–64
    macroscopic appearance, 271
    neoadjuvant therapy, 14–16
MBC. See Male breast cancer (MBC); Metaplastic breast
        carcinomas (MBCs)

Medullary carcinoma, 259
Melan A, 169, 183
Melanoma, 167–170, 183, 184
Mesenchymal stem-like (MSL) groups, 218
Metaplastic breast carcinomas (MBCs), 153, 154, 254,
        255
    adenosquamous carcinoma (see Adenosquamous
        carcinoma)
    clinical features, 154
    on core biopsy, 162–163
    diagnostic features, 162
    differential diagnoses, 161–162
    epidemiology, 154
    genetics of, 163–164
    gross pathology, 154
    histologic subtype, 163
    low-grade fibromatosis-like metaplastic carcinoma,
        160
    low-grade metaplastic carcinomas, 159
    low-grade mucoepidermoid carcinoma, 160
    matrix-producing metaplastic carcinoma, 158–159
    mesenchymal-like differentiation, 160–161
    microscopic pathology, 154–155
    outcome of, 163
    spindle cell carcinoma, 156–158
    squamous cell carcinoma and variants, 155, 156
    treatment and prognosis, 163
Metaplastic carcinoma, 154
    high molecular weight cytokeratins, 197, 199
    matrix-producing, 158–159
    spindle cell, 50, 57, 153, 157, 158
Metastatic carcinoma, 167, 168, 177, 182, 185, 196
Metastatic colonic adenocarcinoma, 169–171
Metastatic leiomyosarcoma, 169, 170, 173
Metastatic lesions
    clear cell ovarian carcinoma, 169, 170
    colonic adenocarcinoma, 169–171
    leiomyosarcoma, 169, 170, 173
    malignant melanoma, 168, 169
    neuroendocrine metastases, 173
    ovarian metastases, 170, 172
    parotid adenocarcinoma, 169–171
    renal cell carcinoma, 169, 170, 172
Metastatic lobular carcinoma, 178, 206
Metastatic lung adenocarcinoma, 184
Metastatic melanoma, 170, 184
Metastatic ovarian adenocarcinoma, 183
Metastatic parotid adenocarcinoma, 169–171
Metastatic renal cell carcinoma, 169, 170, 172, 258
Microbubble contrast-enhanced axillary sentinel node
        core biopsy, 176–177
Microcalcification, 146, 154, 236, 239
    fibrosis and chronic inflammation, 58
    vacuum-assisted core biopsy, 2, 3, 45
        evaluation of, 44
Microglandular adenosis, 58, 233–235, 250–252,
        254–255
Micrometastases, 176, 178, 180, 182
Micropapillary DCIS, 69–70, 266, 268

Miller-Payne score, 20
Minimal common regions (MCR), 216
MNF116, 123, 196
Mondor's disease, 242
MUC1, 109, 118, 120, 210
MUC2, 109, 118, 120
MUC5B, 109
Mucinous spherulosis, 120
Mucocele-like lesions, 51, 57, 109, 112–115, 118
Multinucleated tumor giant cells, 131, 254, 256
Myoepithelial (ME) cells, 235
    diagnostic utility, antibodies of, 201
    EPC, 145
    location of, 138
    role of, 140
    SPC, 146
Myoepithelial markers, 49, 73, 74, 202
    immunohistochemistry for, 84
    luminal and, 251
    p63, 234
Myofibroblastoma, 57, 58, 125–127, 162, 206
Myoid hamartoma, 129, 130

N
Needle core biopsy (NCB), 34, 43, 89, 92, 93, 97, 101,
        162, 198
Neoadjuvant therapy
    axillary lymph nodes, 15–17
    breast, 17–20
    and clinical trials, 27–28
    grading systems of response, 23–26
    histological reporting, 17
    mastectomy specimens, 14–16
    pCR, 23
    posttreatment axillary lymph node status, 20–23
    pretreatment diagnosis, 12
    repeat receptor testing, 26–27
    specimen handling, 12–13
    tumor cellularity changes, 20, 21
    tumor response to, 12
    uses, 11
    wide local excision specimens, 13–14
Nerve sheath tumors, 58
Netherlands Cancer Institute (NKI), 220
Neuroendocrine granules, breast carcinoma, 117, 254
    carcinoid-like, 256
    chromogranin, 254
    ER, 254
    HER2, 254
    invasive breast carcinoma with neuroendocrine
        differentiation, 256, 257
    mucinous and solid papillary carcinomas, 254
    neuroendocrine tumor, poorly differentiated, 256
    neuroendocrine tumor, well differentiated, 256
    neuron-specific enolase, 254
    synaptophysin, 254
Neuroendocrine markers, 146, 183, 204–205, 256
Neuroendocrine metastases, 173

Neuroendocrine tumor, 168, 169, 173
Neurofibromas, 244
Neutral buffered formalin (NBF), 62, 190, 191
Next-generation sequencing, 184, 216, 225
NHS Breast Screening Programme (NHSBSP) guidelines
    DCIS, 67
    PLCIS, 84
Nipple adenoma, 240, 268, 272
Nodular fasciitis, 58, 125, 126, 158, 162
Nodular hidradenoma, 240, 242
Noninvasive papillary carcinomas, 139
    EPC, 143–146
    general considerations, 141–142
    intraductal papillary carcinoma (papillary DCIS),
        142–143
    risk of recurrence, 148
    SPC, 146–148
Non-sentinel nodes, 180, 182
No special type (NST), 154, 156, 157, 163, 271, 272
Nottingham grading system (NGS), 87, 88
Nottingham prognostic index (NPI), 26, 88, 146, 216

O
Occult carcinoma, 194, 195
Occult primary breast carcinoma, 183
One-step nucleic acid amplification (OSNA) system,
        180, 181
Osteoclast-like giant cells, 126
Ovarian carcinoma, 168, 170, 172
Ovarian metastases, 170, 172

P
p53, 83, 84, 164, 201, 254, 259
p63, 158
    immunostaining, 235
    intact layer, 252
    spindle cell carcinoma, 99
Paget's cells, 199, 202
Paget's disease of the nipple, 38, 207, 210, 272
Papillary carcinomas, 137
    benign and malignant papillary lesions, 139–140
    challenges, 139
    diagnosis, reproducible criteria for, 139
    differential diagnosis, 139
    EPC (see Encapsulated papillary carcinoma (EPC))
    epithelial displacement in papillary lesions, 150
    immunohistochemistry of papillary lesions, 149–150
    invasive, 148–149
    in males, histological type, 149
    myoepithelial cells, 138–140
    noninvasive (see Noninvasive papillary carcinomas)
    SPC (see Solid papillary carcinoma (SPC))
Papillary hyperplasia, 110, 113, 269
Papillary lesions, 34, 35, 37–38, 47, 51,
        54–55, 138–140, 150, 161
Parotid adenocarcinoma, 169–171
PAS, 119, 238, 256, 258, 259

Pathological complete response (pCR),
        26, 27, 72, 195, 218, 224–226
    definition of, 23
    high-risk group, 222
    and survival outcomes, 28
PAX8, 169, 172, 183
p120 catenin, 48, 202–204
pCR. *See* Pathological complete response (pCR)
Percutaneous image-guided core needle biopsy, 12
PgR, 73, 132, 159, 169, 249, 250, 254, 259
Phyllodes tumor, 50, 51, 56–57, 102–104
    vs. fibroadenoma, 100–101
    malignant and borderline, 98
    prognostic factors, 105–106
    vs. sarcomas and spindle cell carcinoma,
        99–100
    vacuum-assisted excision, 104
Physiological gynecomastia, 266, 268
Pleomorphic adenoma,
        159, 162, 164, 233, 237, 238
Pleomorphic apocrine LCIS (PALCIS), 80, 81
Pleomorphic invasive ductal carcinoma, 254, 256
Pleomorphic LCIS (PLCIS), 48, 53, 272
    description, 78–81
    nuclei, 79
Preoperative endocrine prognostic index
        (PEPI), 26
Primary breast carcinoma, 167, 169
    neuroendocrine metastases, neuroendocrine
        differentiation, 173
    ovarian metastases, 170, 172
Proliferative breast lesions
    ductal, 34–37
    lobular, 38–40
Prophylactic (risk-reducing) mastectomies, 9
Protein expression, 208
Psammoma bodies, 110, 170, 183
Pseudoangiomatous stromal hyperplasia (PASH), 98,
        126, 162, 266, 267

Q
Quadrantectomy, 2
Quantitative reverse transcriptase-polymerase chain
        reaction (qRT-PCR), 216, 219, 222–224

R
Radial scar, 49, 50, 55–56, 64, 162
Radiation risk, 178
RCB. *See* Residual cancer burden (RCB)
RCC. *See* Renal cell carcinoma (RCC)
Reactive spindle cell nodules, 125
Re-excision and bed biopsies, 5
Renal cell carcinoma (RCC), 169, 170, 172, 258
Residual cancer burden (RCB), 12, 18, 20, 24, 26
Rhabdomyosarcoma, 130
Risk of recurrence (ROR) score, 221, 222

S
S100, 125, 129, 169, 183, 238,
        247, 249, 250, 252, 254
Salivary gland-type malignant lesions. *See* Malignant
        lesions
Sarcomas developing after breast radiotherapy, 134
Scatter pattern, chemotherapy, 18
Schwannomas, 129, 131, 244
Sclerosing adenosis, 45, 47, 49, 75, 238, 239
Scoring core biopsies, 114
Screen-detected carcinoma, 90
Secretory carcinoma, 249, 250
Selective ER modulators (SERMs), 206
Sentinel lymph node (SLN), 12, 177–178
    benign epithelial inclusions, 181
    frozen section and imprint cytology, 180
    immunohistochemistry, 178, 179
    intraoperative molecular assessment, 180–181
    microscopic classification, 178, 179
    pretreatment, 12
    radiation risk, 178
    sampling, 178
Signet ring cell carcinoma, 118–120, 254
Simple mucinous cysts, 110
Single apocrine cyst, 268, 269
SLN biopsy. *See* Sentinel lymph node (SLN)
Sloane project, 61, 66, 69
SMA. *See* Smooth muscle actin (SMA)
Small intestinal metastases, 173
SMMHC. *See* Smooth muscle myosin heavy chain
        (SMMHC)
Smooth muscle actin (SMA), 81, 125, 132, 149, 234, 247
Smooth muscle antigen, 253
Smooth muscle myosin heavy chain (SMMHC), 198,
        199, 201, 202, 208, 211
Solid papillary carcinoma (SPC), 120, 138, 141, 142,
        146–148, 238
    differential diagnosis of, 147
    vs. EPC, 140
    invasive, 146, 147
    myoepithelial cells, 146
    postoperative radiation and endocrine therapy, 148
Solitary fibrous tumor, 126
SPC. *See* Solid papillary carcinoma (SPC)
Spindle cell carcinoma, 57
    CK14 and p63, 157, 158
    electron microscopy, 156
    high-grade, 157
    low-grade, 157, 158
    metaplastic breast carcinomas, 156–158
    phyllodes tumor, sarcomas, 99–100
Spindle cell lipoma, 126, 127, 162
Spindle cell melanoma, 130
Spindle-shaped cells,
        50, 125, 127, 129, 130, 132, 134, 173
Squamous cell carcinoma, 153, 154, 161, 162, 167, 209
    acantholytic/pseudoangiomatous change, 155
    focal estrogen receptor staining, 155, 156

high-grade, 161
keratin formation, 155, 156
low-grade, 161
pure squamous differentiation, 155, 156
Standard operating procedures (SOPs), 192–193
Stereotactic biopsies, 1
Stromal atypia, 100, 102, 103, 105
Stromal sarcoma, 132, 162
Sudan III, 259
Synaptophysin, 72, 150, 169, 173, 183, 204, 205, 254, 256
Synovial sarcoma, 130
Syringomatous adenoma of the nipple, 240, 241

T
TRANSBIG group, 221
Trastuzumab, 27, 28, 207, 222
Triple-negative tumors
acinic cell carcinoma, 249, 251
adenoid cystic carcinoma, 247–249
epithelial-myoepithelial carcinoma, 249, 250, 252
secretory carcinoma, 249, 250
TTF1, 161, 169, 173, 183, 184, 256
Tubular carcinoma, 49, 199, 233–235, 240, 241, 250
Tubular differentiation, 90
Tubule formation, 87, 90, 91

U
Ultrasound, 2, 12, 44, 104, 138
Ultrasound-guided axillary node core biopsy, 176
Usual epithelial hyperplasia, 34–35, 37, 56

V
Vacuum-assisted core biopsy, 45, 47
Vacuum biopsies, 2
Van Nuys grading system, 66
Vimentin, 126, 129, 131, 132, 159

W
Wide local excision, 2, 13–15, 106, 134, 190
Wilms' tumor gene (WT1), 115, 119, 120
core biopsy, 112
cribriform mucinous DCIS, 116
cystic hypersecretory DCIS, 117
demonstration of, 114
mucocele-like lesion, 113
simple mucinous cysts, 110, 111
Wire-guided wide local excision, 2
WT1. *See* Wilms' tumor gene (WT1)

Z
Zymogen granules, 249, 251

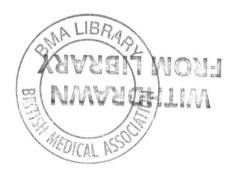

Printed by Printforce, the Netherlands